Germ Cell Tumours V

Springer-Verlag London Ltd.

P. Harnden, J.K. Joffe and W.G. Jones (Eds)

Germ Cell Tumours V

The Proceedings of the Fifth Germ Cell Tumour Conference
Devonshire Hall, University of Leeds
13th – 15th September, 2001

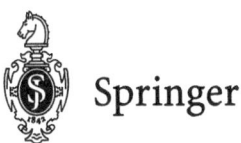

Springer

Patricia Harnden, MD, PhD, FRCPath, MBA
ICRF Cancer Medicine Research Unit
St James's University Hospital, Leeds, UK

Johnathan K. Joffe, MB BS, MD, FRCP
Huddersfield Royal Infirmary
Huddersfield, UK

William G. Jones, MB CHB, FRCR, DMRT
Yorkshire Centre for Cancer Treatments
Cookridge Hospital, Leeds, UK

Front cover illustration: Gain of 12p in the invasive phase of testicular germ cell tumours but not in the precursor lesion, carcinoma in situ (see Oosterhuis et al., chapter 5).
From Rosenberg et al. Overrepresentation of the short arm of chromosome 12 is related to invasive growth of human testicular seminomas and nonseminomas. Oncogene (2000) 19, 5858–62. Reproduced with the permission of Nature Publishing Group.

British Library Cataloguing in Publication Data
Germ Cell Tumour Conference (5th : 2001 : Leeds, England)
    Germ cell tumours V : the proceedings of the Fifth Germ
    Cell Tumour Conference, Devonshire Hall, University of
    Leeds, 13th–15th September, 2001
    1. Germ cells – Tumors – Congresses 2. Oncology – Congresses
    I. Title II. Harnden, P. III. Joffe, J.K. IV. Jones, W.G.
    616.9'94'63
Library of Congress Cataloging-in-Publication Data
A catalog record for this book is available from the Library of Congress.

ISBN 978-1-4471-3283-7   ISBN 978-1-4471-3281-3 (eBook)
DOI 10.1007/978-1-4471-3281-3

a member of BertelsmannSpringer Science+Business Media GmbH
http://www.springer.co.uk

© Springer-Verlag London 2002
Originally published by Springer-Verlag London 2002
Softcover reprint of the hardcover 1st edition 2002

Typeset by Mac Style Ltd, Scarborough, Yorkshire, England

28/3830-543210 Printed on acid-free paper SPIN 10855499

Conference Chairman:

Dr J.K. Joffe, Consultant Medical Oncologist, Huddersfield Royal Infirmary, Huddersfield.

Organising Committee:

Dr J.K. Joffe, Consultant Medical Oncologist, Huddersfield Royal Infirmary, Huddersfield.

Dr P. Harnden, Consultant Pathologist, ICRF Centre for Cancer Research, St James's University Hospital, Leeds.

Dr W.G. Jones, Consultant Clinical Oncologist, Cookridge Hospital, Leeds.

Ms S. Lacey, Conference and Marketing Office, University of Leeds.

Preface

The events of September 11, 2001 in the United States will always be remembered with horror and sadness but also admiration for those who risked, and often lost, their lives attempting to save others. When the Fifth International Germ Cell Tumour Conference began, the US air space was closed and our American friends were unable to join us. We were faced with a programme that now had many gaps. What happened next was an illustration of the sense of community that prevails at the Germ Cell Tumour Conferences. Some of those who could not be there in person, such as Richard Foster and Craig Nichols, sent their slides by email, and we were indebted to those, such as Michael Jewett, Ben Mead and Malcolm Mason, who stepped into the breach to present them. Others gave impromptu, and often thought provoking, talks. The discussion periods were lively and it will come as no surprise to those who regularly attend the meeting that Tim Oliver won the prize for "Most Questions Asked", managing even to ask questions following his own presentations. The quality of the talks was outstanding. There was closer integration of the adult and paediatric sessions than in previous meetings. As a result, the differences and similarities between adult male, female and paediatric germ cell tumours became more apparent. This cross-fertilization of ideas from different groups will no doubt lead to further advances.

As a result of all these efforts, the conference was a great success. As always, the organizing committee, and particularly its chairman Johnathan Joffe, laid the foundation of the conference but the participants made it work. One of the greatest "powers behind the scenes" was Susan Lacey of the University's Conference Office, who supported Jonathan so ably and brought calmness and efficiency to the administration of the conference.

The quality of the manuscripts submitted to this book was such that it made the job of the editors that much easier. Even those who were unable to travel to the conference have contributed, so that this book could be a true representation of the current thinking and research directions in the field of germ cell tumours.

As Bill has known for many years, since he was the driving force behind all of the previous conferences, as Johnathan discovered when he spearheaded the 2001 conference and as Patricia has found during the preparation of the book of proceedings, the organization of an international conference is incompatible with the notion of "free time". We are indebted to our families for their support and understanding.

Patricia Harnden, Johnathan Joffe and Bill Jones

Acknowledgements

The Organising Committee would like to thank the following Organisations and Pharmaceutical Companies for sponsorship of the Fifth International Germ Cell Tumour Conference, Leeds.

Pierre Fabre
Bristol-Myers Squibb
Aventis Pharma
Chugai Pharma
Kyowa Hakko
Amgen
Asta Medica

We are also grateful to the staff at Devonshire Hall, University of Leeds, and Hilary Collins in particular, for their help and graciousness, which made the event not only possible but enjoyable.

The quality of this book is a reflection of each author's hard work, for which we are grateful. As co-ordinating editor, I would like to thank my co-editors, Bill and Johnathan, with a touch of sadness because this may be the last time that we work together on a book. I know that everyone will join me in a vote of thanks to Bill for all he has done for so many years. We wish him well in his retirement and hope that he will continue to support the conference.

Last but not least, I would like to thank Heather Bisby, Wendy Kennedy, Kirsti Miller and Brian Naylor. Without their help and support, this book may have been significantly delayed.

Patricia Harnden

Contents

Section 4: Paediatric Germ Cell Tumours

Section 5: Current Status – Surgery

Section 6: Quality of Life

Section 7: Current Status Non Surgical

Section 1

Genetics and Biology

1. The Genetics of Testicular Germ Cell Tumours

E.A. Rapley[1], G.P. Crockford[2], D.F. Easton[3], M.R. Stratton[1],
D.T. Bishop[2], on behalf of the International Testicular Cancer Linkage
Consortium[4]

*1. Sections of Cancer Genetics, Institute of Cancer Research, Haddow Laboratories, Sutton,
Surrey, SM2 5NG, UK. 2. Imperial Cancer Research Fund Genetic Epidemiology Lab, Ashley
Wing, Leeds, LS97TF, UK. 3. CRC Genetic Epidemiology Unit, Strangeways Research
Laboratories, Worts Causeway, Cambridge, CB1 8RN, UK. 4. International Testicular Cancer
Linkage Consortium members are listed in Table 1.*

Abstract

Testicular Germ Cell Tumours (TGCT) affect 1 in 400 men in the UK. Two per cent of
TGCT cases report another affected family member. The familial relative risk is
estimated to be 8–10 fold for brothers of cases and 4–6 fold for fathers and sons. This
familial relative risk is considerably higher than for most common cancers suggesting
that the contribution of genetic factors to TGCT may be relatively more important
than for other cancers. However, the search by genetic linkage analysis for familial
TGCT susceptibility genes has been confounded by the limited number of large
multiple case families. The International Testicular Cancer Linkage Consortium
family set currently consists of more than 190 families with at least two cases of TGCT.
A genome-wide search conducted on 100 families has yielded strong evidence for a
TGCT susceptibility gene on the X chromosome. This gene appears to predispose to
bilateral TGCT and also possibly to undescended testis. This is the first familial TGCT
gene to be localised and the first cancer susceptibility gene mapped in a genome wide
search using predominantly sib pairs.

1. Testicular Germ Cell Tumours

Testicular germ cell tumours (TGCT) are rare, comprising 2 per cent of all cancers in
men. It is however, the most common malignancy in men aged 15–40 years and
approximately 1700 men in the United Kingdom develop the disease each year [1]. TGCT
has the highest incidence in European populations, with age-standardised rates ranging
from 2 to 9 per 100,000 per year [2]. The incidence of TGCT is increasing. In England
and Wales, it has almost doubled in less than 30 years, from 2.9 cases per 100,000 per year
in 1971 to 5.4 per 100,000 per year in 1997 [3]. A similar trend is observed in almost all
other developed countries [4]. The reason for this increase is not clear.

TGCT are divided into two main histological entities, seminomas and non-
seminomas. Seminomas represent approximately 50 per cent of TGCT and
non-seminomas 40 per cent. The remaining 10 per cent are of mixed histology,
combining both tumour types. The age of onset of the histological groups differs:

seminoma has an older median age of onset (35 years) compared to non-seminoma (28 years). Tumour histology is not necessarily concordant in bilateral disease or in different affected relatives in the same family. It is now generally accepted that TGCTs arise from carcinoma *in situ* or intratubular germ cell neoplasia (ITGCN), the importance of which was first identified by Skakkebæk in 1972 [5]. ITGCN cells express many of the same immunohistochemical markers as primordial germ cells [6] and can be found in the adjacent parenchyma of most TGCT and also before the development of an invasive TGCT. It is believed that all ITGCN will progress to invasiveness with no evidence of spontaneous regression [7].

1.1 Risk Factors

Several consistent and strong risk factors exist for TGCT. The largest case-control study for TGCT has shown that one of the strongest risk factors for testicular cancer is heredity [8, 9]. Patients with TGCT were four times more likely than controls to have a father and eight times more likely to have a brother with the same malignancy [8].

The strongest known risk factor for testicular cancer is a previous TGCT. In men who have testicular cancer the relative risk in the remaining, contralateral testis is estimated to be approximately 25 [10, 11]. Biopsy studies have shown that ITGCN can be found in the contralateral testicle of testicular cancer patients in approximately 5 per cent of cases [12–14] which corresponds well with the expected frequency of second primary TGCT.

The other important risk factor for testicular cancer is undescended testis (UDT) [15–18]. Eight to 10 per cent of men with TGCT have a history of UDT compared with the population rate of 1–2 per cent [9]. Men with unilateral TGCT have an increase risk of TGCT in the normally descended contralateral testis but it is not as high as in the undescended one [9, 17].

A recent study has shown that men with a history of infertility are at an increased risk of developing a TGCT [19, 20]. An analysis according to specific semen characteristics showed that low sperm concentration (standardised incidence ratio 2.3), poor motility of spermatozoa (2.5) and a high proportion of morphologically abnormal spermatozoa (3.0) were all associated with an increased risk of testicular cancer [20].

Malformations or abnormalities of the male genital organs, including inguinal hernia [9], atrophic testes [21], hypospadias [22], hydrocoele [23] and varicocele [24] are among the less consistent and less certain risk factors for TGCT.

1.2 Gonadal Dysgenesis, Klinefelter's Syndrome and Other Rare Genetic Abnormalities

Patients with 46 XY or 45 X/46 XY gonadal dysgenesis are at very high risk (10–50 per cent) of gonadal germ cell tumour (GCT) [25]. Patients with complete androgen insensitivity syndrome are also at increased risk of developing a gonadal GCT [26]. Klinefelter's syndrome (47, XXY) patients have an estimated relative risk of 67 of developing an extragonadal GCT [27]. Eight per cent of males with mediastinal GCT have Klinefelter's syndrome, which is 50 times greater than expected [28]. The incidence of TGCT in Klinefelter's patients is low [27, 29–31] although this may be attributable to the fact that adults with Klinefelter's syndrome have few, if any, residual testicular germ cells [32]. Individuals with Down syndrome have also been reported to have an increased risk of testicular ITGCN and TGCT [33–35].

2. Genetic Susceptibility to Testicular Germ Cell Tumour

Epidemiological studies have shown that there is an eight to ten fold increase in relative risk of TGCT to brothers of patients and a fourfold increased risk to fathers and sons [8, 23, 26]. This relative risk is considerably higher than for most other common cancers, which rarely exceeds four, and strongly suggests that genes may play an important role in TGCT.

Familial cancer predisposition syndromes are often characterised by a younger age of disease onset and higher incidence of bilateral disease. The incidence of bilateral disease is certainly higher among cases with a family history of TGCT (7.3 per cent) compared to that seen in cases with no family history (2.7 per cent) [8]. Forman et al. also calculated that the age of onset in familial cases was significantly lower than that for cases without a family history [8].

The incidence of TGCT varies greatly among different populations and ethnic groups (Figure 1.1). The highest rates occur in Europe, particularly the Nordic countries and the lowest rates typically occur in Asia and Africa. The Maori population of New Zealand with an incidence rate of 7.9 per 100,000 is the only non-European population that has a high incidence of TGCT [37]. There is little change in the incidence of a population with migration, for example the US black population has a low incidence (0.7 per 100,000) of TGCT similar to other African populations while the US white population is similar to other European countries and this pattern contrasts with all common epithelial tumours. This population variation and lack of change in incidence with migration again suggests that genes are important in the aetiology of TGCT.

In summary there are several lines of evidence that support the notion that a gene or genes play an important role in the development of TGCT. The high relative risk is one of the most convincing arguments and is supported by the population variation, the younger age of onset and the high incidence of bilateral disease among familial cases. Indeed the contribution that susceptibility genes make to TGCT overall may be

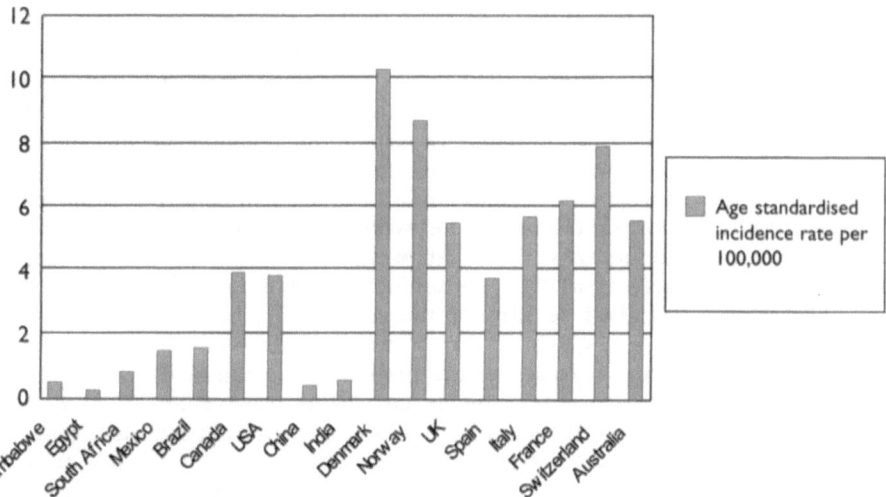

Figure 1.1: Incidence of TGCT in a variety of populations worldwide [1]

substantial. Nicholson and Harland calculated that an underlying genetic susceptibility could account for almost a third of all TGCT cases [38].

3. Mode of Inheritance of a Testicular Germ Cell Tumour Gene

TGCT pedigrees are mainly affected relative pairs so a simple inspection of the pedigrees is not sufficient to establish the mode of inheritance of a TGCT susceptibility gene. In addition, the incidence rates for TGCT have changed greatly and treatment has significantly altered the lethality of the disease in the last generation. Two analyses have been conducted in an effort to determine the mode of inheritance for a TGCT susceptibility gene. One study examined the frequency of bilateral disease [38] and a second performed a segregation analysis on a set of Norwegian and Swedish families [39].

A study by Nicholson and Harland [38] aimed to ascertain the incidence in the general population of genetically predisposed TGCT. Their analysis was based on the incidence of bilateral and unilateral cancer following similar arguments to those used by Knudson [40] for retinoblastoma. They examined the published data on the age of onset of TGCT and the prevalence of bilateral disease in familial and unselected general cases. In unselected cases, bilateral disease occurs approximately 25 times more frequently than by chance alone. Assuming that this high risk of contralateral disease is due entirely to genetic susceptibility, and that this is mediated by a single susceptibility gene, then almost all bilateral cases must be carriers of the susceptible genotype. The higher risk to brothers than fathers of cases, and the high risk of contralateral disease relative to the sibling risk, suggest that this gene is more likely to act recessively. Based on the higher frequency of bilateral disease amongst cases with a family history, Nicholson and Harland estimate that approximately one third of cases occur in predisposed individuals, that the frequency of the susceptibility allele would be 0.05 and the penetrance of the allele would be 0.45.

Segregation analysis is a statistical technique, which attempts to model familial aggregation of disease. Heimdal et al. [39] performed a segregation analysis based on all available patients treated at the Norwegian Radium Hospital and Lund for TGCT from 1981 to 1991. Testicular cancer was reported in first-degree relatives in 30 patients and no family had more than two affected members. They found that a recessive model, with a estimated gene frequency of 0.038, fits the data best. Under this model 7.6 per cent of men would be carriers of the mutant allele but only those that were homozygous would be at high risk of developing TGCT. Homozygous men would have a lifetime risk of developing TGCT of 43 per cent, very close to the model proposed by Nicholson and Harland. In the proband generation, 25 per cent of TGCT cases diagnosed before the age of 35 would be attributed to genetic susceptibility, 14 per cent of cases between 35 and 54 years and 12 per cent of cases above the age of 55. The analysis was potentially sensitive to the variation in incidence rates between parent and proband generations and also to reduced fertility among susceptible men (i.e. the potential fathers of cases in the proband generation). However varying assumptions about the trends in incidence within reasonable limits did not appreciably change the best fitting model and these estimates appear quite robust.

The two approaches used to establish a mode of inheritance for TGCT are quite different in their methodologies and can be regarded as independent support for a recessive mode of inheritance. Both analyses derived a similar common gene frequency and overall lifetime penetrance, although the proportion of TGCT cases due to genetic predisposition is somewhat higher in the Nicholson and Harland model.

It is important to note that neither of these analyses is able to distinguish between a single major gene model and a model with several independent susceptibility genes (i.e. a genetic heterogeneity model). Moreover, neither analysis considered an X-linked mode of inheritance (see below). The segregation analysis did however consider, and reject, a polygenic model of inheritance, under which several susceptibility alleles would act multiplicatively on disease risk [39]. Overall the power of a segregation analysis approach is limited, and only by identifying the susceptibility genes for TGCT will the true model be clarified.

4. The International Testicular Cancer Linkage Consortium

The International Testicular Cancer Linkage Consortium (ITCLC) was formed in 1994 with the aim to pool resources and identify TGCT susceptibility genes. This group now comprises centres all over the world collecting and contributing family material to a central body for genotyping studies and additional collaborators to aid with the identification of the *TGCT1* gene (Table 1). We continue to collect families from current consortium members and hope to attract additional collaborators to increase the family set.

4.1 International Testicular Cancer Linkage Consortium Pedigrees

A total of 193 families with two or more cases of testis cancer have been collected by the ITCLC (Table 1.2). Patients donated samples and information with full informed consent and with local ethical review board approval. Information on clinical status including type of TGCT, age of diagnosis, presence of UDT, and laterality of disease was confirmed by reviewing histological reports and clinical notes

Large TGCT pedigrees like those used to isolate the genes *BRCA1* and *BRCA2* have never been reported and although pedigrees with three, four or five affected members have been described [41, 42], they are rare. Interest in TGCT generated after the publication of our paper describing linkage at Xq27 [43] has resulted in an ascertainment of 11 large TGCT families with 3 or more cases, almost doubling the number in our set in the last 12 months (Figure 1.2). However the majority of TGCT pedigrees are affected relative pairs, most of which are sibs. A breakdown of the family types and sources is given in Table 1.2.

For each pedigree in the consortium set, detailed information on age at diagnosis, histology, laterality, UDT and other relevant medical history is collected. The distribution of age at diagnosis and bilaterality is similar to that from previous studies. Forman et al. [8] found that the age of diagnosis in familial cases was slightly younger than that for sporadic cases (29 years versus 32.5 years). The average age at diagnosis for the cases in the consortium set is 31.6 years, slightly higher than that calculated by Forman and not significantly different from that of population cases [8]. Of 328 cases with known histology, 165 cases had seminoma (mean age of onset = 34.8years) and 163 cases had non-seminoma or mixed histology (mean age of onset = 28.9 years). Histology on each affected case in a family is known for 151 pedigrees. Histology was concordant in 78 pedigrees (39 seminoma and 39 non-seminoma) and discordant in 73 pedigrees. There is a higher frequency of bilateral disease in the ITCLC (6.8 per cent) than sporadic cases (2.6 per cent) and the mean age of the first

Table 1.1: The International Testicular Cancer Linkage Consortium (September 2001)

Institutional Address	Investigators
Institute of Cancer Research, UK	Elizabeth Rapley, Shelia Seal, Rita Barfoot, Nina Persinguhe, Robert Huddart, Colin Cooper, Michael Stratton
Imperial Cancer Research Fund, UK	Gillian Crockford, David Forman, Michael Leahy, Julia Bodmer, R. Timothy D. Oliver, Timothy Bishop
CRC Genetic Epidemiology Unit, Cambridge, UK	Dawn Teare, Douglas Easton
Norwegian Radium Hospital, Oslo, Norway	Ketil Heimdal, Sophie Fossa
Indiana University, Indianapolis, USA and University of Pennsylvania School of Medicine, Philadelphia, USA	L. Einhorn and B. Weber
National Cancer Institute, Rockville, USA	Mark H. Greene and Mary McMaster
Academic Hospital Rotterdam, Netherlands	Leendert H.J. Looijenga
University of Otago, New Zealand	Parry Guilford
University Hospital, Switzerland	Walter Weber and Hans Stoll
Peter MacCallum Cancer Institute, Australia	Kelly Phillips
Phillips University, Marburg, Germany	Axel Heidenreich
Prince of Wales Hospital, Sydney Australia	Kathy Tucker and Michael Friedlander
Toronto General Hospital, Canada	David Hogg and Paul Goss
St James Hospital, Dublin, Ireland	Wilma Ormiston and Peter Daly
Génétique Oncologique EPHE Faculté de Médecine Paris, France	Stéphane Richard
University Hospital, Czech Republic	Radka Kalbacova
Sanger Centre, Cambridge, UK	Jackie Bye and Mark Ross

cancer of these bilateral cases is younger (26.1 years) than either sporadic or familial cases. Of the 319 cases in the set for whom we have information about testicular descent, 40 reported a history of UDT (12.5 per cent). This is somewhat higher than reported in previous sporadic or familial series and suggests that UDT may be a particular feature of genetically susceptible cases.

4.2 Evidence for Genetic Anticipation?

There is a substantial difference in the age at diagnosis between fathers and sons in the ITCLC set (43 years versus 27 years) and this could indicate "genetic anticipation" as suggested by Raghavan [44] and again by Han in a review of 52 father–son pairs documented in the literature [45]. Forman's study [8] also showed a substantial difference between the age of onset in nine father – son pairs (some of which are now included in the ITCLC set) but suggested that selection due to death or infertility of young cases in the paternal generation before they could produce children could entirely explain this difference. The ITCLC set now contains 15 uncle–nephew pairs which would be not subject to the same selection pressures due to death or infertility. This set also shows a noticeable difference between ages of onset in the different generations (39 years versus 25 years). However there are still substantial biases even in the uncle-nephew comparison. Uncles are almost always substantially older; hence in many families an older case can only be observed in the uncle, since the nephew will not have reached that age. It is difficult to decide how to interpret such data and

Table 1.2: Testicular Cancer Pedigrees in International Testicular Cancer Linkage Consortium

Source	Total	Sib pair	Sib trio	Father & son	Cousins Paternal	Maternal	Other	Uncle/Nephew Paternal	Maternal	Other Pairs*	Larger Pedigrees (ped nos)**
ICR (UK)	73	39	2	11	4	3	3	2	3	2	251, 254, 294, 2124
Australia (POWH)	18	6		6		1	1	1		1	102, 114
Canada	5	3		1							122
German	16	12		2			1		1		
ICRF (UK)	44	28	3	5	2		2	2	1		303
Ireland	2						1				159
Norway	25	15					2	4	2		128, 160
USA (NCI)	4	2									400, 424
USA (Indiana & Philadelphia)	2			1	1						
Others	4										2169 (Czech Republic); 500 (France), 194 (Switzerland) 195 (New Zealand),
Total Collected	193	105	5	26	7	4	10	9	7	3	16

* Other pedigree pairs such as grandfather/grandson pairs, 2nd cousins or more complex cousins pairs
** Larger pedigrees given as the pedigree number, please refer to figure 2 for pedigree structure

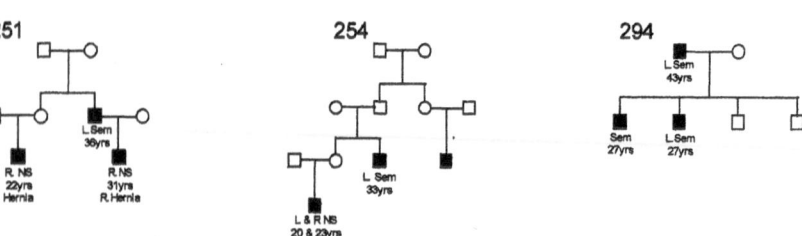

Figure 1.2: Large TGCT pedigrees in ITCLC set. O = female; □ = male; v = affected male; Information on histology of tumour, age of diagnosis and history of undescended testis is shown. Sem = seminoma; NS = non-seminoma and mixed = combined histology tumour.

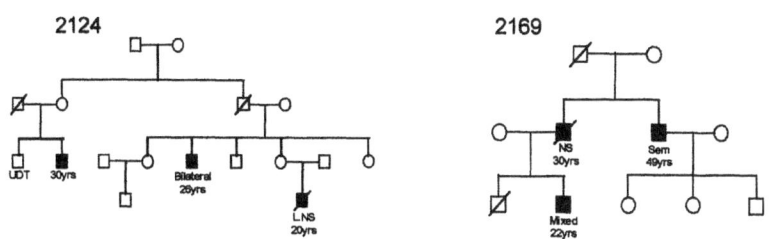

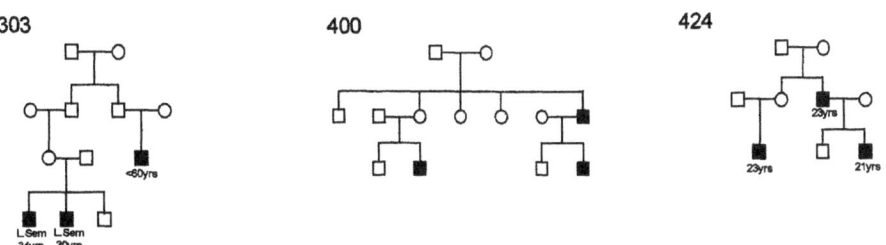

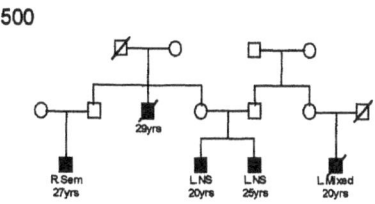

Figure 1.2: (continued)

the answer to this observation may not be resolved until the underlying genetic mechanisms of TGCT are elucidated.

4.3 The Power of the ITCLC Pedigree Set

The ITCLC set of pedigrees represents the largest collection of testicular cancer pedigrees in the world. This set gives us considerable power to detect the presence of TGCT susceptibility genes. We have examined the power to detect such genes with 160 ITCLC families (father–son pedigrees are excluded from the analysis and more recently ascertained pedigrees were not included). Calculations were performed under the best autosomal dominant and autosomal recessive models given by the segregation analysis of Heimdal et al. [39], but allowing for the possibility of genetic heterogeneity. An X-linked component to susceptibility was not considered in this analysis. If there were two autosomal recessive genes each contributing to half of the pedigrees the estimated power to detect linkage (to either locus) with a LOD score >3 was 94 per cent. A LOD score is the conventional measure of evidence for linkage and a score of at least three is considered strong evidence of having mapped a gene. For two dominant autosomal loci contributing equally, the corresponding probability was 41 per cent. Thus, the failure to find LOD scores of this magnitude so far suggests that no single locus can explain more than 50 per cent of the families. In contrast, under a model with four recessive genes existed each contributing to a quarter of the families, the expected LOD score at each locus would only be around 2, so that we would require a set of pedigrees 1.5 times larger (approximately 250 pedigrees) to establish strong evidence for linkage. Under the dominant model, the corresponding expected LOD score if there were four genes each contributing to a quarter of the families would be around 1, so that a set of pedigrees three times larger (approximately 500 pedigrees) would be required. Linkage analysis on the pedigrees genotyped from the ITCLC would suggest that there are more than two TGCT susceptibility genes.

5. Localisation of a Testicular Germ Cell Tumour Gene (TGCT1) to Xq27

Two extensive genome screens on a set of ITCLC pedigrees gave suggestive evidence for linkage at several loci (see later sections), however no region showed statistical significance. The increased risk of TGCT to fathers or sons of cases has been reported to be less than the increased risk to brothers of cases [8, 36]. Since this could be interpreted as evidence of X inheritance we extended the linkage search to include the X chromosome. In these analyses we excluded from genotyping the families that show male to male transmission and hence, *a priori*, are inconsistent with X-linkage. Linkage analysis of the set of families compatible with X-linkage, 80 per cent of which are sib pairs, provided preliminary evidence for a TGCT predisposition locus at Xq27–28 (maximum HLOD score (LOD score under heterogeneity) = 2.01, estimated proportion of linked families α = 0.32) (Table 1.3). Evidence in favour of linkage was observed in families from all contributing groups (data not shown).

We subsequently stratified families according to the presence of at least one bilateral case, the presence of undescended testis, histology and age (Table 1.3). Fifteen families contained at least one case of bilateral disease, all of which are sib pairs except for one family with two affected maternal cousins and one family with

Table 1.3: Hlod score results by model

Data Set		Location (cM)	Maximum HLOD score	Proportion of families linked (α)
All families	(n=99)	183.04	2.01	0.32
Bilaterality	Positive (n=15)	175.28	4.76	1.00
	Negative (n=75)	190.19	1.32	0.32
	Unknown (n=9)	35.28	0.69	1.00
UDT status	Positive (n=19)	184.74	2.50	0.74
	Negative (n=56)	162.39	0.56	0.27
	Unknown (n=24)	8.2	0.76	1.00
Mean age	< = 30 (n=39)	183.61	2.09	0.49
	> 30 (n=35)	189.53	0.58	0.29
Tumour type	Seminoma (n=17)	174.94	1.33	0.60
	NonSeminoma (n=17)	190.99	1.54	0.64

three affected sibs. This subset showed strong evidence of linkage to the locus on Xq27 (HLOD score = 4.76, α = 1.00) and were more likely to be linked to the X chromosome than families without a bilateral case (P = 0.0002). The difference in proportion of linked families when dichotomising by presence/absence of bilateral disease is statistically significant after taking into account multiple testing (P = 0.001 allowing for five tests).

The probability of obtaining the HLOD score of 4.76 or greater by chance in a genome-wide search in at least one of the subgroups examined was estimated by 1000 simulations to be 0.034, equivalent to a LOD score of 3.78 in a genome-wide linkage search using affected sib pairs without subgrouping [46]. This result provides highly significant evidence for a TGCT susceptibility gene on chromosome Xq27, that we have called *TGCT1* [46]. Our results would suggest that about one third of the excess familial TGCT risk to brothers is due to *TGCT1*, with little difference in the residual risks to brothers and sons after this locus has been accounted for.

Families with one or more cases of undescended testis, three of which are non-sib pairs (two uncle nephew and one cousin pedigree), show evidence of linkage to the same region on Xq27 (HLOD score = 2.52, α = 0.73) and are more likely to be linked than families without a case of undescended testis (P = 0.03 for the comparison). Age of onset and histopathology did not discriminate those families that were linked to the X chromosome from those that were not (Table 1.3).

5.1 Minimal TGCT1 Region

Haplotypes were constructed for the 15 families with bilateral tumours (Figure 1.3). Two informative recombinants appear to limit the size of the common interval to *DXS8043-FMR1Di*, a distance of approximately 4cM (although the small size of these two families and the consequent weakness of the linkage information from each mean that both could be linked by chance). There is no segregating haplotype throughout the *DXS8043-FMR1Di* interval that is common to all these families (Figure 1.3). Although there are haplotype similarities between families in the region *DXS548-FMR1di*, the haplotype frequencies are not significantly different to those obtained by genotyping of 762 control males (data not shown).

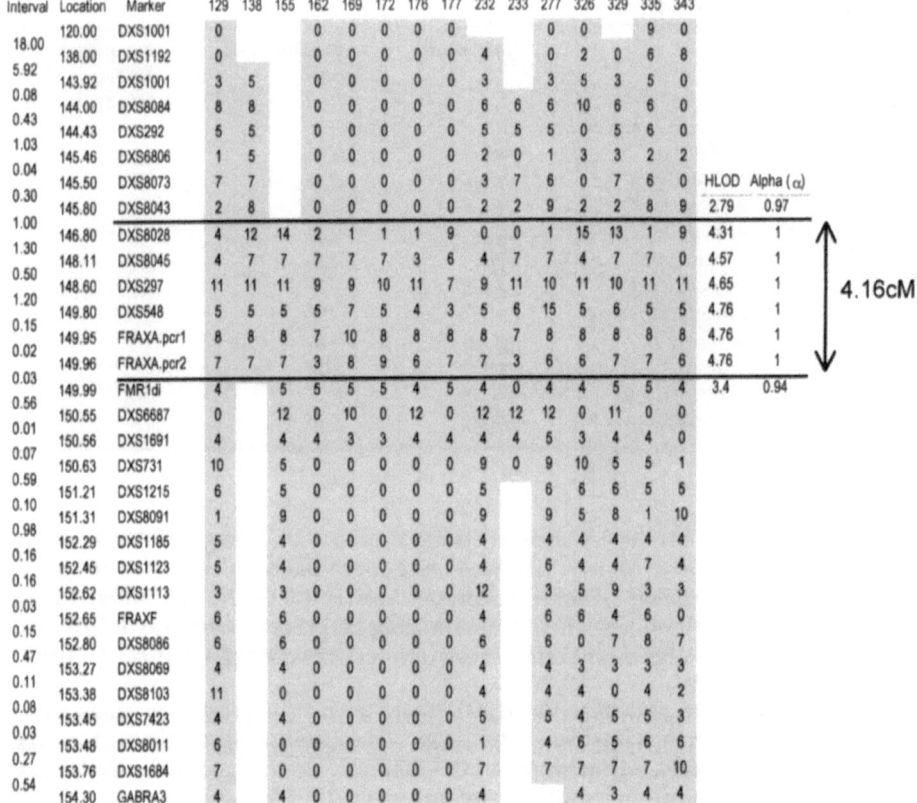

Interval	Location	Marker	129	138	155	162	169	172	176	177	232	233	277	326	329	335	343	HLOD	Alpha (α)
18.00	120.00	DXS1001	0			0	0	0	0	0			0	0		9	0		
5.92	138.00	DXS1192	0			0	0	0	0	0	4		0	2	0	6	8		
0.08	143.92	DXS1001	3	5		0	0	0	0	0	3		3	5	3	5	0		
0.43	144.00	DXS8084	8	8		0	0	0	0	0	6	6	6	10	6	6	0		
1.03	144.43	DXS292	5	5		0	0	0	0	0	5	5	5	0	5	6	0		
0.04	145.46	DXS6806	1	5		0	0	0	0	0	2	0	1	3	3	2	2		
0.30	145.50	DXS8073	7	7		0	0	0	0	0	3	7	6	0	7	6	0		
1.00	145.80	DXS8043	2	8		0	0	0	0	0	2	2	9	2	2	8	9	2.79	0.97
1.30	146.80	DXS8028	4	12	14	2	1	1	1	9	0	0	1	15	13	1	9	4.31	1
0.50	148.11	DXS8045	4	7	7	7	7	7	3	6	4	7	7	4	7	7	0	4.57	1
1.20	148.60	DXS297	11	11	11	9	9	10	11	7	9	11	10	11	10	11	11	4.65	1
0.15	149.80	DXS548	5	5	5	5	7	5	4	3	5	6	15	5	6	5	5	4.76	1
0.02	149.95	FRAXA.pcr1	8	8	8	7	10	8	8	8	8	7	8	8	8	8	8	4.76	1
0.03	149.96	FRAXA.pcr2	7	7	7	3	8	9	6	7	7	3	6	6	7	7	6	4.76	1
0.56	149.99	FMR1di	4		5	5	5	5	4	5	4	0	4	4	5	5	4	3.4	0.94
0.01	150.55	DXS6687	0		12	0	10	0	12	0	12	12	12	0	11	0	0		
0.07	150.56	DXS1691	4		4	4	3	3	4	4	4	4	5	3	4	4	0		
0.59	150.63	DXS731	10		5	0	0	0	0	0	9	0	9	10	5	5	1		
0.10	151.21	DXS1215	6		5	0	0	0	0	0	5		6	6	6	5	5		
0.98	151.31	DXS8091	1		9	0	0	0	0	0	9		9	5	8	1	10		
0.16	152.29	DXS1185	5		4	0	0	0	0	0	4		4	4	4	4	4		
0.16	152.45	DXS1123	5		4	0	0	0	0	0	4		6	4	4	7	4		
0.03	152.62	DXS1113	3		3	0	0	0	0	0	12		3	5	9	3	3		
0.15	152.65	FRAXF	6		6	0	0	0	0	0	4		6	6	4	6	0		
0.47	152.80	DXS8086	6		6	0	0	0	0	0	6		6	0	7	8	7		
0.11	153.27	DXS8069	4		4	0	0	0	0	0	4		4	3	3	3	3		
0.08	153.38	DXS8103	11		0	0	0	0	0	0	4		4	4	0	4	2		
0.03	153.45	DXS7423	4		4	0	0	0	0	0	5		5	4	5	5	3		
0.27	153.48	DXS8011	6		0	0	0	0	0	0	1		4	6	5	6	6		
0.54	153.76	DXS1684	7		0	0	0	0	0	0	7		7	7	7	7	10		
	154.30	GABRA3	4		4	0	0	0	0	0	4		4	3	4	4			

4.16cM

Figure 1.3: Haplotype of 15 bilateral families demonstrating minimal region between the markers DXS8043 and FMR1di. The map shows the 46 markers, which were typed over the length of the X chromosome and the relative distances (cM) between them.

The maximum lod score was between the markers DXS548 and FRAXA.pcr2. Analysis of the haplotypes at this region from the 15 bilateral families did not show a common haplotype between them but demonstrated two recombinants that possibly narrow the region to approximately 4 cM.

The region is currently being sequenced and annotated at the Sanger centre. A complete BAC map now exists for the region and represents approximately 3.3Mb of DNA. As the group at the Sanger centre sequence and annotate this region, we systematically screen every gene identified. This small region is extremely gene poor and there are only two genes from this region described in the literature, the *FMR1* gene, which is responsible for Fragile-X syndrome, and a single exon gene, *Cxorf1* [47].

Individuals with Fragile X syndrome frequently exhibit macroorchidism although histologically the appearances are unremarkable other than for the presence of oedema (OMIM: #309550, *URL*: http://www3.ncbi.nlm.nih.gov/Omim/). There is no evidence for an excess risk of TGCT in Fragile X cases [48]. Fragile X syndrome is generally caused by an expansion of a CGG repeat in the 5' non-coding region and more rarely by large deletions of *FMR1*. We have examined this gene for small deletions, duplications and missense/non-sense mutations by conformational gel electrophoresis (CSGE) in the set of ITCLC pedigrees linked to Xq27 and found no evidence of these types of mutations. The bilateral families were examined for evidence for CGG repeat expansion and all pedigrees were in the normal range (data not shown).

Cxorf1 is a single exon gene expressed only in hippocampus. This gene was also examined by CSGE analysis and no evidence for any mutations in this gene were identified [47].

5.2 How Is TGCT1 Acting as a Predisposition Cancer Gene?

The identification of a gene at Xq27 raises a number of questions. Firstly what is the mechanism for mutation and secondly why is *TGCT1* not associated with extended pedigrees?

TGCT1 is unlikely to be a classical tumour suppressor gene as males only have one X chromosome. A clue to the oncogenic mechanism of *TGCT1* may lie with the association of Klinefelter's syndrome with extragonadal GCT (chapter 2). The majority of Klinefelter's patients have a constitutional karyotype of 47 XXY. The relative risk of mediastinal GCT in Klinefelter's syndrome is 67 and 8 per cent of cases of mediastinal GCT in males have Klinefelter's syndrome [27]. Since Klinefelter's patients carry extra copies of the X chromosome this raises the possibility that two active normal copies of *TGCT1* may be responsible for the increased risk of GCTs in Klinefelter's syndrome.

Pedigrees with bilateral cases of TGCT and/or a history of UDT gave the strongest evidence for linkage to *TGCT1*, but the majority of the pedigrees were sib pairs. The absence of linked families with many affected relatives suggests that the penetrance of *TGCT1* is likely to be low. This observation would suggest that for *TGCT1* to cause TGCT, other modifying factors must also be present and perhaps (given the absence of more distant, affected relatives) may include modifying genes or environmental factors shared between brothers (e.g. maternal environment). Of course the real mechanism may not be known until *TGCT1* is identified.

5.3 Confirmation of Linkage at Xq27 and Recombinant Information

In order to refine our recombinant information and strengthen our linkage result we would like to repeat our observation in a set of 50–100 pedigrees compatible with X linkage and/or a set of 10–20 pedigrees compatible with X linkage and a history of bilateral disease. The small family size means some families including those that we have used to define out minimal gene region may be linked by chance. If we have exhausted all the genes identified in the 4cM interval and cannot identify *TGCT1* we will need to extend our interval to include at least two recombinants. With the current bilateral family set this would extend to a 30 Mb interval between the markers *DXS1001* and *DXS731* (Figure 1.3). Obviously refining this interval may be very important.

In the most recent screen there are only 14 pedigrees compatible with X linkage that have not previously been typed for the Xq27 region. These pedigrees are yet to be extensively evaluated and analysed but provisionally there is no change to the evidence for this locus by these 14 pedigrees and no refinement of the minimal region.

6. The Search for Other Testicular Germ Cell Tumour Genes

To date three genome screens have been performed on a subset of ITCLC pedigrees. Two screens each generated a 20cM marker map and the latest genotyping effort utilised a 10cM marker map. Some pedigrees have only ever been run for candidate

Table 1.4: Number of pedigrees typed and corresponding marker density

Pedigree structure	10 cM map (2000 screen)	20 cM map (ICRF & 1996 screen)	Candidate loci only	Total
Sib pairs	28	50	19	97
Sib trios	2	2	1	5
Cousin pairs	11	8	4	23
Uncle/nephew	5	6	4	15
Father/son	4	0	9	13
Large pedigrees	10	3	0	13
Other relative pairs	1			1
Total	61	69	37	167

regions but will eventually be examined through the entire genome. A breakdown of the number of pedigrees genotyped and the density of the marker map is given in Table 1.4. A summary of the current genotyping protocol and statistical analysis is given in the following section.

6.1 Genotyping

Genomic DNA was prepared from whole blood, from immortalised lymphoblastoid cell lines and from formalin-fixed, paraffin-embedded tumour sections using standard techniques. Methods for genotyping from previous genome screen can be found elsewhere [43, 49, 50]. The current method utilises the LMS-MD10 ABI marker set (Applied Biosystems). Microsatellite markers were amplified in PCR reactions with one primer 5' labelled with a fluorochrome. 1 μl of PCR product was combined with up to twenty other markers as described in the panel configuration for the LMS-MD10 marker set and electrophoresed on ABI3700 DNA sequencers (Applied Biosystems). Gels were analysed using the ABI Genescan and Genotyper software. In addition, some markers were end-labelled with $[\gamma-^{32}P]$ ATP using T4 polynucleotide kinase, electrophoresed on standard denaturing polyacrylamide gels, dried and exposed to X-ray film.

6.2 Statistical Analysis

Linkage analysis was performed with the GENEHUNTER software [51] utilising non-parametric and a variety of formal linkage models reflecting the concerns about the underlying mode of inheritance. Linkage models were based on the segregation analyses performed by Heimdal et al. [39]. A lifetime penetrance of 0.45 and a gene frequency of 0.03 for a recessive model and a lifetime penetrance of 0.14 and gene frequency of 0.003 for the dominant model were assumed. As there has not been a formal segregation analysis involving a sex-linked locus for testis cancer, the autosomal recessive values were assumed for the X chromosome model.

Multipoint analyses were performed based on the Marshfield chromosome maps [52] and/or the Location Data-Base (LDB) [53].

Previous research suggests that there is no single major locus for familial testicular cancer (data not shown). Any analysis of the set of testicular cancer families must therefore be examined under heterogeneity. As such we report LOD scores under heterogeneity (HLOD) and the proportion of families linked (α).

Since familial testicular cancer is heterogeneous, we analysed the families under a number of subgroups based on histology, undescended testis status, age of onset and bilaterality. Families were coded as follows; bilateral if there was one or more cases of bilateral disease or ITGCN in a contralateral testis within the family; UDT if at least one of the affected relatives had a history of UDT (retractile testis or hernia were not counted as UDT); seminoma if at least two affected had seminoma; non-seminoma if at least two affected relatives had non-seminoma (i.e. sibs are concordant for histology); ≤ 30 if the mean age of diagnosis of the affected relatives in the family is less than 30 years and > 30 if the mean age at diagnosis is greater than 30 years.

6.3 "ICRF Screen"

In 1995 Leahy and colleagues [49] published the results of a study of 35 families, 32 sib pairs and 3 sib trios (one trio had only two affected members collected). These families were typed for 220 autosomal microsatellite markers spaced at approximately 20 cM throughout the genome. Six regions gave a LOD score of more than 1.0 on formal linkage analysis or a P value of 0.05 or less using a non-parametric approach (Table 1.5).

6.4 "1996" Screen"

A second genome screen was performed on a total of 41 pedigrees within the ITCLC. Of the 41, four pedigrees (all sibs) had been previously screened on the

Table 1.5: Six Candidate regions for TGCT susceptibility [49]

Approx physical location	Locus symbol	Formal Linkage Analysis				Sib-pair Analysis	
		Dominant model	α	Recessive model	α	Mean sharing	P value
1p36	D1S243	0.80	0.01	0.63	0.2	0.59	0.05
4p14–p13	D4S391	1.01	0.05	1.06	0.1	0.64	0.01
4cen–q13	D4S398	1.74	0	2.29	0.05	0.65	0.002
	D4S392	0.77	0.05	1.25	0.1	0.60	0.03
5q12–21	D5S528	1.83	0	1.62	0.1	0.63	0.002
	D5S409	0.63	0.01	0.62	0.1	0.58	0.05
14q13–q24.3	D14S63	0.46	0.1	0.69	0.2	0.59	0.02
18q21.1–q23	D18S64	0.87	0	0.69	0.2	0.59	0.02
	D18S68	1.10	0.01	1.33	0.1	0.63	0.004
	D18S554	1.94	0	0.137	0.2	0.65	0.0004

Table 1.6: Candidate regions as identified in the 1996 screen

Approx physical location	Locus symbol	Two-point LOD scores			
		Dominant model	α	Recessive model	α
3q25–2	D3S12 82	1.09	0.1	0.84	0.20
	D3S16 01	1.55	0.20	1.94	0.20
	D3S27 48	1.62	0.15	1.51	0.20
	D3S12 65	1.27	0.15	2.00	0.15
5p15	D5S43 2	1.17	0.15	0.90	0.20
5q31	D5S40 06	0.90	0.15	1.07	0.20
9p21	D9S18 06	1.20	0.20	0.89	0.25
11q23–24	D11S1 328	1.28	0.10	1.19	0.20
16q24	D16S5 20	1.42	0.15	1.35	0.20
18q22–23 23	D18S5 8	1.62	0.10	0.88	0.20

ICRF search. Thirty-four pedigrees were sib pairs, 2 were sib trios, five were large pedigrees and the remainder were other types of relative pairs. Approximately 230 microsatellite autosomal and X chromosome markers were typed on this pedigree set. Two – point LOD scores were generated for each marker and a number of potential candidate regions were identified (defined as those loci with a LOD score > 1) (Table 1.6)

This demonstrated two regions in common with the ICRF search, one on chromosome 5 and the other on chromosome 18. All potential candidate regions were examined through for the entire ITCLC pedigree set available at the time.

6.5 A Combined Analysis

A non-parametric linkage analysis combining all the genotyping data from the two genome screens and the additional pedigrees genotyped for candidate regions showed that the strongest (but not statistically significant) evidence for linkage at an autosomal locus was on chromosomes 3, 5 and 18 with some evidence for a locus on chromosome 12 (Table 1.7) [50].

6.6 "2000" Screen

Sixty-one ITCLC pedigrees were analysed in this genome screen. These families were examined under the current genome screening protocol given in section 6.1.

Table 1.7: Candidate regions determined by non-parametric analysis of all genotyping data up to 1995 [50]

Approx. physical location	Locus	ITCLC set (1998) NPL	ICRF screen		1996 screen	
			p value / NPL	p value	NPL	p value
3q25–q26	D3S1282–D3S1265	1.44	0.07 / 0.47	0.31	2.21	0.01
5q13–q14	D5S428–D5S421	1.16	0.12 / 1.92	0.02	–0.14	0.55
12q24	D12S324–D12S357	1.36	0.08 / 1.87	0.03	0.23	0.40
18q12–q21	D18S57–D18S70	1.58	0.05 / 2.23	0.01	0.48	0.31

This screen contained 36 new pedigrees for which there was no genotyping information, 22 pedigrees, which had only been examined through candidate loci, and three large pedigrees for which we decided to generate a denser marker map. Of the 36 new pedigrees, 14 were compatible with X linkage (no male–male transmission).

The statistical analysis for these new data is underway. The data has been combined with previous searches and analysed using GENEHUNTER as described in section 6.2. Results from subgroup analysis are not yet available. Provisional results show evidence for an autosomal locus on chromosome 16p13 near the marker *D16S3046* (maximum HLOD = 1.7 α = 0.43 under a dominant model) and chromosome 18q22 near the marker *D18S462* (Maximum HLOD = 1.73 α = 0.2 under a recessive model). Suggestive evidence for linkage remains for chromosome 3q25 - 26 (Maximum HLOD = 1.18 α = 0.16 under a recessive model) but the result is reduced from previous analyses. A locus on chromosome 14q23–24 (Maximum HLOD = 1.01 α = 0.21 under a recessive model) is also suggested.

Chromosomes without any suggestive evidence for linkage are chromosome 6 (maximum = HLOD 0.9), chromosome 12 (maximum HLOD = 0.22), chromosome 19 (maximum HLOD 0.06) and chromosome 21 (maximum HLOD = 0.06).

7. Conclusions

The localisation of a familial TCGT susceptibility gene at Xq27 is the first strong evidence for such a gene. Our data suggest that *TGCT1* is associated with a higher risk of bilateral TGCT and perhaps undescended testis than other TGCT susceptibility genes. However, it seems unlikely that *TGCT1* is the only TGCT susceptibility gene that predisposes to this syndrome, since there are other families with both bilateral disease and undescended testis which are incompatible with X-linkage. *TGCT1* is the first cancer susceptibility gene to be mapped in a genome wide search predominantly using sib pairs and the third cancer predisposing gene to be mapped to the X chromosome following the report of a prostate cancer susceptibility gene [54] and the association of androgen receptor mutations with familial male breast cancer [55].

Other genes for TGCT must exist and the genome searches provide suggestive evidence for a TGCT locus on chromosome 18 and chromosome 16 and also possibly on chromosomes 3 and 14. Our power calculations (section 4.3) would suggest that there are at least two other TGCT genes. We estimate that approximately one quarter of the entire ITCLC set may be due to *TGCT1*. It is unknown whether additional TGCT genes act independently of *TGCT1* or indeed of one another, so that families may be linked to only one gene or more synergistically. These details will only become clear once the other loci are mapped.

References

1. Ferlay, J, Bray P, Pisani P, and Parkin DM GLOBOCAN 2000: Cancer Incidence, Mortality and Prevalence Worldwide, Version 1. IARC CancerBase No.5. Lyon. 2001. IARCPress.
2. Parkin DM, Pisani P, Ferlay J. Estimates of the worldwide incidence of 25 major cancers in 1990. *Int.J.Cancer* 1999;80:827–41.
3. Power DA, Brown RS, Brock CS, Payne HA, Majeed A, Babb P. Trends in testicular carcinoma in England and Wales, 1971–99. *BJU.Int.* 2001;87:361–5.
4. Bergstrom R, Adami HO, Mohner M et al. Increase in testicular cancer incidence in six European countries: a birth cohort phenomenon. *J.Natl.Cancer Inst.* 1996;88:727–33.
5. Skakkebaek NE. Possible carcinoma-in-situ of the testis. *Lancet* 1972;2:516–7.
6. Jorgensen N, Rajpert-De Meyts E, Graem N, Muller J, Giwercman A, Skakkebaek NE. Expression of immunohistochemical markers for testicular carcinoma in situ by normal human fetal germ cells. *Lab Invest* 1995;72:223–31.
7. Giwercman A, Muller J, Skakkebaek NE. Prevalence of carcinoma in situ and other histopathological abnormalities in testes from 399 men who died suddenly and unexpectedly. *J.Urol.* 1991;145:77–80.
8. Forman D, Oliver RT, Brett AR et al. Familial testicular cancer: a report of the UK family register, estimation of risk and an HLA class 1 sib-pair analysis. *Br.J Cancer* 1992;65:255–62.
9. UK Testicular Cancer Study Group. Aetiology of testicular cancer: association with congenital abnormalities, age at puberty, infertility, and exercise. United Kingdom Testicular Cancer Study Group [see comments]. *BMJ.* 1994;308:1393–9.
10. Osterlind A, Berthelsen JG, Abildgaard N et al. Risk of bilateral testicular germ cell cancer in Denmark: 1960–1984. *J.Natl.Cancer Inst.* 1991;83:1391–5.
11. Wanderas EH, Fossa SD, Tretli S. Risk of a second germ cell cancer after treatment of a primary germ cell cancer in 2201 Norwegian male patients. *Eur.J.Cancer* 1997;33:244–52.
12. von der MH, Rorth M, Walbom-Jorgensen S et al. Carcinoma in situ of contralateral testis in patients with testicular germ cell cancer: study of 27 cases in 500 patients. *Br.Med.J.(Clin.Res.Ed)* 1986;293:1398–401.
13. Dieckmann KP. Loy V. Prevalence of contralateral testicular intraepithelial neoplasia in patients with testicular germ cell neoplasms. *J.Clin.Oncol.* 1996;14:3126–32.
14. Loy V. Dieckmann KP. Prevalence of contralateral testicular intraepithelial neoplasia (carcinoma in situ) in patients with testicular germ cell tumour. Results of the German multicentre study. *Eur.Urol.* 1993;23:120–2.
15. Brown LM, Pottern LM, Hoover RN. Testicular cancer in young men: the search for causes of the epidemic increase in the United States. *J.Epidemiol.Community.Health* 1987;41:349–54.
16. Swerdlow AJ, Huttly SR, Smith PG. Testicular cancer and antecedent diseases. *Br.J Cancer* 1987;55:97–103.
17. Swerdlow A.J. Prenatal and familiar associations of testicular cancer. Huttly S.R.A., Smith P. G. Britih Journal of Cancer 55, 571–577. 1987. Ref Type: Generic
18. Swerdlow AJ, Higgins CD, Pike MC. Risk of testicular cancer in cohort of boys with cryptorchidism. *BMJ* 1997;314:150711.
19. Moller H, Skakkebaek NE. Risk of testicular cancer in subfertile men: case-control study. *BMJ* 1999;318:559–62.
20. Jacobsen R, Bostofte E, Engholm G et al. Risk of testicular cancer in men with abnormal semen characteristics: cohort study. *BMJ* 2000;321:789–92.
21. Harland SJ, Cook PA, Fossa SD et al. Intratubular germ cell neoplasia of the contralateral testis in testicular cancer: defining a high risk group. *J.Urol.* 1998;160:1353–7.

22. Prener A, Engholm G, Jensen OM. Genital anomalies and risk for testicular cancer in Danish men. *Epidemiology* 1996;7:14–9.
23. Tollerud DJ, Blattner WA, Fraser MC *et al.* Familial testicular cancer and urogenital developmental anomalies. *Cancer* 1985;55:1849–54.
24. Karagas MR, Weiss NS, Strader CH, Daling JR. Elevated intrascrotal temperature and the incidence of testicular cancer in noncryptorchid men. *Am.J.Epidemiol.* 1989;129:1104–9.
25. Verp MS,.Simpson JL. Abnormal sexual differentiation and neoplasia.
26. Collins GM, Kim DU, Logrono R, Rickert RR, Zablow A, Breen JL. Pure seminoma arising in androgen insensitivity syndrome (testicular feminization syndrome): a case report and review of the literature. *Mod.Pathol.* 1993;6:89–93.
27. Hasle H, Mellemgaard A, Nielsen J, Hansen J. Cancer incidence in men with Klinefelter syndrome. *Br.J.Cancer* 1995;71:416–20.
28. Hasle H, Jacobsen BB, Asschenfeldt P, Andersen K. Mediastinal germ cell tumour associated with Klinefelter syndrome. A report of case and review of the literature. *Eur.J.Pediatr.* 1992;151:735–9.
29. Okada H, Fujioka H, Tatsumi N *et al.* Klinefelter's syndrome in the male infertility clinic. *Hum.Reprod.* 1999;14:946–52.
30. Reddy SR, Svec F, Richardson P. Seminoma of the testis in a patient with 48, XXYY variant of Klinefelter's syndrome. *South.Med.J.* 1991;84:773–5.
31. Carroll PR, Morse MJ, Koduru PP, Chaganti RS. Testicular germ cell tumor in patient with Klinefelter syndrome. *Urology.* 1988;31:72–4.
32. Muller J, Skakkebaek NE, Ratcliffe SG. Quantified testicular histology in boys with sex chromosome abnormalities. *Int.J.Androl* 1995;18:57–62.
33. Satge D, Sommelet D, Geneix A, Nishi M, Malet P, Vekemans M. A tumor profile in Down syndrome. *Am.J.Med.Genet.* 1998;78:207–16.
34. Satge D, Sasco AJ, Cure H, Leduc B, Sommelet D, Vekemans MJ. An excess of testicular germ cell tumors in Down's syndrome: three case reports and a review of the literature. *Cancer* 1997;80:929–35.
35. Dieckmann KP, Rube C, Henke RP. Association of Down's syndrome and testicular cancer. *J Urol.* 1997;157:1701–4.
36. Heimdal K, Olsson H, Tretli S, Flodgren P, Borresen AL, Fossa SD. Familial testicular cancer in Norway and southern Sweden. *Br.J.Cancer* 1996;73:964–9.
37. Wilkinson TJ, Colls BM, Schluter PJ. Increased incidence of germ cell testicular cancer in New Zealand Maoris. *Br.J.Cancer* 1992;65:769–71.
38. Nicholson PW, Harland SJ. Inheritance and testicular cancer. *Br.J.Cancer* 1995;71:421–6.
39. Heimdal K, Olsson H, Tretli S, Fossa SD, Borresen AL, Bishop DT. A segregation analysis of testicular cancer based on Norwegian and Swedish families. *Br.J.Cancer* 1997;75:1084–7.
40. Knudson AG, Jr. Mutation and cancer: statistical study of retinoblastoma. *Proc.Natl.Acad.Sci.U.S.A* 1971;68:820–3.
41. Goss PE, Bulbul MA. Familial testicular cancer in five members of a cancer-prone kindred. *Cancer* 1990;66:2044–6.
42. Gedde-Dahl TJ, Hannisdal E, Klepp OH *et al.* Testicular neoplasms occurring in four brothers. A search for a genetic predisposition. *Cancer* 1985;55:2005–9.
43. Rapley EA, Crockford GP, Teare D *et al.* Localization to Xq27 of a susceptibility gene for testicular germ-cell tumours. *Nat.Genet 2000.Feb.;24.(2.):197–200.* 2000;24:197–200.
44. Raghavan D, Jelihovsky T, Fox RM. Father-son testicular malignancy. Does genetic anticipation occur? *Cancer* 1980;45:1005–9.
45. Han S, Peschel RE. Father-son testicular tumors: evidence for genetic anticipation? A case report and review of the literature. *Cancer* 2000;88:2319–25.
46. Lander E,.Kruglyak L. Genetic dissection of complex traits: guidelines for interpreting and reporting linkage results. *Nat.Genet.* 1995;11:241–7.
47. Redolfi E, Montagna C, Mumm S *et al.* Identification of CXorf1, a novel intronless gene in Xq27.3, expressed in human hippocampus. *DNA Cell Biol.* 1998;17:1009–16.
48. Phelan MC, Stevenson RE, Collins JL, Trent HE. Fragile X syndrome and neoplasia. *Am.J.Med.Genet.* 1988;30:77–82.
49. Leahy MG, Tonks S, Moses JH *et al.* Candidate regions for a testicular cancer susceptibility gene. *Hum.Mol.Genet.* 1995;4:1551–5.
50. Candidate regions for testicular cancer susceptibility genes. The International Testicular Cancer Linkage Consortium. *APMIS* 1998;106:64–70.
51. Kruglyak L, Daly MJ, Reeve-Daly MP, Lander ES. Parametric and nonparametric linkage analysis: a unified multipoint approach. *Am.J.Hum.Genet.* 1996;58:1347–63.
52. Broman KW, Murray JC, Sheffield VC, White RL, Weber JL. Comprehensive human genetic maps: individual and sex-specific variation in recombination. *Am J Hum Genet* 1998;63:861–9.

53. Morton NE, Collins A, Lawerence S, Shields DC. Algorithms for a location database. *Ann Hum Gene* 1992;56:223–32.
54. Xu J, Meyers D, Freije D *et al*. Evidence for a prostate cancer susceptibility locus on the X chromosome. *Nat.Genet.* 1998;20:175–9.
55. Wooster R, Mangion J, Eeles R *et al*. A germline mutation in the androgen receptor gene in two brothers with breast cancer and Reifenstein syndrome. *Nat.Genet.* 1992;2:132–4.

2. Advances in the Understanding of Germ Cell Tumour Biology

Jane Houldsworth*, V.V.V.S. Murty†, George J. Bosl‡,
R.S.K. Chaganti*‡

Cell Biology Program* and Department of Medicine‡, Memorial Sloan-Kettering Cancer Center, and Department of Pathology†, College of Physicians and Surgeons of Columbia University, New York

Genetic Mechanisms of Germ Cell Tumour Origin and Progression

Traditional karyotypic analysis of adult male germ cell tumours (GCTs) performed in this and other laboratories revealed several chromosome abnormalities that may have roles in the aetiology and progression of this disease [1–3].

Over-representation of 12p

One chromosome abnormality includes the almost invariable presence of extra copies of the short arm of chromosome 12, manifested either as an isochromosome i(12p), or as tandem duplications embedded within marker chromosomes [4]. This abnormality has become a molecular marker for GCTs aiding in the diagnosis of some midline carcinomas of uncertain histology [5]. Since this chromosomal marker has been observed in early GCTs, it has been suggested that this genetic lesion is amongst the first associated with transformation of a germ cell. Analysis of GCT-derived cell lines and GCT biopsies has indicated CCND2 mapped to 12p13 that encodes cyclin D2, is a good candidate for the target over-represented gene [6, 7]. In addition to over-representation of the entire short arm, few tumours have exhibited a sub-regional amplification of the 12p11.2–12 region, thought to play a role in GCT progression [8, 9]. Release of the draft human genome sequence and recent technological developments have provided a more comprehensive approach to identifying target amplified genes, especially when the regions of interest are in the range of 20–40 Mbp. This approach initially utilizes publicly available databases to provide a coverage of 12p with known genes and expressed sequence tags (ESTs) (both unassigned and assigned to Unigene clusters). In order to identify over-represented sequences, tumour DNAs are subjected to array-comparative genomic hybridization (A-CGH), using microarrays generated from the 12p cDNAs/ESTs. In this method, tumour and placenta control DNAs are differentially labeled, co-hybridized to microarrays, and appropriate software determines the relative abundance of each 12p sequence in the respective tumour DNA. Similarly, over-expressed 12p sequences are identified by differentially hybridizing tumour and normal testis RNA. For an amplified region, the relevant target gene should be both over-represented and over-expressed. This approach now in progress, permits a more comprehensive manner in which to identify genes on 12p that have important roles in GCT aetiology and progression.

Deletion of 12q

Recognition of recurrent deletion of 12q in GCTs is suggestive for the presence of loss of function genes [2, 10]. Molecular characterization of the 12q cytogenetic deletions by restriction fragment length polymorphism (RFLP) analyses has mapped two regions of high frequency of loss of heterozygosity (LOH) at 12q13 and 12q22 [11]. These deletions occurred in all GCT histologies, suggesting the presence of candidate tumour suppressor genes (TSGs) important to germ cell tumourigenesis on this chromosomal arm. Characteristically, TSGs are inactivated by a combination of genetic (intragenic mutations, LOH, homozygous deletions) and/or epigenetic (hypermethylation) mechanisms [12]. In GCTs, no known TSG has been mapped to the sites of 12q deletions. To identify such a TSG, high-resolution deletion and physical maps of the regions have been constructed which have further restricted the common regions of deletions at the 12q13 and the 12q22 loci [13, 14]. Annotation of the sequence generated from these regions has identified a number of candidate genes at the 12q13 (ALK1, ALK4, TR3, and KRT7) and 12q22 (KITLG, LUM, DCN, RAIDD, BTG1, ELK3, PCTK2, NEDD1, and APAF1) regions. Extensive search for somatic mutations in primary tumours and cell lines in these genes has failed to reveal any pathogenic changes [15]. Thus, these data suggest that mutational inactivation is not a common mechanism of tumour suppression at 12q in GCTs and that other inactivating mechanisms may be operating. Roles for non-mutational gene inactivation mechanisms such as haplo-insufficiency and promoter hypermethy-lation in cancer biology are emerging [16, 17]. To identify the role of such mechanisms in the 12q22 region in GCTs, we studied the steady state levels of gene expression in GCT specimens and derived cell lines. A number of genes mapped to this region showed a complete lack of or down-regulated expression, while others did not exhibit detectable changes in expression. This type of gene expression profile involving a number of genes on a large chromosomal domain may be consistent with an epigenetic inactivation mechanism. Domain-wide gene silencing by clustered organization of imprinted genes has been shown in two related neurological disorders Prader-Willi and Angelman syndromes [18], and in the cancer prone Beckwith-Wiedemann syndrome [19, 20].

Epigenetic modifications resulting from aberrant DNA hypermethylation has been increasingly shown to play an important role in a wide variety of human tumours [17]. To understand whether the mechanism of down-regulated expression of the 12q22 candidate genes represents an epigenetic phenomenon due to hypermethylation of promoter regions, GCT cell lines were treated with the demethylating agent 5-azacytidine (5-aza), which allows re-expression of genes by partial reversion of the methylation. In the GCT cell lines, 5-aza treatment resulted in re-activation of gene expression in a number of genes but had no effect on others. Since recovery of gene expression was observed for a number of genes by 5-aza treatment, a large chromosomal domain inactivated by hypermethylation is indicated. Thus, LOH accompanied by down-regulated gene expression and re-activation upon treatment with a demethylating agent, suggests that the mechanism of tumour suppression at 12q22 is epigenetic. This hypothesis, if confirmed experimentally, may have marked implications in the understanding of the biology of GCTs.

Initiation of Embryonal-like Lineage Differentiation

Adult male GCTs are unique in their display of histopathologies that resemble different stages of human development [7]. *In vitro*, embryonal carcinoma-derived cell lines exhibit varying capacities for differentiation and lineage commitment, with the most widely characterized being NTera2/Clone D1 (NT2/D1) [21]. These cell lines are an invaluable *in vitro* resource in which molecular events regulating differentiation itself, and cell fate/lineage decision can be studied. For NT2/D1, pluripotentiality of the cell line has been established for both known mammalian morphogens such as all-*trans*-retinoic acid (RA) and members of the bone-morphogenetic protein family (BMP-2, BMP-4, BMP-7), and for other agents such as hexamethylene bisacetamide (HMBA) [22–25]. While changes in the levels of select mRNAs have been described during these differentiation programs, global perspectives of the expression patterns of such cell lines during the different programs may lead to the identification of genes that play important roles in lineage decision/cell fate. To this end, comprehensive expression profiling of the NT2/D1 cell line was performed in triplicate during RA-induced differentiation along a predominantly neuronal lineage using oligonucleotide microarray hybridization (Affymetrix). Of the over 12,000 human transcripts represented on the array, 953 exhibited a change (predominantly an increase) in level of expression during the differentiation program. Within these, k-means clustering recognized several clusters of transcripts that may play early roles in the differentiation program, versus later occurring ones possibly more involved with lineage decision. As expected, changes in the levels of transcripts encoded by genes known to be involved in the response of cells to RA such as the retinoid receptors and cofactors, as well as those involved in the cellular metabolism of retinoids, were observed. In addition, transcripts whose function could be directly implicated in cell cycle control consistent with growth arrest were also found to alter during the differentiation program. Alterations were also revealed in the expression of genes, amongst others, whose products function in affecting cytoskeleton remodeling (at signal transduction and structural levels) and glycolytic/oxidative pathways of energy metabolism respectively. Examination of markers for cell lineage indicated the loss of a stem cell phenotype, with the induction of lineage markers consistent with transition to neuronal progenitor cells expressing patterning markers compatible with posterior hindbrain fates, followed by the appearance of immature postmitotic neurons with an evolving synaptic apparatus. Thus, global analysis of gene expression allows monitoring of cell fate and differentiation of embryonal carcinoma cells *in vitro* and comparison with profiles of differentiation programs induced by other morphogens and in other embryonal carcinoma cell lines, may well identify candidate genes ranging from master regulators of differentiation to molecular inducers of specific differentiation programs.

Biological Mechanisms of GCT Resistance

GCTs serve as a good model for a curable malignancy. However, the high cure rate obscures the clinical finding that 20–30 per cent of patients who present with metastatic disease will succumb to their disease [26]. In the past few years, we have embarked upon a series of studies aimed at identifying pathways by which resistance is achieved in GCTs. These studies have involved the combining of cellular, molecular, and genome and transcript scanning technologies. The molecular participants in these pathways may represent powerful markers of clinical resistance and/or provide insights on novel treatment approaches.

TP53 Mutation

The relative paucity of *TP53* mutations in male GCTs has been recognized for some time now [27, 28], and in recent years, we had identified one subset of clinically resistant GCTs that exhibited mutations and/or deletions in *TP53* [29]. More recently, we have scanned the entire coding region of *TP53* for mutations using an oligonucleotide microarray GeneChip p53 assay (Affymetrix). Application of this assay to a panel of 16 clinically-resistant GCTs has revealed additional mutations than those detected by traditional single strand conformation polymorphism (SSCP) analysis, but was not successful in detecting deletions greater than one base pair. Thus, the estimated frequency of *TP53* mutations within resistant GCT patients may be somewhat higher than previously noted by us [29]. Subsequent *in vitro* studies revealed a relative resistance to the induction of apoptosis and cell death by cisplatin of a GCT cell line harbouring a *TP53* mutation (228A) derived from a tumour which failed to respond completely to cisplatin-based chemotherapy, compared with a GCT cell line with wild type *TP53* (218A) derived from a tumour which responded completely [29]. Thus, in this disease, *TP53* mutation is a harbinger of a poor clinical outcome to a cisplatin-based treatment regimen and subversion of the presumably p53-dependent apoptotic response to therapy represents one biological pathway by which resistance is achieved. In order to molecularly characterize the cellular response in GCTs following cisplatin exposure, a profiling study of GCT cell lines was recently initiated to identify transcripts either present/absent inherently in the respective cell lines, or up-/down-regulated following cisplatin exposure. Initially our studies focused on the chemosensitive GCT cell line 218A. In triplicate, the relative expression of over 12,000 human transcripts was profiled both prior to and during cisplatin treatment, using oligonucleotide microarrays (Affymetrix). Little or no transcriptional response to cisplatin was detected until three hours into treatment, and then many fewer transcripts were up-regulated than down-regulated. Few up-regulated transcripts comprised genes previously known to be p53-regulated transcriptional targets following genotoxic damage. A few (*TOB1, BTG3*) were genes known to function as cell growth inhibitors following either stress or differentiation signals [30, 31]. Comparison of the transcript responses between GCT cell lines will identify genes whose up- or down-regulation is effective in inducing the apoptotic response in the chemosensitive cell line but ineffective or subverted in chemoresistant GCT cell lines. These comparative studies will also aid in identifying potential pathways that can be exploited as targets for new therapeutic agents in chemoresistant GCTs and in other tumour systems.

Gene Amplification

We have observed by CGH and reported unique, highly amplified DNA regions in resistant GCT, a genetic abnormality often associated with tumour progression and resistance to therapy [9]. While good candidate genes exist for some of the identified regions, a more comprehensive assay to identify amplified sequences is required. To this end, DNAs extracted from a panel of 13 GCTs that exhibited clinical resistance to cisplatin-based chemotherapy and from a panel of six sensitive GCTs comprising the primary specimen from patients treated with cisplatin-based chemotherapy and whose retroperitoneal lymph node dissection revealed no evidence of viable disease, were submitted to A-CGH. In this case, cDNA/EST microarrays with genome-wide coverage were utilized. While low-level gain of cDNAs/ESTs was detected in both resistant and sensitive GCTs, as predicted from our previous CGH study, only higher-level gene amplification at chromosomal sites other than 12p was detected in resistant GCTs. Four previously amplified sites by conventional CGH were confirmed by A-CGH, while another four were not, indicating the lack of cDNAs/ESTs mapped to this chromosomal site on the array. In addition, seven new sites of amplification were detected, possibly representing small amplicons below the detectable size limit of conventional CGH. These data have confirmed our previous observation of the association of high-level gene amplification in cisplatin-resistant GCT specimens [9]. As yet, the identity of the amplified genes remains largely unknown in three recurrently amplified regions due to lack of full coverage of mapped sequences on the microarrays. Construction of region-specific microarrays as described for 12p, would aid in the identification of amplified and over-expressed target genes in the recurrently amplified regions that have been confirmed in a larger panel of tumours.

Differentiation

While differentiated elements within GCTs (immature and mature teratoma) do not generally impact on overall survival, they do represent a histological subtype with documented poor response to therapy [26]. Pluripotential embryonal carcinoma cell lines such as NT2/D1 as described above, comprise a model system in which the effect of differentiation on the cellular response to cisplatin can be studied. Exposure of the undifferentiated NT2/D1 cell line to cisplatin revealed a typical sensitive cellular response (decline in viable cell count and increase in number of cells undergoing apoptosis), while the RA-differentiated culture exhibited a relatively resistant response. An induction of p53 and p53-responsive genes was observed in undifferentiated cells, with a much-attenuated response in RA-differentiated cells. Again, molecular profiling of the response of these two cell types to cisplatin may reveal a molecular understanding of the role in drug resistance of this biological mechanism inherent to GCTs. These studies are currently in progress.

Concluding Comments

In the quest of understanding the biology of these unique tumours, application of recent cellular, molecular, and genome and transcript scanning technologies to experimental studies has been insightful. Progress has been made on several aspects of the disease, including the prominent role of chromosome 12 in GCT aetiology and progression, the use of GCT-derived cell lines as powerful model systems for identifying genes with important functions during normal human development, and the identification of genetic and biological mechanisms whereby resistance to chemotherapy is achieved. Further experimental approaches should help in unraveling the unique biology of these fascinating tumours.

References

1. Rodriguez E, Mathew S, Reuter V, Ilson DH, Bosl GJ, Chaganti RS. Cytogenetic analysis of 124 prospectively ascertained male germ cell tumors. *Cancer Res* 1992;52:2285-2291
2. Chaganti RSK, Murty VVVS, Bosl GJ. Molecular genetics of male germ cell tumors. In: Vogelzang NJ, Shipley WU, Scardino PT, Coffey DS (eds). *Comprehensive Textbook of Genitourinary Oncology*. Baltimore: Williams and Wilkins, pp 932-940, 1996
3. Chaganti RSK, Rodriguez E, Bosl GJ. Cytogenetics of male germ-cell tumors. *Urol Clin N Amer* 1993;20:55-66
4. Chaganti RSK, Houldsworth J, Bosl GJ. Molecular biology of adult male germ cell tumors. In: Vogelzang NJ, Scardino PT, Shipley WU, Coffey DS (eds). *Comprehensive Textbook of Genitourinary Oncology*, 2nd edn. Philadelphia: Lippincott, Williams and Wilkins, pp 891-896, 2000
5. Motzer RJ, Rodriguez E, Reuter VE, Bosl GJ, Mazumdar M, Chaganti RSK. Molecular and cytogenetic studies in the diagnosis of patients with poorly differentiated carcinomas of unknown primary site. *J Clin Oncol* 1995;13:274-82
6. Houldsworth J, Reuter V, Bosl GJ, Chaganti RSK. Aberrant expression of cyclin D2 is an early event in human male germ cell tumorigenesis. *Cell Growth Differ* 1997;8:293-299
7. Chaganti RSK, Houldsworth J. Genetics and biology of adult human male germ cell tumors. *Cancer Res* 2000;60:1475-1482
8. Mostert MC, Verkerk AJ, van de Pol M, et al. Identification of the critical region of 12p over-representation in testicular germ cell tumors of adolescents and adults. *Oncogene* 1998;16:2617-2627
9. Rao PH, Houldsworth J, Palanisamy N, et al. Chromosomal amplification is associated with cisplatin resistance of human male germ cell tumors. *Cancer Res* 1998;58:4260-4263
10. Murty VVVS, Chaganti RSK. A genetic perspective of male germ cell tumors. *Seminars Oncol* 1998;25:1-13
11. Murty VVVS, Houldsworth J, Baldwin S, et al. Allelic deletions in the long arm of chromosome 12 identify sites of candidate tumor suppressor genes in male germ cell tumors. *Proc Natl Acad Sci USA* 1992;89:11006-11011
12. Ponder BA. Cancer genetics. *Nature* 2001;411:336-341
13. Murty VVVS, Renault B, Falk CT, Bosl GJ, Kucherlapati R, Chaganti RSK. Physical mapping of a commonly deleted region, the site of a candidate tumor suppressor gene, at 12q22 in human male germ cell tumors. *Genomics* 1996;35:562-570
14. Murty VVVS, Montgomery K, Dutta S, et al. A 3-Mb high-resolution BAC, PAC contig of 12q22 encompassing the 830 kb consensus minimal deletion in male germ cell tumors. *Genome Res* 1999;9:662-671
15. Bala S, Oliver H, Renault B, et al. Genetic analysis of the APAF1 gene in male germ cell tumors. *Genes Chroms Cancer* 2000;28:258-268
16. Fero ML, Randel E, Gurley KE, Roberts JM, Kemp CJ. The murine gene p27Kip1 is haplo-insufficient for tumour suppression. *Nature* 1998;396:177-180
17. Baylin SB, Herman JG. DNA hypermethylation in tumorigenesis: epigenetics joins genetics. *Trends Genet* 2000;16:168-174
18. Shemer R, Hershko AY, Perk J, et al. The imprinting box of the Prader-Willi/Angelman syndrome domain. *Nature Genet* 2000;26:440-443
19. Engemann S, Strodicke M, Paulsen M, et al. Sequence and functional comparison in the Beckwith-Wiedemann region: implications for a novel imprinting centre and extended imprinting. *Hum Mol Genet* 2000;9:2691-2706
20. Maher ER, Reik W. Beckwith-Wiedemann syndrome: imprinting in clusters revisited. *J Clin Invest* 2000;105:247-252
21. Andrews PW. Teratocarcinomas and human embryology: pluirpotent human EC cell lines. A review. *APMIS* 1998;106:158-168
22. Andrews PW, Nudelman E, Hakomori S-I, Fenderson BA. Different patterns of glycolipid antigens are expressed following differentiation of TERA-2 human embryonal carcinoma cells induced by retinoic acid, hexamethylene bisacetamide (HMBA) or bromodeoxyuridine (BudR). *Differ* 1990;43:131-138
23. Andrews PW, Damjanov I, Berends J, et al. Inhibition of proliferation and induction of differentiation of pluripotent human embryonal carcinoma cells by osteogenic protein-1 (or bone morphogenetic protein-7). *Lab Invest* 1994;71:243-251
24. Caricasole A, Ward-Van Oostwaard D, Zeinstra L, Van Den Eijnden-Van Raaij A, Mummery C. Bone morphogenetic proteins (BMPs) induce epithelial differentiation of NT2D1 human embryonal carcinoma cells. *Int J Dev Biol* 2000;44:443-450
25. Houldsworth J, Reuter VE, Bosl GJ, Chaganti RSK. ID gene expression varies with lineage during differentiation of pluripotential male germ cell tumor cell lines. *Cell Tissue Res* 2001;303:371-379

26. Bosl GJ, Motzer RJ. Testicular germ-cell cancer. *New Engl J Med* 1997;337:242–253
27. Heimdal K, Lothe LA, Lystad S, Holm R, Fossa SD, Borresen AL. No germline TP53 mutations detected in familial and bilateral testicular cancer. *Genes Chroms Cancer* 1993;6:92–97
28. Peng H-Q, Hogg D, Malkin D, et al. Mutations of the p53 gene do not occur in testis cancer. *Cancer Res* 1993;53:3574–3578
29. Houldsworth J, Xiao H, Murty VVVS, et al. Human male germ cell tumor resistance to cisplatin is linked to TP53 gene mutation. *Oncogene* 1998;16:2345–2349
30. Tirone F. The gene PC3(TIS21/BTG2), prototype member of the PC3/BTG/TOB family: regulator in control of cell growth, differentiation, and DNA repair? *J Cell Physiol* 2001;187:155–165
31. Matsuda S, Rouault J, Magaud J, Berthet C. In search of a function for the TIS21/PC3/BTG1/TOB family. *FEBS Lett* 2001;497:67–72

3. A Notch-related Gene Located on the Long Arm of Human Chromosome 12

David Adamah, Paul J. Gokhale, James Walsh, Peter W. Andrews

The Department of Biomedical Science, University of Sheffield, Western Bank, Sheffield S10 2TN

Family and cytogenetic studies of testicular germ cell tumours (TGCT) suggest a strong genetic component in the aetiology of these tumours. We have focused upon genes that may play a key regulatory role in the development of germ cells. Following studies in the nematode worm, Caenorhabditis elegans [1], we have investigated the Notch gene family. Initial results indicate that members of the Notch family are expressed by primordial germ cells, and by seminoma and intratubular germ cell neoplasia, consistent with a possible role in tumour development (unpublished results).

We have also identified a novel gene that, although not a classical *Notch* gene, does contain the Lin/Notch motifs hitherto only seen in the *Notch* family. This gene maps to human chromosome 12q23, close to the location of a possible tumour suppresser gene suggested by studies of LOH in TGCT patients [2]. This gene encodes a message of approximately 6kb, and coincides, at least in part, with a gene predicted by the human genome project. The gene is expressed in clinical samples of seminoma and in human EC cell lines. It is, therefore, a candidate gene that may play a role in TGCT development.

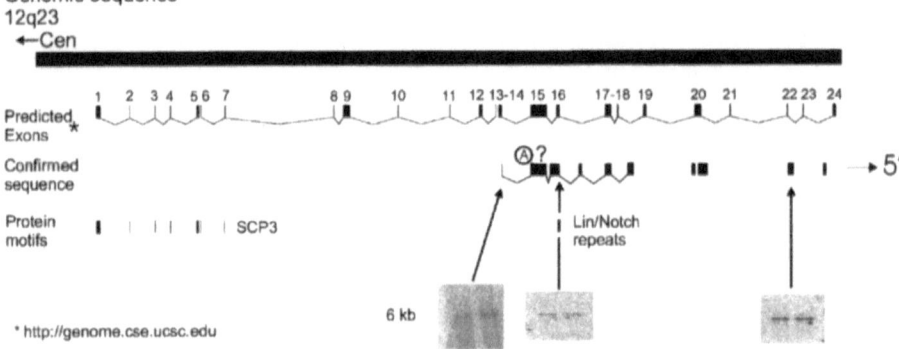

Figure 3.1: Schematic diagram of a candidate gene involved in formation of TGCT. Twenty-four exons were predicted and map to 12q23. The mRNA sequence confirmed by experiment mapped to 12q23. There is partial correspondence with the predicted sequence: exons 16 and 22 appear to be expanded, 18, 21, 23 are missing. There appears to be additional exon sequences between exons 16, 17, 18 and 19. Exon 20 appears to be split in two and expanded. A poly A site was initially predicted at exon 15. Exons that are definately part of the same sequence are joined by lines. Several parts of the predicted sequence were used to probe northern blotting, each recognising a transcript of approximately 6 kb. Exons 1–7 and exon 16 from the predicated sequence encode protein mofits, homologous to synaptonemal complex protein 3 and Lin/Notch repeats.

Acknowledgements

Supported in part by a grant from Yorkshire Cancer Research and studentship from the Commonwealth Universities Association (David Adamah).

References

1. Berry, L.W., Westlund, B., Schedl, T. Germ line tumour formation caused by activation of *Glp-1*, a Caenorhabditis elegans member of the *Notch* family of receptors. *Development* 124, 925–936, 1997
2. Murty VV, Montgomery K, Dutta S, Bala S, Renault B, Bosl GJ, Kucherlapati R, Chaganti RS. A 3-Mb high-resolution BAC/PAC contig of 12q22 encompassing the 830-kb consensus minimal deletion in male germ cell tumors. *Genome Research* 9:662–671, 1999

4. Investigating Gain of 12p Material in Testicular Germ Cell Tumours and Its Apparent Absence in Carcinoma in situ

B. Summersgill, O. Jafer, H. Goker, S. Rodriguez, R. Huddart, J. Shipley

Institute Cancer Research, Sutton, Surrey UK

Adult and adolescent testicular germ cell tumours (TGCT) are consistently associated with gain of 12p material, involving an isochromosome 12p [i(12p)] in around 80 per cent of cases. In some, high level gain or amplification corresponding to the sub-region of 12p at 12p11–12 has been found, indicating at least one region of 12p which harbours a gene or genes important in the development of TGCT.

We have determined the stage at which gain of 12p appears critical in TGCT development. Carcinoma in situ (CIS) or intratubular germ cell neoplasia is generally considered as the precursor lesion of adult TGCTs. CGH analysis of microdissected CIS with interphase FISH analysis of CIS and associated TGCT was undertaken. Neither gain nor amplification of 12p material was detected at the CIS stage indicating that most CIS cells do not contain this change [1]. This is consistent with recent independent work [2, 3] but different to earlier studies [4–8]. We identified shared imbalances in CIS and associated invasive disease, including gain of material from chromosomes 1, 5, 7, 8, 12q and X and loss of material from chromosome 18. Our results suggest that gain and amplification of 12p material are associated with either progression of CIS to invasive TGCT or further progression of the invasive disease.

As gain of 12p material appears central to TGCT development, we have applied interphase FISH analysis to invasive cases with 12p amplicons in order to define a region harbouring critical genes on 12p. This has defined the smallest overlapping region of amplification. Our results were coincident with similar work from Looijenga's group in Rotterdam [9, 2]. Cell lines derived from GCT were also screened for 12p amplification as a potential resource for more detailed analyses. Only one cell line was identified with an increased gene dosage in the 12p11-p12 region but the dosage was very subtle (10 copies of the entire 12p versus 2–3 additional copies of the 12p11-p12 region) [10]. Two hundred and fifty cDNA clones from chromosome 12, including all known genes mapping to the 12p amplicon region, have been collected and arrayed onto microscope slides in addition to a 5,500 Geneset which includes many known oncogenes. Microarray analyses are ongoing with both DNA and RNA from cases with and without amplicons. Preliminary expression profiling of five cases has revealed a number of genes and expressed sequences from the amplicon region (such as PI3KC2G, SIAT8, KRAS2, SURB7, and I.M.A.G.E. ID – 685807, 1234105, 453328, 1501595, 142964), which are consistently overexpressed relative to normal testicular tissue and fibroblasts. This approach will facilitate identifying genes involved in the progression of testicular germ cell tumours.

References

1. Summersgill B, Osin P, Lu YJ, Huddart R, Shipley J, Chromosome imbalances associated with carcinoma in situ and associated testicular germ cell tumour of adolescents and adults. *Br J Cancer*, 2001;85:213–20
2. Roelofs H, Mostert MC, Pompe K et al. Restricted 12p amplification and RAS mutation in human germ cell tumors of the adult testis, *Am J Pathol*, 2000, 157:1155–66
3. Rosenberg C, Van Gurp RJHLM, Geelen E, Oosterhuis JW, Looijenga LHJ. Overrepresentation of the short arm of chromosome 12 is related to invasive growth of human testicular seminomas and nonseminomas. *Oncogene* 2000;19:5858–62
4. Vos AM, Oosterhuis JW, De Jong B, Buist J, Koops HS, Cytogentics of carcinoma in situ of the testis, *Cancer Genet. Cytogenet*, 1990;46:75–81
5. van Echten J, van Gurp RJHLM, Stoepker M, Looijenga HL, de Jong B, Oosterhuis JW. Cytogenetic evidence that carcinoma in situ is the precursor lesion for invasive testicular germ cell tumors. *Cancer Genet Cytogenet*, 1995;85:133–7
6. Meng FJ, Giwercman A, Skakkebaek NE. Investigation of carcinoma in situ cells of testis by quantification of argyrophilic nucleolar organizer region associated proteins (AgNORs). *J Pathol*, 1998;186:235–239
7. Looijenga LH, Rosenberg C, van Gurp RJ et al. Comparative genomic hybridization of microdissected samples from different stages in the development of a seminoma and a non-seminoma. *Br J Cancer*, 2000;83:729–36
8. Chaganti RS, Houldsworth J. Genetic and biology of adult testicular germ cell tumours. *Cancer Res* 2000;60:1475–82
9. Mostert MC, Verkerk AJ, van de Pol M et al. Identification of the critical region of 12p ove representation in testicular germ cell tumors of adolescents and adults. *Oncogene*, 1998;16:2671–672
10. Summersgill B, Jafer O, Wnag R et al. Definition of chromosome aberration in testicular germ cell tumour cell lines by 24-colour karyotyping and complementary molecular cytogenetic analysis, *Cancer Genet Cytogenet*. 2001;128:120–29

5. Overrepresentation of the Short Arm of Chromosome 12 Is Related to Invasive Growth of Testicular Seminomas and Non-seminomas

J.W. Oosterhuis[1], R.J.H.L.M. van Gurp[1], C. Rosenberg[2], L.H.J. Looijenga[1]

1. Pathology/Laboratory for Experimental Patho-Oncology, University Hospital Rotterdam/Daniel,Josephine Nefkens Institute, Erasmus University Rotterdam, Building Be, room 430b, Dr. Molewaterplein 50, 3015 GE Rotterdam, 2. Department of Cytochemistry and Cytometry, Leiden University Medical Center, Leiden, the Netherlands.

Abstract

Relative overrepresentation of the short of chromosome 12, mostly as isochromosomes (i(12p)), is considered to be characteristic for testicular germ cell tumours (TGCTs). Here we show that gain of 12p is not one of the initiating events in the development of TGCTs, but is related to invasive growth.

Introduction

Testicular germ cell tumours of adolescents and adults (TGCTs), i.e., seminomas and non-seminomas, represent the most common malignancy in young Caucasian men [1]. Epidemiological [2], morphological [3] and immunohistochemical [4–8] characteristics suggest that the initiating event in the pathogenesis of TGCTs may occur during intra-uterine development. Carcinoma in situ (CIS) or intratubular germ cell neoplasia (ITGCN) [9] is the precursor lesion to invasive TGCTs. TGCTs [10] and CIS [11] are aneuploid, and invasive TGCTs are characterized by additional copies of the short arm of chromosome 12 [12]. This is mostly due to the formation of isochromosomes (i12p), first described in 1982 [13]. The presence of gain of 12p in CIS has not been established [14–16], mainly because of the limited availability of interpretable cases.

Materials and Methods

The tumours included in this study were collected in collaboration with urologists and pathologists in the South-Western part of the Netherlands from patients who had not received chemotherapy or radiotherapy. Representative samples of the tumour and adjacent parenchyma were snap frozen. The rest was sampled and fixed overnight in 10 per cent buffered formalin for paraffin embedding. The tumours were diagnosed according to the World Health Organization (WHO) classification of testicular tumours [17]. CIS was identified by direct staining for alkaline phosphatase enzyme reactivity [18]. Chromosomal analysis, fluorescent *in situ* hybridization (FISH), comparative genomic hybridization (CGH), and micro-dissection were performed as previously described [16, 19–21].

Results and Discussion

We examined four seminomas and seven non-seminomas and their corresponding CIS for overrepresentation of the short arm of chromosome 12, by FISH and CGH. Prior to CGH, CIS cells were purified using micro-dissection, and DNA was amplified. Out of the 16 morphologically different invasive tumour components investigated (four seminomas, four embryonal carcinomas, six teratomas, and two yolk sac tumours), all except one teratoma showed gain of 12p using CGH. FISH confirmed the CGH results in all four seminomas and three out of the four embryonal carcinomas. In contrast, none of the CIS cells showed additional copies of the short arm of chromosome 12 by either technique (front cover). Our data demonstrate that gain of 12p is not an initiating event in the pathogenesis of TGCTs, but related to invasive growth.

Using the same approach, we investigated the presence of gain of 12p in three gonadoblastomas and matched dysgerminomas. These are the putative counterparts of CIS and seminoma of the dysgenetic gonad [22, 23]. As found for the tumours in

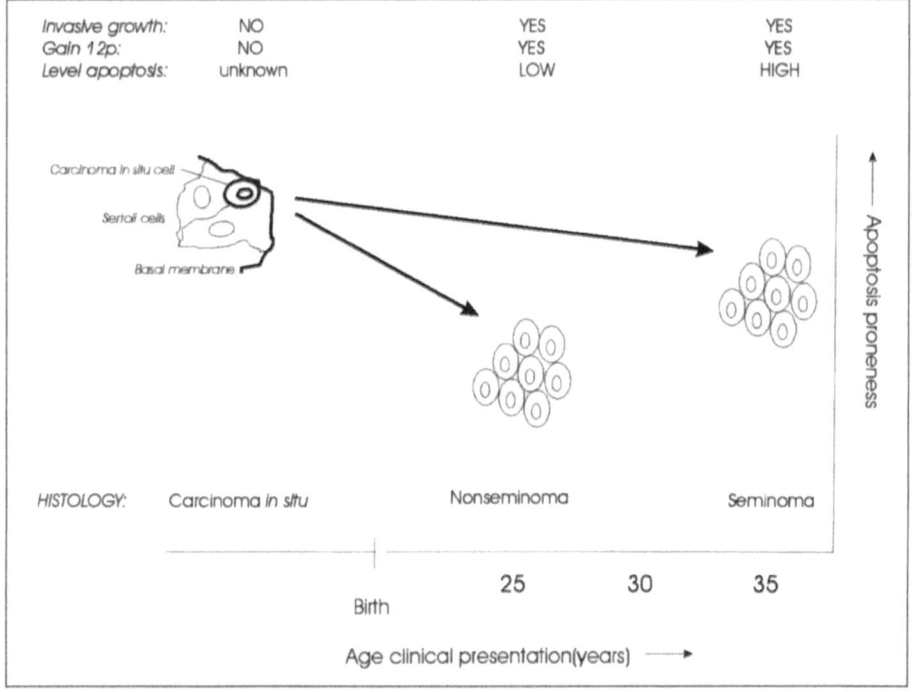

Figure 5.1: A schematic model indicating the supposed role of gain of 12p in the development of TGCTs.

the adult testis, gain of 12p was restricted to the invasive dysgerminomas components (Stoop *et al.*, in prep).

We attempted to further identify the relevant genes on 12p involved in the development of invasive TGCTs. We investigated a subset of TGCTs, mainly seminomas, which show high levels of amplification of a restricted region of 12p, cytogenetically identified as 12p11.2–12.1. These tumours contained no i(12p), showed a lower level of apoptosis, and presented clinically at an earlier age than seminomas without this restricted 12p-amplification [19, 24]. CIS cells adjacent to these seminomas did not share this restricted 12p amplification [19]. Our hypothesis is that gain of 12p is associated with suppression of apoptotic cell death, which confers a survival advantage to CIS cells as they start to become invasive, i.e., leave the micro-environment of the seminiferous tubules.

Conclusion

Our data demonstrate that gain of 12p is not an initiating event in the development of TGCTs but is related to invasive behaviour. The association between the presence of restricted 12p-amplification, levels of apoptosis and patient age at diagnosis, allows a more straightforward approach to the identification of relevant genes.

The work was financially supported by the Dutch Cancer Society

References

1. Pottern ML, Morris Brwn L, Devesa SS. Epidemiology and pathogenesis of testicular cancer. In: Ernsthoff MS, Heaney JA, Peschel RE, editors. *Testicular and Penile Cancer.* Oxford: Blackwell Science, 1998:2–10
2. Møller H. Decreased testicular cancer risk in men born in wartime. *J Natl Cancer Inst* 1989; 81(21):1668–9
3. Gondos B. Ultrastructure of developing and malignant germ cells. *Eur Urol* 1993;23:68–75.
4. Jørgensen N, Giwercman A, Müller J, Skakkebæk NE. Immunohistochemical markers of carcinoma in situ of the testis also expressed in normal infantile germ cells. *Histopathol* 1993;22:373–378
5. Rajpert-De Meyts E, Skakkebæk NE. Expression of the c-kit protein product in carcinoma-in-situ and invasive testicular germ cell tumours. *Int J Androl* 1994;17:85–92
6. Jørgensen N, Rajpert-De Meyts E, Graem N, Müller J, Giwercman A, Skakkebæk NE. Expression of immunohistochemical markers for testicular carcinoma in situ by normal fetal germ cells. *Lab Invest* 1995;72:223–231
7. De Meyts ER, Jorgensen N, Muller J, Skakkebaek NE. Prolonged expression of the c-kit receptor in germ cells of intersex fetal testes. *Journal of Pathology.* 1996;178:166–169
8. Roelofs H, Manes T, Millan JL, Oosterhuis JW, Looijenga LHJ. Heterogeneity in alkaline phosphatase isozyme expression in human testicular germ cell tumours. An enzyme-/immunohistochemical and molecular analysis. *J Pathol* 1999;189:236–244
9. Skakkebæk NE. Possible carcinoma-in-situ of the testis. *Lancet* 1972:516–517
10. Oosterhuis JW, Castedo SMMJ, De Jong B et al. Ploidy of primary germ cell tumours of the testis. Pathogenetic and clinical relevance. *Lab Invest* 1989;60:14–20
11. De Graaff WE, Oosterhuis JW, De Jong B et al. Ploidy of testicular carcinoma in situ. *Lab Invest* 1992;66:166–168
12. Van Echten-Arends J, Oosterhuis JW, Looijenga LHJ et al. No recurrent structural abnormalities in germ cell tumours of the adult testis apart from i(12p). *Genes Chromosom & Cancer* 1995;14:133–144
13. Atkin NB, Baker MC. Specific chromosome change, i(12p), in testicular tumours? *Lancet* 1982;8311:1340
14. Van Echten-Arends J, Stoepker M, Leegte B, Looijenga LHJ, De Jong B, Oosterhuis JW. Cytogenetic evidence that carcinoma in situ is the precursor lesion for invasive testicular germ cell tumours. *Cancer Genet Cytogenet* 1994;77:194

15. Looijenga LHJ, Gillis AJM, Van Putten WLJ, Oosterhuis JW. In situ numeric analysis of centromeric regions of chromosomes 1, 12, and 15 of seminomas, nonseminomatous germ cell tumours, and carcinoma in situ of human testis. *Lab Invest* 1993;68:211–219

16. Looijenga LHJ, Rosenberg C, Van Gurp RJHLM et al. Comparative genomic hybridization of microdissected samples from different stages in the development of a seminoma and nonseminoma. *J Pathol* 2000;19:187–192

17. Mostofi FK, Sesterhenn IA. *Histological typing of testis tumours.* 2nd ed. Berlin: Springer, 1998

18. Mosselman S, Looijenga LHJ, Gillis AJM, et al. Aberrant platelet-derived growth factor a-receptor transcript as a diagnostic marker for early human germ cell tumours of the adult testis. *Proc Natl Acad Sci USA* 1996;93:2884–2888

19. Roelofs H, Mostert MC, Pompe K et al. Restricted 12p-amplification and RAS mutation in human germ cell tumours of the adult testis. *Am J Pathol* 2000;157(4):1155–1166

20. Rosenberg C, Van Gurp RJHLM, Geelen E, Oosterhuis JW, Looijenga LHJ. Overrepresentation of the short arm of chromosome 12 is related to invasive growth of human testicular seminomas and nonseminomas. *Oncogene* 2000;19:5858–5862

21. Stoop H, Van Gurp RHJLM, De Krijger R et al. Reactivity of germ cell maturation stage-specific markers in spermatocytic seminoma: diagnostic and etiological implications. *Lab Invest* 2001; 81:919–928

22. Scully RE. Gonadoblastoma/ A review of 74 cases. *Cancer* 1970;25:1340–1356

23. Jørgensen N, Muller J, Jaubert F, Clausen OP, Skakkebaek NE. Heterogeneity of gonadoblastoma germ cells: similarities with immature germ cells, spermatogonia and testicular carcinoma in situ cells. *Histopathol* 1997;30(2):177–86

24. Mostert MC, Verkerk AJMH, Van de Pol M et al. Identification of the crucial region of 12p overrepresentation in testicular germ cell tumours of adolescents and adults. *Oncogene* 1998;16:2617–2627

6. Reactivity of Germ Cell Maturation Stage-specific Markers in Classical and Spermatocytic Seminoma

L.H.J. Looijenga, H. Stoop, R. J.H.L.M. van Gurp, R.de Krijger,
J. W. Oosterhuis

Pathology/Laboratory for Experimental Patho-Oncology, University Hospital Rotterdam/Daniel, Josephine Nefkens Institute, Erasmus University Rotterdam, Building Be, room 430b, Dr. Molewaterplein 50, 3015 GE Rotterdam, The Netherlands

Abstract

This paper presents data supporting the model that classical seminoma originates from a primordial germ cell/gonocyte in which maturation is blocked. Although spermatocytic seminoma might also originate from an embryonic germ cell, it retains the capacity to undergo further maturation, including partial meiosis. Moreover, we identified immunohistochemical markers helpful in the diagnosis of spermatocytic seminomas.

Introduction

It is generally accepted that classical seminoma and spermatocytic seminomas have a separate pathogenesis, although their cell of origin is still a matter of debate [1]. Epidemiological data [2], as well as morphological [3] and immunohistochemical [4–8] characteristics suggest that classical seminomas originate from a primordial germ cell/gonocyte, and that the initiating event in their pathogenesis may occur during intra-uterine development. Mainly on the basis of morphological analysis, it has been suggested that spermatocytic seminomas originate from a spermatocyte [9–14]. These tumours are less frequent than classical seminoma, arise at an older age, and rarely metastasize [15, 16]. However bilateral spermatocytic seminomas are relatively frequent which might argue against spermatocytes as cells of origin.

Here we summarize the available data on the usefulness of various types of markers to distinguish classical seminoma from spermatocytic seminoma and present the results of a number of new immunohistochemical markers. The data will be discussed in the context of the possible cell of origin of these two tumour types.

Materials and Methods

The tumours included in this study were collected in collaboration with urologists and pathologists in the South-Western part of the Netherlands, from patients who had not received chemotherapy or irradiation. Representative samples were snap frozen and the remaining specimen was sampled and fixed overnight in 10 per cent buffered formalin and embedded in paraffin. The tumours were diagnosed according to the World Health Organization (WHO) classification for testicular tumours [17]. Immunohistochemistry, expression studies and chromosomal analysis were performed as described before [18, 19].

Results and Discussion

A summary of the published data on different types of markers in classical seminoma and spermatocytic seminoma is given in Table 6.1. The most striking observation is that these markers are either positive in both types of tumours, or are only positive in classical seminoma. None of the available markers specifically stain spermatocytic seminomas, which limits their diagnostic usefulness because of the possibility of false negative results. In terms of histogenesis, it is of interest that glycogen, c-KIT, GCAP/PLAP, and OCT4 (De Leeuw *et al.*, in prep.) are found in both seminoma and primordial germ cells/gonocytes, but not in spermatocytic seminoma. OCT4 in particular is a marker of pluripotency [20]. Although both types of seminoma are positive for VASA, spermatocytic seminomas show a much stronger intensity than found in normal spermatocytes up to the spermatid stage [21] (Zeeman et al., submitted). The RNA markers *HIWI* and the 1.5 kb transcript of the PDGF alpha-receptor are specifically positive in seminoma [22] (Qiao et al., submitted). Because of the lack of a specific positive marker for spermatocytic seminoma, we investigated several markers that are associated with specific stages of normal germ cell maturation. We selected these markers based on the hypothesis that the cells of spermatocytic seminoma show characteristics of cells that undergo meiosis. These markers included *SCP1* (synaptonemal complex protein 1, found in cells undergoing meiosis, in particular meiotic prophase) [23,24], *SSX* (synovial sarcoma on X chromosome, mainly found in spermatogonia, see Figure 6.1A) [25], and *XPA* (xeroderma pigmentosum type A, predominantly present in pachytene spermatocytes) [19]. The SCP1 specific antibodies can only be used on frozen material. None of the 25 classical seminomas, but all 13 spermatocytic seminomas were positive (see Figure 6.1B). These three antibodies can therefore be used diagnostically to distinguish classical seminoma from spermatocytic seminoma, as they provide a positive marker of the latter. These results also support the contention that spermatocytic seminoma cells can undergo partial meiosis, explaining the presence of small (diploid), intermediate (tetraploid) and large (hypertetraploid) nuclei [9, 11–13, 16, 26–30]. Interestingly, c-KIT negative/SSX positive

Table 6.1: Overview of different markers tested on classical and spermatocytic seminomas

Markers	Classical seminoma	Spermatocytic seminoma
Fap1, Fas/FasL, lectins, VASA, XIST (a), 43-9F, telomerase, KI-A10	+	+
Glycogen, c-KIT, GCAP/PLAP, OCT4, TRA-1-60/81, HIWI (a), PDGFaR 1.5 (a), HERV-K, gain 12p (b)	+	−
Cytokeratin, CD30	+/−	−
SCP1 (c), SSX, XPA, gain chromosome 9 (b)	−	+

From references 5, 8, 17, 19, 22, 29, 31-41; (a) are RNA markers, (b) are chromosomal markers and (c) can only be used on frozen tissue sections.

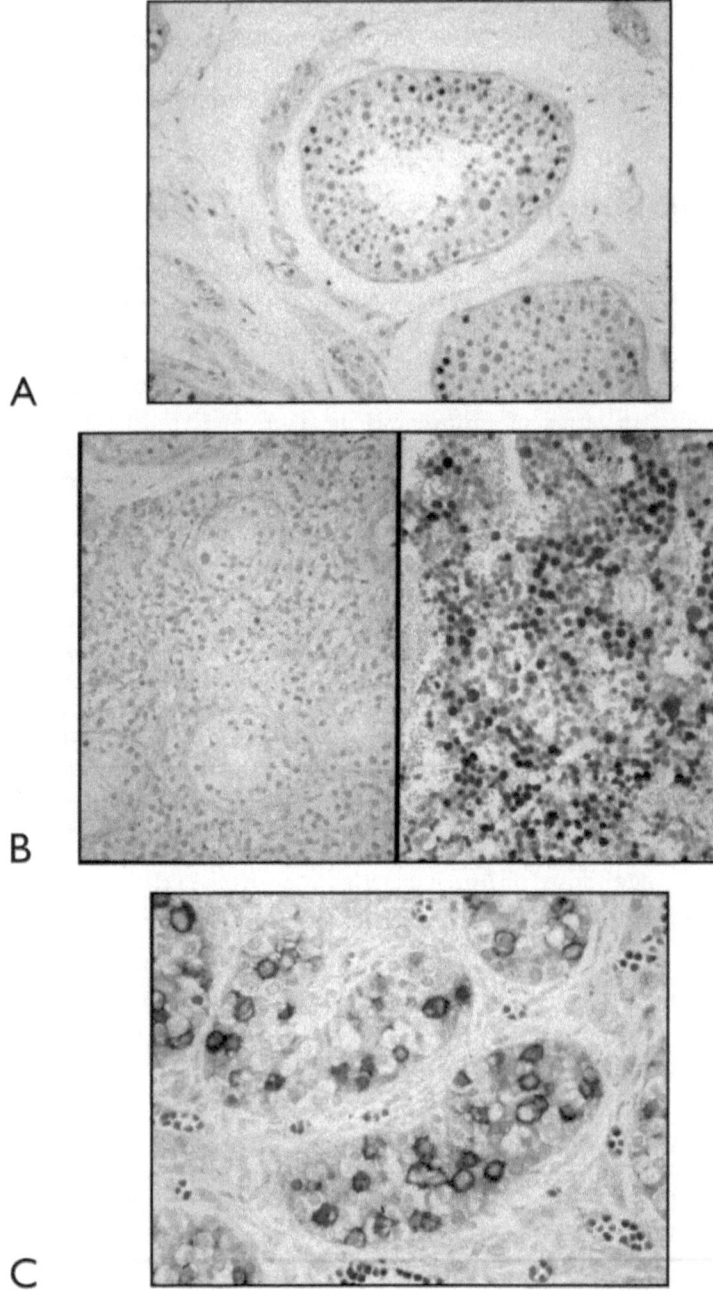

Figure 6.1: Representative example of immunohistochemistry of A). a normal testis (left panel), B). classical seminoma (left panel) and a spermatocytic seminoma (right panel) using an antibody specific for SSX. Note the positive staining in both spermatogonia/spermatocytes and spermatocytic seminoma; C). an embryonic testis of 17 weeks of development stained for SSX (originally red) and c-KIT (originally blue). There are germ cells positive for SSX and negative for c-KIT, which might be the cell of origin of spermatocytic seminoma.

embryonic germ cells are identifiable in testes at 17 weeks of development (see Figure 6.1C). These cells could be the cells of origin of spermatocytic seminoma, as previously suggested by studies of chromosomal constitution [29]. This could explain the occurrence of bilateral tumours, despite the generally benign behaviour of these spermatocytic seminomas.

Conclusion

We have demonstrated that spermatocytic seminomas can be specifically diagnosed based on immunohistochemistry using antibodies directed against SCP1, SSX and XPA. The results imply that the pathogenesis of spermatocytic seminoma may be initiated during embryonic development, although the cells are still capable of further maturation, including partial meiosis.

The Dutch Cancer Society financially supported this work

References

1. Looijenga LHJ, Oosterhuis J.W. Pathogenesis of testicular germ cell tumours. *Rev of Reproduction* 1999;4:90–100
2. Møller H. Decreased testicular cancer risk in men born in wartime. *J Natl Cancer Inst* 1989;81:1668–9
3. Gondos B. Ultrastructure of developing and malignant germ cells. *Eur Urol* 1993;23:68–75
4. Jørgensen N, Giwercman A, Müller J, Skakkebæk NE. Immunohistochemical markers of carcinoma in situ of the testis also expressed in normal infantile germ cells. *Histopathol* 1993;22:373–378
5. Rajpert-De Meyts E, Skakkebæk NE. Expression of the c-kit protein product in carcinoma-in-situ and invasive testicular germ cell tumours. *Int J Androl* 1994;17:85-92
6. Jørgensen N, Rajpert-De Meyts E, Graem N, Müller J, Giwercman A, Skakkebæk NE. Expression of immunohistochemical markers for testicular carcinoma in situ by normal fetal germ cells. *Lab Invest* 1995;72:223-231
7. De Meyts ER, Jørgensen N, Møller J, Skakkebaek NE. Prolonged expression of the c-kit receptor in germ cells of intersex fetal testes. *J Pathol* 1996;178:166–169
8. Roelofs H, Manes T, Millan JL, Oosterhuis JW, Looijenga LHJ. Heterogeneity in alkaline phosphatase isozyme expression in human testicular germ cell tumours. An enzyme-/immunochemical and molecular analysis. *J Pathol* 1999;189:236–244
9. Rosai J, Khodadoust K, Silber I. Spermatocytic seminoma. *Cancer* 1969;24:103–116
10. Talerman A. Spermatocytic seminoma. *J Urol* 1974;112:212-6
11. Talerman A. Spermatocytic seminoma. *Cancer* 1980;45:2169–2176
12. Romanenko AM, Persidskii YV. Ultrastructure and histogenesis of spermatocytic seminoma. *Voprosi Onkologii* 1983;19:61–66
13. Talerman A, Fu YS, Okagaki T. Spermatocytic seminoma. Ultrastructural and micro spectrophotometric observations. *Lab Invest* 1984;51:343–349
14. Muller J, Skakkebaek NE, Parkinson MC. The spermatocytic seminoma: views on pathogenesis. *Int J Androl* 1987;10:147-56
15. Burke AP, Mostofi FK. Spermatocytic seminoma. A clinicopathologic study of 79 cases. *J Urol Path* 1993;1:21–32
16. Eble JN. Spermatocytic seminoma. *Hum Pathol* 1994;25:1035–1042
17. Mostofi FK, Sesterhenn IA. *Histological typing of testis tumours.* 2nd ed. Berlin: Springer, 1998
18. Roelofs H, Mostert MC, Pompe K et al. Restricted 12p-amplification and RAS mutation in human germ cell tumours of the adult testis. *Am J Pathol* 2000;157:1155–1166
19. Stoop H, Van Gurp RJHLM, De Krijger R et al. Reactivity of germ cell maturation stage-specific markers in spermatocytic seminoma: diagnostic and etiological implications. *Lab Invest* 2001;81:919–928
20. Pesce M, Scholer HR. Oct-4: control of totipotency and germline determination. *Mol Reprod Dev* 2000;55:452-7

21. Castrillon DH, Quade BJ, Wang TY, Quigley C, Crum CP. The human VASA gene is specifically expressed in the germ cell lineage. *Proc Natl Acad Sci U S A* 2000;97:9585–9590
22. Palumba C, Van Roozendaal K, Gillis AJM et al. Expression of the PDGF alpha-receptor 1.5 kb transcript, OCT-4 and c-KIT in human normal and malignant tissues. Implications for early diagnosis of testicular germ cell tumours and understanding regulatory mechanisms. *J Pathol* 2001;in press
23. Meuwissen RL, Offenberg HH, Dietrich AJ, Riesewijk A, van Iersel M, Heyting C. A coiled-coil related protein specific for synapsed regions of meiotic prophase chromosomes. *Embo J* 1992;11:5091–100
24. Tureci O, Sahin U, Zwick C, Koslowski M, Seitz G, Pfreundschuh M. Identification of a meiosis-specific protein as a member of the class of cancer/testis antigens. *Proc Natl Acad Sci U S A* 1998;95:5211–6
25. Dos Santos NR, Torensma R, de Vries TJ et al. Heterogeneous expression of the SSX cancer/testis antigens in human melanoma lesions and cell lines. *Cancer Res* 2000;60:1654–62
26. Kysela B, Matoska J. Flow cytometry analysis of ploidy and proliferation activity in classicalal and spermatocytic seminoma. *Neoplasma.* 1991;38:3–11
27. Takahashi H. Cytometric analysis of testicular seminoma and spermatocytic seminoma. *Acta Pathol Japon* 1993;43:121–129
28. Looijenga LHJ, Olie RA, Van der Gaag I et al. Seminomas of the canine testis; counterpart of spermatocytic seminoma of men? *Lab Invest* 1994;71:490–496
29. Rosenberg C, Mostert MC, Bakker Schut T et al. Chromosomal constitution of human spermatocytic seminomas: comparative genomic hybridization suppored by conventional and interphase cytogenetics. *Genes Chromosom & Cancer* 1998;23:286–291
30. Kraggerud SM, Berner A, Bryne M, Pettersen EO, Fossa SD. Spermatocytic seminoma as compared to classicalal seminoma: an immunohistochemical and DNA flow cytometric study. *APMIS* 1999;107:297–302
31. Kosmehl H, Langbein L, Katenkamp D. Lectin histochemistry of human testicular germ cell tumours. *Neoplasma.* 1989;36:29–39
32. Giwercman A, Andrews PW, Jørgensen N, Müller J, Graem N, Skakkebæk NE. Immunohistochemical expression of embryonal marker tra-1-60 in carcinoma in situ and germ cell tumours of the testis. *Cancer* 1993;72:1308–1314
33. Hittmair A, Rogatsch H, Hobisch A, Mikuz G, Feichtinger H. CD30 expression in seminoma. *Hum Pathol* 1996;27:1166–71
34. Rajpert-De Meyts E, Kvist M, Skakkebæk NE. Heterogeneity of expression of immunohistochemical tumour markers in testicular carcinoma in situ: Pathogenetic relevance. *Virchows Arch Int J Pathol* 1996;428:133–139
35. Looijenga LH, Gillis AJ, van Gurp RJ, Verkerk AJ, Oosterhuis JW. X inactivation in human testicular tumours. XIST expression and androgen receptor methylation status. *Am J Pathol* 1997;151:581–90
36. Herbst H, Sauter M, Kuhler-Obbarius C, Loning T, Mueller-Lantzsch N. Human endogenous retrovirus (HERV)-K transcripts in germ cell and trophoblastic tumours. *APMIS* 1998;106:216–20
37. Heidenreich A, Sesterhenn IA, Mostofi FK, Moul JW. Immunohistochemical expression of monoclonal antibody 43-9F in testicular germ cell tumours. *Int J Androl* 1998;21:283–8
38. Kersemaekers AMVW, P.C., Oosterhuis JW, Looijenga LHJ. Involvement of the Fas/FasL-pathway in the pathogenesis of germ cell tumours of the adult testis. *J Pathol* 2001;in press
39. Delgado R, Rathi A, Albores-Saavedra J, Gazdar AF. Expression of the RNA component of human telomerase in adult testicular germ cell neoplasia. *Cancer* 1999;86:1802–11
40. Rudolph P, Kellner U, Schmidt D, Kirchner V, Talerman A, Harms D, et al. Ki-A10, a germ cell nuclear antigen retained in a subset of germ cell- derived tumours. *Am J Pathol* 1999;154:795–803
41. Dekker I, Rozeboom T, Delemarre J, Dam A, Oosterhuis JW. Placental-like alkaline phosphatase and DNA flow cytometry in spermatocytic seminoma. *Cancer* 1992;69:993–996

7. Expression of Human Endogenous Retroviruses HERV-K/HTDV in Germ Cell Tumours: Possible Biological Role and Clinical Application

A. Kleiman[1], N. Senyuta.,[1] A. Trjakin[1], T. Vinogradova[2],
A. Karseladze[1], V. Gurtsrvitch[1], S. Tjulandin[1]

1. *N.N. Blokhin Cancer Research Center, RAMS, Moscow, Russia; 2. Shemyakin-Ovchinnikov Institute of Bio-Organic Chemistry, RAS, Moscow, Russia*

The most biologically active human endogenous retroviruses (HERV) are the provirus HERV-K/HTDV (human teratocarcinoma divided viruses) family, which have open reading frames for all viral proteins – Gag, Prt, Pol, Env. The expression of HERV-K/HTDV proviruses is strictly associated with germ cell tumours (GCTs) [1, 2] and 62.5 to 80 per cent of patients with GCTs have antibodies (Abs) to Gag and/or Env HERV-K/HTDV proteins [3, 4]. HERV-K/HTDV proviruses also code the accessory protein cORF [5]. The function of cORF is to regulate splicing and transport of unspliced proviral mRNA into the cytoplasm [6]. Only the cORF protein, and no other HERV-K/HTDV proteins, is capable of cell transformation [7].

Aims

We set out to 1) study the expression of cORF in GCTs of different morphology, as well as in normal testicular parenchyma and placenta and 2) investigate the possibility of using Abs to HERV-K/HTDV proteins as additional diagnostic and prognostic markers of GCTs

Materials and Methods

We investigated cORF HERV-K/HTDV transcription by RT-PCR with specific primers to cORF HERV-K/HTDV in 16 GCTs (seven seminomas, three embryonal carcinomas, three combined tumours, three teratoma differentiated, one of which had immature foci), nine samples of parenchyma adjacent to tumour, two of normal testicular parenchyma and two of placenta. Antibody titers to Gag and Env HERV-K/HTDV proteins were determined by immunofluorescence in 310 patients with different types of GCT prior to treatment. We also monitored specific Abs titers in 142 GCT patients during and after treatment.

Results

cORF HERV-K/HTDV was transcribed in all types of GCTs except differentiated teratomas. cORF mRNA was found in six of nine samples of parenchyma adjacent to tumour, correlating with the presence of intratubular germ cell neoplasia (ITGCN) or invasive foci. cORF mRNA cORF was not detected in the samples of normal testis parenchyma or placenta.

Antibodies to Gag and/or Env HERV-K/HTDV proteins were detected in 209 of the 310 (67.4 per cent) GCT patients prior to treatment, regardless of GCT subtype and including patients with teratoma differentiated. The presence or absence of antibodies did not correlate with the IGCCCG prognostic classification.

Monitoring of antibody titers in 142 patients showed a decrease in titers in the majority of seropositive patients, correlating with response to treatment. Patients whose titers remained stable during chemotherapy suffered disease progression or early relapse. The presence of antiviral antibodies in patients with non-seminomatous GCTs after chemotherapy was strictly associated with the presence of viable tumour cells in residual masses. In 32 patients, antibodies to Gag and Env HERV-K/HTDV proteins were the only serological markers of tumour as AFP and HCG were not elevated.

Conclusion

The role of the expression of HERV-K/HTDV proviruses in the pathogenesis of GCTs is still unclear. The hypothesis that cORF is involved in the multi-stage process of gonocyte transformation needs further investigation. Antibodies to Gag and Env HERV-K/HTDV may be used as additional serological markers for monitoring GCT patients.

This work was supported by a grant from RFFI (94–04–49371)

References

1. Herbst H, Sauter M, Muller-Lantzsch N. Expression of human endogenous retrovirus K element in germ cell and trophoblastic tumors *Am J Pathol* 1996;149:1727–1735
2. Roelofs H, van Gurp R, Oosterhius J, Looijenga L. Detection of human endogenous retrovirus type K-specific transcripts in testicular parenchyma and testicular germ cell tumor of adolescents and adults: clinical and biological implications *Am J Pathol* 1998;153:1277–1282
3. Boller K, Janssen O, Schuldes H, Tonjes RR, Kurth R. Characterization of the antibody response specific for the human endogenous retrovirus HTDV/HERV-K *J Virol* 1997;71:4581–4588
4. Sauter M, Roemer K, Best B et al. Specificity of antibodies directed against Env protein of human endogenous retroviruses in patients with germ cell tumors *Cancer Res* 1996;56:4362–4365
5. Lower R, Tonjjes RR, Korbmacher C, Kurth R, Lower J. Identification of Rev-related protein by analysis of spliced transcripts of the human endogenous retroviruses HTDV/HERV-K *J Virol* 1994;69:141–149
6. Magin C, Lower R, Lower J. cORF and RcRE, the Rev/Rex and RRE/RxRE homologues of the human endogenous retrovirus family HTDV/HERV-K. *J. Virol* 1999;73:9496–9507
7. Boese A, Sauter M, Galli U et al. Human endogenous retrovirus protein cORF supports cell transformation and associates with the promyelocytic leukemia zink finger protein. *Oncogene* 2000;19:4328–4336

8. No Association Between HLA Class II Genes and Testicular Germ Tumour (TGCT) with Genotyping of the HLA-Region on Chromosome 6p21 and Haplotype Sharing Analysis

M.F. Lutke Holzik[1], D.J.A. Sonneveld[1], H.J. Hoekstra[1], I.M. Nolte[2], M. Bruinenberg[2], W.T.A. van der Graaf[3], D.Th. Sleijfer[3], R.H. Sijmons[4], C.H.C.M. Buys[4], G.J. Te Meerman[2]

Departments of 1. Surgical oncology, 2. Medical biology, 3. Medical oncology, 4. Clinical genetics, Groningen University Hopsital, The Netherlands

Association with HLA, in particular class II genes (DQB1, DRB1), has been suggested as one of the genetic factors involved in TGCT development [1]. The present study used a marker haplotyping method in trios (parents or spouse and child) to replicate the previous findings, obtained through HLA typing.

Methods

We genotyped the HLA-region on chromosome 6p21 in TGCT patients for a set of 15 closely linked microsatellite markers. As each allele of the many genes in this region is likely present on only a few haplotypes from the quite limited set of conserved founder haplotypes [2], we can study association to all genes in the region. We analyzed the results by single marker association, transmission disequilibrium test (TDT) and haplotype sharing analysis to find a possible association between genes in the HLA class II region and TGCT. Haplotype sharing analysis derives extra information from phase in addition to single marker tests [3].

Patients

One hundred and fifty one TGCT patients (87 per cent nonseminomas, 13 per cent seminomas) treated at the Groningen University Hospital in the Netherlands, along with parent (n = 108) or spouse (n = 43) controls, were genotyped for 15 microsatellite markers in the HLA-region (particularly class II).

Results

In both patients and controls strong linkage disequilibrium was observed in the genotyped region indicating that similar haplotypes are likely to be identical by descent. However, association analysis as well as the TDT did not show significant results. Haplotype sharing analysis did not show qualitative or quantitative differences in haplotype sharing between patients and controls. The sample size in the present investigation was about three times higher than previously reported [1], which implies that there was substantial power to replicate previous findings.

Conclusion

The present genotyping study could not confirm the previous reported association between HLA class II genes and TGCT. As the HLA alleles for which associations were reported are also prevalent in the Dutch populations, these associations are likely to be either non-existent or much weaker than reported. Further research focusing on other candidate loci should be performed to identify possible TGCT susceptibility genes.

References

1. Ozdemir E, Kakehi Y, Mishina M et al. High-resolution HLA-DRB1 and DQB1 genotyping in Japanese patients with testicular germ cell carcinoma. *Br J Cancer* 1997;76:1348–1352
2. Sonneveld DJA, Schaapveld M, Sleijfer DTh, et al. Geographic clustering of testicular cancer incidence in the northern part of the Netherlands. *Br J Cancer* 1999;81:1262–1267
3. Beckmann L, Fischer C, Deck K-G, Nolte IM, Meerman GJ, Chang-Claude J. Exploring haplotype sharing methods in general and isolated populations to detect gene(s) of a complex genetic trait. *Genetic Epidemiol* 2001;in press

9. RT-PCR for AFP, HCG, GCAP and PDGF-1 To Detect Circulating Tumour Cells in Testicular Germ Cell Tumours

A. Heidenreich

Department of Urology, Philipps-Universität, Baldingerstrasse, 35043 Marburg, Germany

Introduction and objectives

Clinical staging in low volume testicular germ cell tumours (TGCTs) is inadequate with regard to the correct prediction of final pathological retroperitoneal lymph node status. Serum tumour markers are positive in only about 60 per cent of all patients and imaging modalities such as CT scan or MRI have a false negative rate of 25 per cent and a false positive rate of up to 10 per cent [1] and markers such as Ki-67, PCNA, p53, Bcl-2, E-cadherin and cathepsin D are not helpful [2, 3]. It is therefore impossible to adopt an individualized therapeutic approach for patients with low volume TGCT, stratified for risk. Reverse transcriptase (RT) polymerase chain reaction (PCR) is highly sensitive in detecting circulating tumour cells from patients with prostate cancer, melanoma, and hepatic carcinoma [4, 5]. We evaluated the clinical significance of the presence of specific PCR-positive mRNA markers in the peripheral blood of patients with TGCT.

Patients and methods

Total RNA was extracted from cell lines TERA-2 for HCG, GCAP and PDGF-1 and from HepG2 for AFP to optimize RT-PCR conditions and serial dilution experiments were conducted to assess RT-PCR sensitivity. We then obtained total RNA from the peripheral blood of 30 patients with organ confined or pathological stage IIA/B TGCT, 20 patients with benign testicular disease and 20 healthy volunteers. The PCR products were analyzed by gel electrophoresis and direct sequencing.

Results

Assay sensitivity was one TERA-2 or HepG2 cell per 10^6 peripheral blood lymphocytes. RT-PCR for AFP, HCG, GCAP mRNA was negative in healthy controls and patients with benign disease; PDGF-1 mRNA was detected in 20 per cent of healthy controls and in 40 per cent of patients with testicular disease. Prior to orchiectomy, positive RT-PCR results were demonstrated in 57 per cent of clinical stage I TGCT and in 60 per cent of stage IIA/B TGCT. None of the patients had positive RT-PCR results following adjuvant or inductive chemotherapy.

Conclusion

Our data indicate a positive correlation between RT-PCR findings and the presence of circulating tumour cells in TGCT. PDGF-1 mRNA was not specific for patients with TGCT, but RT-PCR for AFP, HCG and GCAP mRNA may be a useful adjunct to clinical staging. Ongoing studies will determine the clinical utility of RT–PCR in the diagnosis and monitoring of TGCT patients.

Funded by the German Research Council He 2618/2–1

References

1. McLeod DG, Weiss RB, Stablein DM et al. Staging relationships and outcome in early stage testicular cancer: a report from the Testicular Cancer Intergroup Study. *J Urol* 1991;145:1178
2. Heidenreich A, Mostofi K, Sesterhenn IA, Moul JW. Prognostic factors to predict patients at low risk and at high risk for metastasis in clinical stage I nonseminomatous germ cell tumors. *Cancer* 1998;82:1002
3. Heidenreich A, Sesterhenn IA, Moul JW. Editorial comment: prognostic risk factors in low stage testicular germ cell tumors. *Cancer* 1998;79:1641
4. Corey E, Corey M. Detection of disseminated prostate cells by reverse transcriptase polymerase chain reaction: technical and clinical aspects. *Int J Cancer* 77:655, 1998
5. Fey MF, Kulozik AE, Hansen-Hagge TE, Tobler A. The polymerase chain reaction: a new tool for the detection of minimal residual disease in hematological malignancies. *Eur J Cancer* 27:89, 1991

10. The Prognostic Significance of Tumour Infiltrating Lymphocyte Count in Stage I Testicular Seminoma Managed by Surveillance

Chris Parker, Michael Milosevic, Padraig Warde, Tony Panzarella, Diponkar Banerjee, Michael Jewett, Charles Catton, Mary Gospodarowicz

Princess Margaret Hospital, Toronto, Canada

Introduction

The number and type of tumour infiltrating lymphocytes (TILs) have been reported to be significant determinants of outcome for a variety of malignancies, consistent with the concept that an active host immune response may inhibit tumor progression. Testicular seminoma is typically associated with a lymphocytic infiltrate, but although this infiltrate is notable for its intensity, the existence of a functional anti-tumour role has been questioned [1]. In an updated analysis of our previous seminoma surveillance study [2], we have studied the prognostic role of the TIL count.

Methods

Two hundred and three patients with stage I testicular seminoma, presenting between 1981 and 1993, were managed by surveillance according to the Princess Margaret Hospital protocol. Fifty-three were excluded from the current analysis (5 spermatocytic seminoma, 48 paraffin blocks unobtainable), leaving a total of 150 cases. TIL count was assessed from the orchidectomy specimen by an experienced genitourinary pathologist (DB), and classified, according to his judgement, as high, intermediate or low.

Results

At a median follow-up of 9.4 years, 30 of the 150 men had developed recurrent seminoma. The actuarial risk of relapse at 10 years was 21 per cent (standard error 2.3 per cent). On univariate analysis, a higher risk of relapse was associated with young age (33 years or less, $p = 0.002$), tumour diameter over 6 cm ($p = 0.03$), lymphatic or vascular invasion ($p = 0.04$), tumour invasion of rete testis ($p = 0.05$), and lower TIL count ($p = 0.02$). The 10-year actuarial risk of relapse was 44 per cent, 22 per cent and 9 per cent in men with low, intermediate and high TIL counts, respectively. Significant predictors of risk of relapse on multivariate analysis were young age (hazard ratio: 4.7; 95 per cent confidence intervals: 1.7–12.2; $p = 0.002$) and tumour diameter greater than 6 cm (HR: 2.8; CI: 1.2–6.5; $p = 0.01$). The hazard ratio for the risk of relapse in cases with a low rather than an intermediate TIL count, or an intermediate rather than a high TIL count, was 1.8 (CI: 0.96 to 3.44; $p = 0.07$).

Discussion

The potential implications of this study are not limited to identifying or refuting the existence of another prognostic factor. Rather, the data generate the hypothesis that the activity of the anti-tumour immune response may be a determinant of outcome in testicular seminoma managed by surveillance. Limitations of the study include the modest number of events for analysis, and the use of a qualitative, rather than a quantitative, assessment of TIL count. Future studies should use quantitative methods and multiple observers, and include the type, and location, as well as the number of TILs. In conclusion, the functional role and prognostic significance of the lymphocytic infiltrate in testicular seminoma warrant further study.

References

1. Bols B, Jensen L, Jensen A, Braendstrup O. Immunopathology of in situ seminoma. *Int J Exp Pathol* 2000;81:211–7
2. Warde P, Gospodarowicz M, Banerjee D, et al. Prognostic factors for relapse in stage I testicular seminoma treated with surveillance. *J Urol* 1997;157:1705–9

11. HIV Related Testicular Cancer

T. Powles, M. Bower, M. Nelson, R.T.D. Oliver

Chelsea and Westminster and St Bartholomew's Hospitals, London, UK

Introduction

There have been conflicting reports since 1985 as to the frequency and nature of HIV related testicular (HT) cancer. Two recent reports, and another large series confirm that testicular cancer is more common compared to age matched controls (relative risk 3.9), and seminoma occurs more frequently than non seminoma [1, 2].

We present new data, and review the literature to understand more about the disease process and outcome.

Patients and Methods

The notes of 12 patients with HT cancer were reviewed. Eleven had seminoma and one a combined germ cell tumour. We focused on the 11 patients with seminoma. At diagnosis, the median age was 33 yrs (range 23–45) and the median CD4 count 211/mm3 (range 17–450/mm3). Three of the patients were already taking antiretroviral therapy, a further 5 started treatment subsequently.

Results

These are presented in the table.

Discussion

Unlike most HIV related malignancies, no viral oncogene has been implicated in the development of Seminoma but there may be a role for immune surveillance. We speculate that an HIV related loss of immune surveillance leads to an acceleration of invasive disease from intratubular germ cell neoplasia. If this is the case, individuals with HIV related seminoma should present at a younger age. A median age of between 30 and 33 in both our series, and another larger meta-analysis study [3] suggests this might be the case.

The two largest studies published to date reviewed 26 and 15 patients respectively. The larger study consisted of predominantly intravenous drug users, and showed no increase in the incidence of seminoma. Both studies showed the presentation of the disease and its response to treatment was similar to the HIV negative population. Mortality was related to the HIV rather than testicular cancer [4, 5].

Stage	n	Age	Prior AIDS	CD4 count	Treatment	Response	HIV deaths
I	6	37	50%	235	surveillance	No relapse at 5 yrs	50%
II	4	33	50%	185	Chemo	No relapse at 8 yrs	25%
III	1	23	0%	522	Chemo	No relapse at 9 yrs	0%

The data presented in our study is similar, with good response rates. A large proportion of patients had stage II disease due to retroperitoneal lymphadenopathy. It is important to confirm this is related to the testicular cancer rather than HIV by confirmatory biopsy, rising markers or progression of disease on CT.

There is uncertainty as to the aetiology of this disease in the HAART era and there is a need for a multicentre database for these patients.

References

1 Vaccher E., Spina M., Tirelli U. Clinical aspects and management of Hodgkin's disease and other tumour in HIV-infected individuals. *Eur J Cancer* 2001;37:1306–15

2 Lyter DW, Kingsley LA, Rinaldo CR. Bryant J. Malignancies in the multicentre AIDS cohort study 1984–1994. in proc 3ASCO, # 852: Philadelphia 1996, 305

3 Morten F, Biggar J, Engels E. Association of cancer with AIDS related immunosupression in adults. *JAMA* 2001;285:1736–44

4 Leibovitch , Baniel J, Rowland R, Smith E Malignant testicular cancer in immunosuppressed patients *J Urol* 1996;155:1938–1942

5 Timmerman M, Northfelt D, Small E Malignant germ cell tumours in men infected with the HIV virus *J Clin Oncol* 1995;13:1391–1397

6 Bernadi D, Salvioni R, Vaccher E. Testicular germ cell tumours and HIV infection. *J Clin Oncol* 1995;13: 2705–2711

12. Microinvasive Testicular Germ Cell Tumours: Prevalence in Stage I Tumours

F.E. von Eyben[1], G.K. Jacobsen[2]

1. Center of Tobacco Research, Odense, 2. Department of Pathology, Copenhagen University Hospital in Gentofte, Copenhagen, Denmark

Background

Microinvasive testicular germ cell tumour (GCT) is defined as invasion of the interstitium by malignant germ cells without palpable tumour formation [1]. Microinvasive GCTs can also accompany overt tumours.

Patients

Stage I patients with seminoma or non-seminomatous testicular GCTs treated by surveillance in two Danish national studies, whose pathology had been reviewed, and who had been monitored by measurement of serum lactate dehydrogenase isoenzyme 1 catalytic concentration [2, 3].

Methods

One of us (GKJ) reviewed the overt tumours and the remaining testis for the presence of intratubular germ cell neoplasia (ITGCN) and microinvasive GCT [4, 5].

Results

Eighty of the 99 seminoma patients had ITGCN and 8 had microinvasive GCT. Sixty eight of the 104 non-seminoma patients had ITGCN and 24 had microinvasive GCT. Seminoma was associated with ITGCN more often than non-seminoma ($p = 0.02$). In contrast, non- seminoma was associated with microinvasive GCTs more often than seminoma tumour ($p = 0.005$).

Discussion

Ten to 20 per cent of patients with stage I testicular GCTs have associated microinvasive tumours, which may represent the intermediate step between ITGCN and macroscopically overt tumours. Further analyses of ITGCN, microinvasive and overt tumours may elucidate the genetic mechanisms of early invasion, tumour formation and differentiation.

References

1. von Eyben FE, Mikulowski P, Busch C. Microinvasive germ cell tumors of the testis. *J Urol* 1981;126:842–4
2. von Eyben FE, Madsen EL, Blaabjerg O et al. Serum lactate dehydrogenase isoenzyme 1 and relapse in patients with nonseminomatous testicular germ cell tumors clinical stage I. *Acta Oncol* 2001;40:536–40
3. von Eyben FE, Madsen EL, Blaabjerg O et al. Serum lactate dehydrogenase isoenzyme 1 in patients with seminoma stage I followed with surveillance. *Acta Oncol* 2001;in press.
4. Jacobsen GK, Rørth M, Østerlind K et al. Histopathological features in stage I non seminomatous testicular germ cell tumours correlated to relapse. *APMIS* 1990;98:377–82
5. Jacobsen GK, von der Maase H, Specht L et al. Histopathological features in stage I seminoma treated with orchidectomy only. *J Urologic Pathology* 1995;3:85–94

13. Serum Lactate Dehydrogenase Isoenzyme 1 in Patients with Testicular Seminoma or Nonseminoma Stage I: Two Nationwide Danish Studies of Surveillance

F.E. von Eyben[1], G.K. Jacobsen[2], L. Specht[3], P.H. Petersen[4], E.L. Madsen[5], O. Blaabjerg[4], M. Rørth[3], H. von der Maase[6], for the DATECA study group

1 Center of Tobacco Research, Odense, 2 Department of Pathology, Copenhagen University Hospital in Gentofte, 3 Department of Oncology, National University Hospital in Copenhagen, 4 Department of Clinical Chemistry, Odense University Hospital, 5 Department of Oncology, Sønderborg Hospital, 6 Department of Oncology, Århus University Hospital, Denmark

Background

The use of surveillance in patients with stage I testicular germ cell tumours is increasing internationally. The aim of this study was to elucidate pathological and clinical aspects of serum lactate dehydrogenase isoenzyme 1 catalytic concentration in this setting.

Patients

Two Danish nationwide studies of surveillance for patients with non-seminoma in 1980–1984 and with seminoma in 1985–1988 [1, 2].

Methods

Serum lactate dehydrogenase isoenzyme 1 (S-LD-1) was measured preoperatively in 68 patients with non-seminoma and 110 with seminoma, selected randomly [3, 4]. The histology of the tumours was revised according to the WHO classification, with a semiquantitative assessment of tumour size, mitotic rate, and extent of necrosis [5, 6]. The patients were monitored for 5 years. Correlations were analyzed with non-parametric statistics, and the survival of subgroups using the logrank test.

Results

For patients with seminoma, S-LD-1 related to the size of the tumour (p = 0.0006) and the extent of the necrosis (p < 0.00001). For patients with non-seminoma, S-LD-1 related to the size of the tumour (p = 0.0002) but not to the extent of necrosis (p = 0.19). A raised S-LD-1 implied an increased risk of relapse for patients with non-seminoma (p = 0.003) but not for those with seminoma (p = 0.79).

Discussion

Although an isolated raised S-LD-1 was more frequently seen in patients with stage I seminoma, it was not predictive of relapse in these patients, whereas this was the case for patients with non-seminoma on surveillance.

References

1. Rørth M, Jacobsen GK, von der Maase H, Madsen EL, Nielsen OS, Pedersen MSH et al. Surveillance alone versus radiotherapy after orchiectomy for clinical stage I nonseminomatous testicular cancer. *J Clin Oncol.* 1991;9:1543–8
2. von der Maase H, Specht L, Jacobsen GK, Jacobsen A, Madsen EL, Pedersen M et al. Surveillance following orchiectomy for seminoma of the testis. *Eur J Cancer* 1993;29A:1931–4
3. von Eyben FE, Madsen EL, Blaabjerg O, Petersen PH, von der Maase H, Jacobsen GK et al. Serum lactate dehydrogenase isoenzyme 1 and relapse in patients with nonseminomatous testicular germ cell tumours clinical stage I. *Acta Oncol* 2001;40:536–40
4. von Eyben FE, Madsen EL, Blaabjerg O, Petersen PH, Jacobsen GK, Specht L et al. Serum lactate dehydrogenase isoenzyme 1 in patients with seminoma stage I followed with surveillance. *Acta Oncol* 2001;in press.
5. Jacobsen GK, Rørth M, Østerlind K, von der Maase H, Jacobsen M, Madsen EL et al. Histopathological features in stage I non-seminomatous testicular germ cell tumours correlated to relapse. *APMIS* 1990;98:377–82
6. Jacobsen GK, von der Maase H, Specht L, Jakobsen A, Madsen EL, Pedersen M et al. Histopathological features in stage I seminoma treated with orchidectomy only. *J Urologic Pathology* 1995;3:85–94

14. The Atrophy Hypothesis and Development of Malignant Germ Cell Cancers of the Testis

R.T.D. Oliver

St Bartholomew's and Royal London School of Medicine Queen Mary College, University of London, West Smithfield, EC1A 7BE

Introduction

It is now beyond doubt that intra-uterine environment and in particular maternal natural oestrogen levels as well as the levels of ingested environmental chemical xeno-oestrogen ingestion can influence the risk of the foetus subsequently developing a malignant germ cell cancer after puberty [1]. It is also clear that a major component of this intrauterine effect is because excess intra-uterine oestrogens contribute to the development of defects in descent of the testis into the scrotum. More controversial is the contribution of intra-uterine events to the neoplastic transformation of intra-tubular germ cells relative to the contribution of post-pubertal events [2]. It is the aim of this brief review to focus on the role of post pubertal testicular atrophic factors in the neoplastic transformation of prepubertally primed but not transformed spermatogonia.

There are four stages in the post pubertal atrophy hypothesis for development of germ cell cancers. 1. Atrophic damage reduces feed back inhibition of the hypothalamus leading to increased gonadotrophin stimulus of the diminished number of normal germ cells. 2. If these germ cells have been primed in utero by excess oestrogen exposure, these fast cycling germ cells become prone to fuse at the tetraploid pachytene spermatocyte stage, fail to undergo meiosis and but switch to mitosis. 3. The resulting tetraploid cell is genetically unstable, loses chromosomes and clonally evolves to seminoma with a median DNA content of 3.6N and then to non-seminoma with a median DNA content of 2.7N under the selection pressure of immune surveillance against antigenic targets expressed on the malignant cell such as endogenous retroviral proteins. 4. Further genetic events in the unstable subtetraploid cells are responsible for clonal development of metastases and then death.

Evidence for the Four Stages of Germ Cell Cancer Development

Atrophy as the Final Common Pathway for Initiation

The contention that normally functioning post pubertal testis can undergo atrophy and then be associated with the development of a germ cell cancer is supported by anecdotal cases where men in early post pubertal life have large families and then notice shrinkage of the testis and, at time of presentation with testis cancer, have bilateral atrophic testes and azoospermia. In epidemiological studies, variants of this pattern of development have been reported in 20 per cent of cases compared to 5 per cent in the control population [3]. The best evidence for one cause of this process comes from a study of post pubertal men infected by mumps virus in an epidemic where 40 per cent developed orchitis, one in three of those with orchitis developed atrophy and two of those with atrophy developed testis cancer giving a rate of 1 in 250 compared to the 3.5 per 10,000 predicted for the 5 years of the follow up [4]. Whether other viruses can do the same is unclear. Equally, given the demonstration that heating the scrotum alone can also induce atrophy [5] and that sedentary life style, traumatic injury to the testis and previous chemical exposure increase the risk of germ cell cancer [3,6], it is clear that viruses are not the only factors that could initiate atrophy. The strongest evidence for the atrophy induced final pathway being active even after a first testis tumour is the demonstration that post orchidectomy FSH level predicts for risk of subsequent tumour in the contralateral testis [7].

Tetraploidisation as Initial Transformation Event

The evidence that tetraploidisation is critical for the initiation of germ cell cancer comes from the study by Muller and Skakkebaek [8] who showed that isolated neoplastic intratubular cells discovered in men with infertility or cryptorchidism were tetraploid. The data from Oosterhuis's group [9] demonstrates that in the testis where a cancer has developed, the neoplastic intratubular cells have lost some DNA but still have levels higher than in the associated tumours. In combined tumours containing both seminoma and non-seminoma, in some tumours there was a gradient of reduction in DNA content between neoplastic intratubular cells, seminoma areas and non-seminoma areas, but in other tumours there were two clones of neoplastic intratubular cells, with the one with the lower DNA content nearest to the non-seminoma areas [9]. There are some cytogenetic data suggesting that specific chromosome losses are associated with the transition from seminoma to non-seminoma [9]. The strongest evidence of a possible mechanism whereby the tetraploid pachytene spermatocyte switches from meiosis to mitosis comes from the observations of Chaganti and his group [10, 11]. They showed that one of the earliest molecular changes in the neoplastic transformation of spermatogonia was expression of Cyclin D2 and they speculated that this was acting as an oncogene stimulating the tetraploid pachytene cell to undergo mitosis. There is simultaneous expression of c-KIT proto-oncogene, a receptor for stem cell factors [12], and this helps to favour further expansion of the transformed clone.

Escape from Immune Surveillance and Progression to Non-seminomas

The strongest support for immune surveillance playing a role in the development of germ cell cancer comes from the observations that prognosis in seminoma is influenced by the degree of lymphoid infiltrate. The evidence that the incidence of seminoma but not non-seminoma is increased in immuno-suppressed HIV infected individuals whereas use of mutagenic chemical immuno-suppressive drugs in transplant recipients increases the proportion of non-seminomas [13] provides support for the concept that mutagenic clonal escape from immune surveillance could be a factor in the evolution from seminoma to non-seminoma. As yet little work has been done on possible antigenic targets for immune-surveillance. Antibodies against endogenous retrovirus proteins are present universally in germ cell tumour patients

Table 14.1: Combined Tumours as as Intermediate Prognosis Subgroup of Testicular Germ Cell Tumours (modified from reference 15)

	Seminoma n = 248	Combined Seminoma/ Non-Seminoma n = 116	Non-Seminoma n = 241
Median age stage 1	36 years	31 years	29 years
Median age metastatic patients	42 years	37 years	29 years
Proportion presenting in stage 1	79%	51%	41%
Relapse stage 1 surveillance	23%	31%	38%

but disappear with successful treatment [14]. This suggests further study of these proteins could be worth pursuing.

Clonal Development of Metastatic Disease

The low frequency and slow speed with which metastases develop in seminomas compared to non-seminomas (Table 14.1) provides some support for the contention of a clonal component in the development of the terminal manifestations of germ cell cancer. There is some evidence that external environmental influences such as a smoking habit affected the development of metastases in patients with seminoma whereas familial genetics as manifested by a past occurrence of cancer in first degree relative played a more important role in the early steps of transformation and increased the frequency with which pure non-seminomas developed metastases [15].

Differences in frequency of HLA class II DR antigens in stage I [1] and metastatic non-seminoma and between seminoma and non-seminoma provide possible evidence that host genetic plays a role in this process [16].

Conclusion

With more than 70 per cent of germ cell cancer patients presenting with atrophic changes in the normal testis as manifested by a subfertile sperm count compared to 20–30 per cent in the normal population (and in the minority without a low sperm count there are atrophic areas associated with areas of intratubular neoplasia), it is clear that the atrophy induced gonadotrophin drive, albeit initiated by multiple different factors, is the final common pathway for germ cell cancer development. Furthermore the evidence reviewed provides unequivocal support for the concept that a major part of this development takes place after puberty, though there is clear evidence that intra-uterine events are also important. The evidence that the tetraploid pachytene spermatocyte is the target for the initial transforming event is increasingly accepted as is the step-wise progression from intratubular neoplasia to seminoma and non-seminoma, associated with loss of DNA after initiation via expression of cyclin D2 and c-KIT. These observations provide strong support for the view that there should be different therapeutic approaches to seminoma and non-seminoma. The renewed interest in immune surveillance issues developing out of the increasing clear evidence for an increase in seminoma in immuno-suppressed HIV individuals highlights an important area in need of further research and provides justification for continued pursuit of clinical trials of testis conservation.

References

1. Rajpert-De Meyts E, Giwercman A, Skakkebaek NE. Carcinoma in-situ of the Testis- A Precursor of Testicular Germ Cell Cancer: Biological and Clinical Aspects. Comprehensive Textbook of Genitourinary Oncology (Ed: NJ Vogelzang, PT Scardino, WU Shipley, DS Coffey 2000:897–908

2. Oliver RTD. Atrophy, hormones, genes and viruses in aetiology of germ cell tumours. In: *Cancer Surveys*; 1990. p. 263–268

3. Forman D, Chilvers C, Oliver R, Pike M. The aetiology of testicular cancer: association with congenital abnormalities, age at puberty, infertility and exercise. *Br Med J* 1994;308:1393–1399

4. Beard CM, Benson RC, Kelalis PP. The incidence and outcome of mumps orchitis in Rochester, Minnesota 1935-1974. *Mayo Clinic Proceedings* 1977;52:3–7

5. Mieusset R, Bujan L. The potential of mild testicular heating as a safe, effective and reversible contraceptive method for men. *Int J Androl* 1994;17:186–191

6. Chilvers CEO, Forman D, Oliver RTD et al. Social, behavioural and medical factors in the aetiology of testicular cancer - results from the UK study. *Br J Cancer* 1994;70:513–520

7. Hoff Wanderas E, Fossa SD, Heilo A, Stenwig AE, Norman N. Serum Follicle Stimulating Hormone –Predictor of Cancer in the Remaining Testis in Patients with Unilateral Testicular Cancer. *Br J Urol* 1990;66:315–317

8. Muller J, Skakkebaek NE. Microspectrophotometric DNA measurements of carcinoma-in-situ germ cells in the testis. *Int J Androl* 1981;4:211–221

9. Ooesterhuis JW, Gillis AJM, Putten WJLv, Jong Bd, Looijenga LHJ. Interphase cytogenetics of carcinoma in situ of the testis. *Eur J Urol* 1993;23:16–22

10. Murty VVVS, Houldsworth J, Baldwin S et al. Allelic deletions in the long arm of chromosome 12 identify sites of candidate tumour suppressor genes in male germ cell tumours. *Proc Natl Acad Sci USA* 1992;89:11006–11010

11. Houldsworth J, Reuter V, Bosl GJ, Chaganti RS. Aberrant expression of cyclin D2 is an early event in human male germ cell tumorigenesis. *Cell Growth Differ* 1997;8:293–

12. Rajpert-De Meyts E, Skakkebaek NE. Expression of the c-kit protein product in carcinoma in situ and invasive testicular germ cell tumours. *Int J Androl* 1994;17:85–92

13. Leibovitch I, Baniel J, Rowland RG, Smith ER, Jr., Ludlow JK, Donohue JP. Malignant testicular neoplasms in immunosuppressed patients. *J Urol* 1996;155:1938–42

14. Boller K, Janssen O, Schuldes H, Tonjes RR, Kurth R. Characterisation of the antibody response specific for the human endogenous retrovirus HTDV/HERV-K. *J Virol* 1997;71:4581–8

15. Oliver RTD, Leahy M, Ong J. Combined seminoma/non-seminoma should be considered as intermediate grade germ cell cancer (GCC). *Eur J Cancer* 1995;31A:1392–1394

16. Oliver RTD. HLA phenotype and clinicopathological behaviour of germ cell tumours – possible evidence for clonal evolution from seminomas to nonseminomas. *Int J Androl* 1987;10:85–93

Section 2

Why Do Treatments Fail? Implications for Clinical Trial Strategy

15. Prognosis and Prognostic Factors

M.K. Gospodarowicz and B. O'Sullivan

Department of Radiation Oncology, Princess Margaret Hospital, University Health Network, University of Toronto, Toronto, Canada

Introduction

The management of patients or clinical practice has four main components. These are prophylaxis, diagnosis, treatment, and prognosis [1]. Appraisal of a patient's prognosis is part of everyday practice and studies of prognostic factors are integral to cancer research. However, the science of prognosis is rarely considered in a structured manner in cancer. Therefore, as in all areas of research, common definitions are required to allow communication of knowledge and new ideas.

Cancer is a heterogeneous group of diseases characterized by growth, invasion and metastasis. To consider management of an individual cancer case, the fundamental pieces of information required include the site of origin, e.g., testis or lung, and morphological type (histology), e.g., seminoma, or squamous cell carcinoma. In addition, the outcome in a cancer patient depends on a variety of variables referred to as "prognostic factors". These are defined as "variables that can account for some of the heterogeneity associated with the expected course and outcome of a disease" [2].

Knowledge of prognostic factors helps to understand the progress of disease (Table 15.1). We are seldom able to study the natural history of cancer, because some form of intervention is commonly applied in the hope that it will ameliorate the course of the disease. Treatment may have different goals, e.g., cure, avoidance or delay of symptoms, or prolongation of survival. Thus, the natural history of disease refers to the probable course of disease in a given patient, or groups of patients, defined by a set of prognostic factors and observed in the context of an intervention. Knowledge about prognostic factors is used in everyday patient care and in clinical research. To compare treatment outcomes among groups of patients, prognostic factors should be equally distributed, otherwise apparent differences in outcome could be explained entirely by a failure to compare "like with like", and not result from a putative effect of treatment. Therefore, knowledge of prognostic factors is essential for the interpretation of study results, and for the design of future studies. To answer a specific therapeutic question, it may be desirable to limit the patients studied to those characterized by selected prognostic variables [3]. In addition to clinical practice and research, knowledge of prognostic factors is essential to cancer control programs, because it permits inference to be applied broadly to other groups of individuals who may be at risk for cancer or benefit from educational or treatment related programs.

Table 15.1: Application of prognostic factors

Learning about the natural history of disease
Patient care
Select appropriate diagnostic tests
Select an appropriate treatment plan
Predicting the outcome for individual patient
Informed consent
Assessing the outcome of therapeutic intervention
Selecting appropriate follow-up monitoring
Patient and care giver education
Research
Prognostic stratification
– To improve the efficiency of research design and data analysis
– To enhance the confidence of prediction
– To demarcate phenomena for scientific explanation
Designing future studies
– Identification of subgroups with poor outcomes for experimental therapy
– Identification of groups with excellent outcomes for simplified therapy
– Identification of candidates for organ preservation trials
Cancer Control Programs
Planning of resource requirements
Assessing the impact of screening programs
Introduction and monitoring of clinical practice guidelines
Monitoring of results
Public education
Explaining variation in the observed outcome

Classifications of Prognostic Factors

Even before the anatomical extent of disease (stage) became the most widely adopted prognostic factor, it was appreciated that this was not the only factor affecting outcome in cancer patients. In recent years, with the availability of new cellular, molecular and genetic factors, a renewed interest in prognostic factors in cancer has materialized. Both the American Joint Committee on Cancer (AJCC) and the International Union against Cancer (UICC) held meetings to discuss the optimal incorporation of prognostic factors, other than the anatomical disease extent, into a new prognostic system [4]. Following initial deliberations, the AJCC published criteria for the interpretation of prognostic factors into an improved prognostic system that would enhance the existing TNM classification [5]. These criteria stipulated that to be included in a prognostic model, a putative prognostic factor had to be significant, independent, and clinically important. The AJCC proposal focused on the future use of molecular markers. The UICC TNM – Prognostic Factor Project Committee embarked on a broad review of the state of the knowledge of all types of prognostic factors, in the early 1990s [6, 7]. In the continuing effort of the UICC, the second edition of "Prognostic Factors in Cancer" proposed approaches to classifying the prognostic factors based on their relevance to clinical practice.

Subject Based Classification

Characteristically, most researcher regard prognostic factors to be those that directly relate to the given tumour. Examples include tumour histology, grade, depth of invasion, or the presence of metastasis. However, other factors not directly related to the tumour also affect the course of disease. To comprehensively review these factors, we divided them into three groups: those that relate to disease or *tumour*, those that relate to the *host* or patient, and those that relate to the *environment* in which we find the patient [8].

Tumour Related Prognostic Factors

Tumour related prognostic factors are those related to the presence of the tumour or its effect on the host. Common tumour related prognostic factors include pathology, anatomical disease extent, and biology. The most important disease related prognostic factor is anatomical extent of disease that is classified according to the UICC TNM system [9]. In addition, other factors that describe disease include tumour bulk, the number of involved sites, involvement of specific organs [10]. Tumour characteristics that influence the outcome include histological type, e.g., seminoma or choriocarcinoma histology in germ cell testis tumours, and diffuse large cell histology in lymphoma [11, 12]. Tumour markers such as AFP and HCG are used in everyday practice and strongly correlate with tumour bulk [13, 14]. Hormone receptors, biochemical markers, expression of proliferation-related factors and, increasingly, molecular tumour characteristics have been shown to affect outcomes for a variety of cancers [15, 16].

Host Related Prognostic Factors

Patient or host related prognostic factors include inherent demographic characteristics such as age, gender and ethnicity and other factors that may be acquired such as performance status, co-morbid conditions and immune status [17–21]. Although usually not related to the presence of the tumour, these factors may have a profound impact on the outcome.

Environment Related Prognostic Factors

Environment related prognostic factors (Table 15.2) comprise those that operate external to the patient. In an ideal setting, these should lend themselves to be modified to benefit an individual patient's outcome. This may also apply to groups of patients if specific health care policies are introduced to ensure the highest standards in a community. The corollary also holds: failure to address these factors may prejudice outcome. Interestingly, these factors are possibly the only ones that lend themselves to a realistic opportunity for immediate modification in the interest of improved outcomes. Environment related prognostic factors could be specific to an individual patient (socio-economic status, choice of treatment, quality of treatment), or more frequently to groups of patients residing in the same geographical area, (access to care, distance from medical facility, health care policy of the region, etc)

Table 15.2: Examples of Environment Related Prognostic Factors

	Related to treatment	Education	Quality
Physician	Choice of physician or specialty • Quality of diagnosis • Accuracy of staging Choice of treatment Expertise of physician – "narrow experts" Timeliness of treatment Ageism	Ignorance of medical profession Access to internet Knowledge, education of the patient Participation in clinical trials Participation in continuing education	Quality of treatment Skill of the physician Treatment verification
Health Care System	Access to appropriate diagnostic methods Access to care • Distance • Waiting Lists Monopoly control of access to care Availability of publicly funded screening programs	Continuing medical education Lack of audit of local results Access to internet Development of practice guidelines Dissemination of new knowledge	Quality of equipment Quality management in treatment facility Maintenance of health records Availability of universal health insurance Quality of diagnostic services Implementation of screening programs Promotion of error free environment
Society Focus	Preference for unconventional therapies Socioeconomic status Distance from cancer center Insurance status Access to transportation, car, etc. Ageism	Literacy Access to information	Access to affordable health insurance Nutritional status of the population

[22–27]. The impact of some of these factors may be profound. Most studies dealing with prognostic factors deal exclusively with tumour related attributes with the exception of age and gender that are easily available and therefore studied in many tumours [28].

Among the environment related factors, expertise and quality have a high potential of impact on outcomes. The expertise of treating physician is a prognostic factor as it affects the outcome in cancer patients. There is increasing evidence that for many cancers, centers that do not treat a certain "critical mass" of patients may not achieve the optimal treatment outcome. This finding has been observed in several studies of advanced testicular germ cell cancer in the United Kingdom and Europe, and also differences in outcome have been observed when the outcomes in SEER data have been compared to the outcome achieved by the expert group at the Memorial Hospital [29–31]. There is much evidence that specialization in cancer care improves the outcomes [23]. Referral to a multidisciplinary team improved survival of patients with ovarian cancer in Scotland [32]. Gillis et al., in a study conducted in a geographically defined area, showed a 9 per cent higher 5–year survival and 8 per cent higher 10–year survival for patients with breast cancer cared for by a specialist surgeon rather than by non-specialists [25].

Quality of treatment is under the direct control of the treating physician, but factors such as the presence of local real time audit of treatment plans, tumour boards to validate staging and treatment decisions, and the completeness and accuracy of health records, all contribute to outcomes. The constraints on access to care in some health care systems may indirectly have a negative impact on the quality of care provided by individual physicians. Similar to industry, in medicine the presence of national and institutional quality improvement initiatives is likely to lead to better results and increased patient satisfaction. Human errors in medicine are common and are responsible for a substantial morbidity and mortality associated with medical care. In oncology, the errors may involve the diagnosis or the treatment of cancer. The introduction of audit and the use of new technology based applications to support human ability are being introduced to lower the error rates.

Prognostic Factor Groupings

While a classification into the three subject based categories may be a useful working model, the distinction between these groupings of prognostic factors is not always clear and many prognostic factors overlap these categories. For example, performance status may be related to the tumour (which is causing debilitating symptoms), or, when compromised due to coexistent illness could be a host related prognostic factor. Similarly, the quality of treatment is a host related factor if it relates to patient compliance, but is usually an environment related factor relating to access to optimal medical care.

Several prognostic factors, each individually giving predictions with relatively low accuracy, may be combined to provide a single variable of high accuracy. Such a variable is called a prognostic index. When T, N, and M categories in the TNM classification are combined, they form a stage grouping, in reality a specific prognostic index focusing mainly on anatomical disease extent. An example of such a prognostic index is the International Prognostic Classification of Germ Cell Testis Tumours.

Clinical Relevance Based Classification

The assessment of prognostic factors allows for a prediction of a probable outcome and is a first step in a determination of treatment plan. The goals may include a variety of outcomes: cure, response with prospects of long-term disease control, or symptom relief only, etc. To consider the relevance of prognostic factors in clinical practice, the prognostic factors in this book are placed in the three distinct categories: essential, additional, and new and promising factors. The essential factors are those that are fundamental to decisions about the goals and choice of treatment, including details of selection of treatment modality, and specific interventions. The additional factors allow finer prognostication, but do not add to the decision making process. They may be used to communicate prognosis, but do not influence treatment choice. Finally, new and promising factors, are those that shed new light about the biology of disease, but for which currently there is, at best, incomplete evidence of an independent effect on outcome or prognosis. For some, evidence may exist about the prognostic impact of these new factors, but conflicting data may exist, or they are not currently in common usage for selecting treatment, or communicating the prognosis. Factors included under the essential, additional and new and promising categories are certain to change with time. With progress in the understanding of the biology of cancer, the ability to discriminate between localized and disseminated disease, and the introduction of new and more effective treatment methods, new factors may be required to select the optimal treatment. Our ability to predict the outcome in the future may be enhanced by molecular tumour characteristics.

Essential Prognostic Factors

The most important essential factor is anatomical disease extent. The fundamental importance of disease extent had been recognized more than 70 years ago with the first attempts at staging classifications. The formal development of a systematic classification of the anatomical extent of disease using the TNM system is attributed to Pierre Denoix and the International Union against Cancer (UICC) through its TNM Project [33]. The TNM Classification has been translated into many languages and is accepted as the international language to describe anatomical extent of cancer. Today, the AJCC and the UICC TNM classifications are identical to facilitate worldwide communication about cancer [34]. However, factors other than anatomical extent of disease are also essential to the management of cancer. Tumour pathology also embraces domains beyond the diagnosis of malignancy, histological type, or microscopical disease extent recognized in the staging classification. It includes the associated histological features of cancer such as tumour grade and the presence of small vessel invasion [35]. Newer imaging methods allow improved measurement of tumour bulk, an important addition to the description of anatomical disease extent. Tumour markers used in germ cell testis tumours, prostate cancer and ovarian cancer provide another dimension in measuring tumour burden [10, 13]. Patient age, a host related factor, is integral to decision making in thyroid cancer and Hodgkin's disease, but does not influence the choice of treatment in most other cancers [36-37].

Additional Prognostic Factors

There are additional attributes that allow refinements in predicting outcome, although they are not currently used in the decision making process. More detailed histological features add to prognostic precision. These include patterns of invasion, phenotype, and surrogate indices for tumour proliferation such as percentage S-phase, expression of Ki-67 or MiB-1 antigens, and PCNA. However, they are usually not required to generate a treatment plan [38–40]. Most host related factors including performance status, co-morbid conditions and the function of vital organs influence the suitability for surgery, chemotherapy or radiotherapy. Therefore, they indirectly have an impact on outcome. The environment-related factors, although rarely considered in an individual case, have a profound impact on the outcome of groups of patients or on patient populations. The choice of an inferior treatment plan, poor quality of diagnostic tests, or treatment has potential to compromise the outcome [23]. Treatment of germ cell testis cancer in a specialized unit, or breast cancer by specialist surgeon resulted in an improved survival in population-based studies in Scotland [25, 26]. Similar findings were observed in surgery for colorectal cancer [41]. As noted earlier, the environment related factors paradoxically lend themselves to modification with the opportunity for profound gain, in contrast to the other factors that are permanently set by the disease.

New and Promising Prognostic Factors

The expansion of molecular biology has provided a wealth of new molecules, and more opportunities to study new prognostic factors. Molecular factors may be used to predict response to a treatment modality, or they present a target for therapy. Another category includes factors that predict for the presence of occult distant metastases. Examples include, polymerase chain reaction (PCR) for cells expressing prostatic specific membrane antigen (PSMA), or the presence of high levels of cell cycle associated proteins, angiogenesis related factors, etc. The numerous candidate prognostic factors allow prediction of the natural or treated history of the specific cancer. Most molecular factors fit into this new and promising category. Among them are the cell cycle associated proteins Rb, p53, p27, etc., the cellular adhesion molecules CD44, e-cadherin, etc., the proliferation antigens Ki-67, MiB-1, and the expression of protein products of translocations [42–46]. Further understanding of tumour biology may allow for greater accuracy and more specific prognostic ability, and in addition provide new and interesting targets for treatment.

A combination of the subject based and clinical relevance based classifications may be used to summarize in simple terms the prognostic factors for individual cancers for a selected management scenario as illustrated in Table 15.3.

Table 15.3: Examples of Prognostic Factors in Cancer

Prognostic factors	Tumor related	Host related	Environment related
Essential	Anatomical disease extent Histological grade	Age	Availability of access to a radiotherapy facility
Additional	Tumor bulk Tumor marker level	Race Gender Cardiac function	Expertise of a surgeon
New and promising	p53 CD44	Germline p53	Access to information

Management Scenarios – Freezing the Prognosis

Prognosis is not static and always changes with time and is affected by a large number of factors that may or may not be disease related. It is essential to be able to capture prognosis at a given time. This is essential to formulate goals and plans for a specific intervention and to be able to discuss these issues with the patients and their support team. In addition, while prognosis changes with time, it also changes with the management decisions made. Thus, to determine the prognosis at a given time and in a given context, it is necessary to freeze the context in time. This is considered a management scenario. A management scenario comprises the prognostic attributes existing at the time, and is influenced by the choice of the planned intervention, and the outcome of interest. (Figure 15.1) Intervention is axiomatic in cancer care and in most instances, it will affect the outcome.

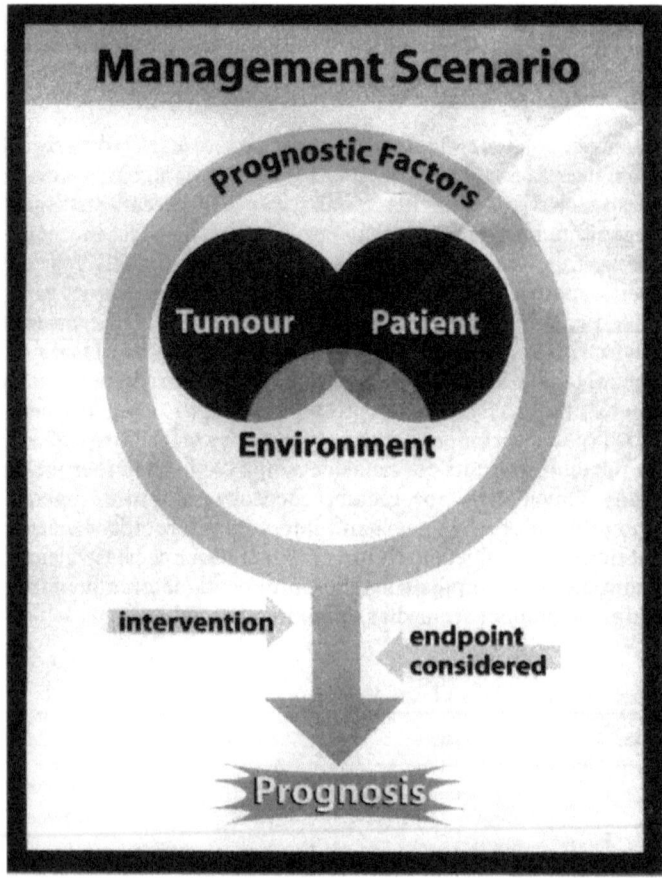

Figure 15.1: Representation of the interaction among the three domains of prognostic factors (tumour, host and environment). The prognostic factors are expressed in the context of the proposed therapeutic intervention and for a given endpoint of interest, e.g., survival, response, local tumour control, organ preservation, etc. In addition, the prognosis itself must be interpreted in the context of both the treatment (because it may change the prognosis) and the endpoint (which must be relevant to the prognosis).

Since the prognosis differs with a given scenario, prognostic factors should be considered within a given context or scenario. Most commonly, prognostic factors are considered at diagnosis before a definitive treatment plan is formulated. Prognostic factors differ with choice of intervention. As treatment interventions have a major impact on the outcome, it is important to discuss prognostic factors in the context of a specific treatment plan or therapeutic intervention. Prognostic factors of value for survival prediction may not be of value for another outcome. Therefore, when considering prognostic factors, the endpoint or the outcome of interest must be a part of management scenario in determining the prognosis.

Endpoints Relevant To Consider in Cancer Patients

It is important to focus again on the main purposes of prognostic factors, whether it is to facilitate the choice of treatment or communication about cancer. As noted earlier, they allow prediction of outcomes. The relevant endpoints to consider in cancer include probability of cure, duration of survival, likelihood of response to treatment, probability of relapse, time to relapse, likelihood of local tumour control, likelihood of organ preservation, possibility for symptom relief, etc. Therefore, the outcomes may be very heterogeneous. Some prognostic factors facilitate prediction of more than one outcome, while others predict selected outcomes only. Consequently, prognostic factors should be always considered in the context of the outcome of interest. For example, the presence of small vessel invasion in non-seminomatous germ cell tumour predicts for distant failure, while its absence reduces this probability. This knowledge permits clinicians to select patients for additional intervention. Another example is the size of retroperitoneal mass in seminoma that predicts for a distant treatment failure, but not for survival.

Response to Treatment and Prognosis

Tumour response is an early endpoint in the assessment of treatment effectiveness. The formally agreed upon criteria for classification of tumour response were introduced in late 1970s by the UICC and the WHO [47]. The four categories of response (complete response, partial response, stable disease and progressive disease) were originally proposed in the WHO handbook and retained in the recently published NCI guidelines [48]. The above criteria were developed to assess the effects of drug therapy, but they may easily be applied to the outcomes of surgical or radiotherapy interventions. Response to treatment, whether to chemotherapy, radiotherapy or surgery, has often been listed as an important prognostic factor. Indeed, as discussed below, complete tumour resection with negative margins could be considered as a complete response to surgical intervention, while positive resection margins could be considered as a partial response to surgical intervention. A response to treatment, however, is an early outcome in cancer. Knowledge of response can be incorporated into the next scenario in patient management. The extent of response is a surrogate for the anatomical extent of disease after the completion of therapy and as such is a prognostic factor for further outcome. Positive response to treatment is almost always associated with a better outcome. Since the knowledge of response is not available until after treatment is completed, it should not be considered a prognostic factor for the scenario that preceded it. Therefore it may be used to predict outcome of the scenario, which follows the response assessment, and this is likely to be unfavorable for the non-responders.

Time Dependent Prognostic Factors

Time dependent prognostic factors are variables which become available over the time course of the patient's disease. While they may be very predictive of outcome, they are also problematic because they risk disturbing the context of relevant disease outcome evaluation and decision-making. This is because it may be impossible to separate real 'causality' in the relationship between a time dependent factor and an outcome of interest from a mere 'association' caused by another factor common to them both. If the latter is the case, and it is not known whether there is 'causality', one is left uncertain whether influencing the time dependent variable can have any effect on the course of the disease. Alternatively, one could incorrectly dismiss a causal association where one in fact exists because of a belief that the methodology for its evaluation was flawed. Therefore, if not undertaken carefully, the clinical interpretation of time dependent prognostic factors may be incorrect. In some cases, prognostic factors associated with a subsequent scenario have been considered together with prognostic factors at diagnosis. For example, the post-chemotherapy serum marker levels may be considered as prognostic factors in germ cell testis tumours. In truth, the serum marker nadir is a surrogate for response to chemotherapy and as such belongs to a different management scenario occurring subsequently.

Generally, time dependent prognostic factors are entered into a Cox regression model in an attempt to adjust for the time bias in assessing the prognostic value of a specific covariate. Most often, these factors are a mathematical representation of disease progression or regression over time but cannot be used to prognosticate about later outcomes at the time of an earlier scenario (e.g. time of diagnosis or initial treatment) since they have not had the opportunity to manifest yet.

Application of Prognostic Factors

Prognostic factors are used in daily clinical practice, in research and in cancer control. In everyday clinical practice, the influence of prognostic factors dominates all the steps in decision-making and the comprehensive management of patients with cancer including selection of the primary goal of management, the most appropriate treatment modality, and the adjustment of treatment according to disease severity. Knowledge of prognostic factors allows clinicians to select treatment options that allow preservation of organs or function without compromising cure and survival. An example of such a situation is in seminoma where the prognostic factors for local control, and hence testis-sparing approaches, may differ from those for the risk of distant failure and disease-specific survival. The availability of prognostic factor information is very helpful in population based studies of the outcomes of treatment of cancer, especially if they focus on specific groups of patients. Measurement of the cost efficacy of cancer treatment has to include economic analysis of new treatment strategies and their impact on the health of the population. Cancer control efforts include population screening programs that require assessment of the prognostic factor in cancers detected by screening as an early endpoint of the effectiveness of such interventions. The implementation of clinical practice guidelines is hoped to improve the quality of decision making and in turn improve the outcomes in cancer patients. Knowledge of prognostic factors is required to evaluate the compliance with practice guidelines, before examining their impact.

Prognostic Factors and Milieu

The prognostic factors that are defined as essential for decision-making depend on their relevance to the issues in cancer care in a particular milieu. What is important to cancer patient care in Toronto, or Paris may not be relevant to a cancer patient in a small African village. The main issues in the developing countries are related to cancer prevention and early detection. Factors that predict for organ preservation and those that contribute to finesse in defining the prognosis may not be important in places with limited diagnostic equipment, and where funding for evaluation of assessment of response to treatment is not available. Therefore the list of essential, additional, and new and promising factors may vary depending on the milieu where the patient and health care professional are located. It is important to note that progress in such situations does not require new discovery, but merely economic development, education, and a process to ensure access.

Future Research into Prognostic Factors

To be relevant to clinical practice, prognostic factors must either have a significant impact on cancer outcome, or be used to select treatment methods. It is likely that with progress in treatment, and improved outcomes, prognostic factors will be more relevant for selection of treatment. An example is seen in the germ cell testis tumours. The prognosis of patients with stage I is excellent and knowledge of the individual patient or disease characteristics is not required to predict the cure. However, knowledge of prognostic factors is required to minimize the impact of treatment. Patients with favorable prognostic factors have a high probability of being cured with orchiectomy alone, while those with unfavorable factors such as small vessel invasion are at a high risk of harboring occult metastatic disease and have an option of receiving adjuvant chemotherapy. Improved staging methods, and especially more accurate characterization of microscopical disease extent will allow more homogeneous grouping of patients with similar disease characteristics, and the tumour related prognostic factors for an individual disease may change. Knowledge of genetic factors will further add to the improved prediction of outcome and greater individualization of therapeutic interventions. However, grouping of patients into similar categories will continue to be required to assess the impact of new technology of patient assessment and new therapies on the outcome.

References

1. Rizzi DA. Medical prognosis – some fundamentals. *Theor Med* 1993;14:365–75
2. Stockler M, Boyd N, Tannock I. *Guide to studies of diagnostic tests, prognostic factors, and treatments*, in Tannock I, Hill R (eds.): The basic science of oncology (ed. 3rd). Toronto, McGraw-Hill, 1998, pp. 466–492
3. Byar DP. *Identification of prognostic factors*, in Buyse ME, Staquet MJ, Sylvester RJ (eds.): Cancer Clinical Trials. New York, Oxford University Press, 1984, pp. 423–443

4. Yarbro JW, Page DL, Fielding LP, et al. American Joint Committee on Cancer prognostic factors consensus conference. *Cancer* 1999;86:2436–46
5. Burke HB, Henson DE. Criteria for prognostic factors and for an enhanced prognostic system. *Cancer* 1993;72:3131–3135
6. Hermanek P, Gospodarowicz M, Henson D, et al. Prognostic Factors in Cancer, in UICC (ed.): (ed. 1st). Heidelberg, Springer, 1995
7. Hermanek P. Prognostic factor research in oncology. *J Clin Epidemiol* 1999;52:371–4
8. Hermanek P, Hutter RVP, Sobin LH. Prognostic grouping: the next step in tumour classification. *J Cancer Res Clin Oncol* 1990;116:513–516
9. Sobin LH, Fleming ID. TNM Classification of Malignant Tumors, fifth edition (1997). Union Internationale Contre le Cancer and the American Joint Committee on Cancer. Cancer 80:1803–4, 1997
10. Sabbatini P, Larson SM, Kremer A, et al. Prognostic significance of extent of disease in bone in patients with androgen-independent prostate cancer. *J Clin Oncol* 1999;17:948–57
11. Gelb AB. Renal cell carcinoma: current prognostic factors. Union Internationale Contre le Cancer (UICC) and the American Joint Committee on Cancer (AJCC). Cancer 80:981–6, 1997
12. Shipp M. Prognostic factors in non-Hodgkin's lymphoma *Curr Opin Oncol* 1992;4:856–62
13. Mead GM, Stenning SP. The International Germ Cell Consensus Classification: a new prognostic factor-based staging classification for metastatic germ cell tumours. *Clin Oncol (R Coll Radiol)* 1997;9:207–9
14. Sassine AM, Schulman C. Clinical use of prostate-specific antigen in the staging of patients with prostatic carcinoma. *Eur Urol* 1993;23:348–51
15. Brien TP, Depowski PL, Sheehan CE, et al. Prognostic factors in gastric cancer. *Mod Pathol* 1998;11:870–7
16. Kramer MH, Hermans J, Wijburg E, et al. Clinical relevance of BCL2, BCL6, and MYC rearrangements in diffuse large B-cell lymphoma. *Blood* 1998;92:3152–62
17. Dolan R, Vaughan C, Fuleihan N. Metachronous cancer: prognostic factors including prior irradiation. *Otolaryngol Head Neck Surg* 1998;119:619–23
18. Aviles A, Yanez J, Lopez T, et al. Malnutrition as an adverse prognostic factor in patients with diffuse large cell lymphoma. *Arch Med Res* 1995;26:31–4.
19. Siu LL, Shepherd FA, Murray N, et al. Influence of age on the treatment of limited-stage small-cell lung cancer. *J Clin Oncol* 1996;14:821–8
20. Moul JW, Douglas TH, McCarthy WF, et al. Black race is an adverse prognostic factor for prostate cancer recurrence following radical prostatectomy in an equal access health care setting. *J Urol* 1996;155:1667–73
21. DeMario MD, Liebowitz DN. Lymphomas in the immunocompromised patient. *Semin Oncol* 1998;25:492-502
22. Feldman JG, Saunders M, Carter AC, et al. The effects of patient delay and symptoms other than a lump on survival in breast cancer. *Cancer* 1983;51:1226–9
23. Selby P, Gillis C, Haward R. Benefits from specialised cancer care. *Lancet* 1996;348:313–8
24. Paszat LF, Mackillop WJ, Groome PA, et al. Radiotherapy for breast cancer in Ontario: rate variation associated with region, age and income. *Clin Invest Med* 1998;21:125–34
25. Gillis CR, Hole DJ. Survival outcome of care by specialist surgeons in breast cancer: a study of 3786 patients in the west of Scotland. *BMJ* 1996;312:145–8
26. Harding MJ, Paul J, Gillis CR, et al. Management of malignant teratoma: does referral to a specialist unit matter? *Lancet* 1993;341:999–1002
27. Mackillop WJ, Zhang-Salomons J, Groome PA, et al. Socioeconomic status and cancer survival in Ontario. *J Clin Oncol* 1997;15:1680–9
28. Fielding LP, Fenoglio-Preiser CM, Freedman LS. The future of prognostic factors in outcome prediction for patients with cancer. *Cancer* 1992;70:2367–77
29. Collette L, Sylvester RJ, Stenning SP, et al. Impact of the treating institution on survival of patients with "poor- prognosis" metastatic nonseminoma. European Organization for Research and Treatment of Cancer Genito-Urinary Tract Cancer Collaborative Group and the Medical Research Council Testicular Cancer Working Party. *J Natl Cancer Inst* 1999;91:839–46
30. Feuer EJ, Sheinfeld J, Bosl GJ. Does size matter? Association between number of patients treated and patient outcome in metastatic testicular cancer. *J Natl Cancer Inst* 1999;91:816–8
31. Aass N, Klepp O, Cavallin-Stahl E, et al. Prognostic factors in unselected patients with nonseminomatous metastatic testicular cancer: a multicenter experience. *J Clin Oncol* 1991;9:818–26
32. Junor EJ, Hole DJ, Gillis CR. Management of ovarian cancer: referral to a multidisciplinary team matters. *Br J Cancer* 70:363–70, 1994
33. Gospodarowicz M, Benedet L, Hutter R, et al. History and international developments in cancer staging. *Cancer Prevention and Control* 1998;2:262-268

34. Fleming I, Cooper J, Henson D, et al. AJCC Cancer Staging Manual, (ed. 5th). Philadelphia, JB Lippincott, 1997
35. Moul JW, Heidenreich A. Prognostic factors in low-stage nonseminomatous testicular cancer. *Oncology (Huntingt)* 1996;10:1359–68, 1374
36. Tsang RW, Brierley JD, Simpson WJ, et al. The effects of surgery, radioiodine, and external radiation therapy on the clinical outcome of patients with differentiated thyroid carcinoma. *Cancer* 1998;82:375–88
37. Gospodarowicz MK, Sutcliffe SB, Clark RM, et al. Analysis of supradiaphragmatic clinical stage I and II Hodgkin's disease treated with radiation alone. *Int J Radiat Oncol Biol Phys* 1992;22:859–65
38. Gisselbrecht C, Gaulard P, Lepage E, et al. Prognostic significance of T-cell phenotype in aggressive non-Hodgkin's lymphomas. Groupe d'Etudes des Lymphomes de l'Adulte (GELA). *Blood* 1998;92:76–82
39. Sunderland MC, McGuire WL. Prognostic indicators in invasive breast cancer. *Surg Clin North Am* 1990;70:989–1004
40. Delahunt B. Histopathologic prognostic indicators for renal cell carcinoma. *Semin Diagn Pathol* 1998;15:68–76
41. McArdle CS, Hole D. Impact of variability among surgeons on postoperative morbidity and mortality and ultimate survival *BMJ* 1991;302:1501–5
42. Aaltomaa S, Lipponen P, Ala-Opas M, et al. Alpha-catenin expression has prognostic value in local and locally advanced prostate cancer. *Br J Cancer* 1999;80:477–82
43. Gascoyne RD, Aoun P, Wu D, et al. Prognostic significance of anaplastic lymphoma kinase (ALK) protein expression in adults with anaplastic large cell lymphoma. *Blood* 1999;93:3913–3921
44. Gascoyne RD, Adomat SA, Krajewski S, et al. Prognostic significance of Bcl-2 protein expression and Bcl-2 gene rearrangement in diffuse aggressive non-Hodgkin's lymphoma. *Blood* 1997;90:244–51
45. Grignon DJ, Caplan R, Sarkar FH, et al. p53 status and prognosis of locally advanced prostatic adenocarcinoma: a study based on RTOG 8610. *J Natl Cancer Inst* 1997;89:158–65
46. Stauder R, Eisterer W, Thaler J, et al. CD44 variant isoforms in non-Hodgkin's lymphoma: a new independent prognostic factor. *Blood* 1995;85:2885–99
47. WHO handbook for reporting results of cancer treatment. Geneva (Switzerland), World Health Organization Offset Publication, 1979
48. Therasse P, Arbuck SG, Eisenhauer EA, et al. New guidelines to evaluate the response to treatment in solid tumors. *J Natl Cancer Inst* 2000;92:205–16

16. Role of the Human Apurinic Endonuclease Ape1/ref–1 in Germ Cell Tumours

M.R. Kelley[1,2], D. Wang[1], S-H. Jung[4], J. Shen[4], T.H. Albright[3], L.H. Einhorn[4], K.A. Robertson[1]

1. Department of Pediatrics, Section of Hematology/Oncology, Herman B Wells Center for Pediatric Research, 2. Department of Biochemistry and Molecular Biology, 3. Department of Pathology, 4. Department of Medicine, Indiana University School of Medicine, 702 Barnhill Dr., Indianapolis, IN 46077

Summary

The human AP endonuclease (Ape1 or ref–1) DNA base excision repair (BER) enzyme is a multifunctional protein impacting on a wide variety of important cellular functions including oxidative signaling, transcription factor regulation, and cell-cycle control. It acts on mutagenic apurinic (AP) or baseless sites in DNA as a critical member of the DNA BER repair pathway. Moreover, Ape1 stimulates the DNA binding activity of transcription factors (Fos-Jun, NFkB, Myb, ATF/CREB family, HIF–1a, HLF, PAX, and p53) through a redox mechanism and thus represents a novel component of signal transduction processes that regulate eukaryotic gene expression. Ape1 has also been shown to be closely linked to apoptosis associated with thioredoxin, and altered levels of Ape1 have been found in some cancers. In a continuation of our previous studies that demonstrated an elevation of Ape1 in germ cell tumours (GCTs), we have determined in the cases we have studied (teratomas) that the level of Ape1 in the cytoplasm is elevated in those patients that ultimately relapse compared to those that remain disease-free. These results lead us to conclude that cytoplasmic Ape1 may function as a marker for patients who may not be responsive to standard GCT treatments and eventually relapse. However, the function of Ape1 in the cytoplasm is unknown at this time and is a focus of our continuing studies, as is the study of Ape1 expression in other GCT subgroups.

Introduction

The DNA Base Excision Repair (BER) pathway is responsible for the repair of alkylation and oxidative DNA damage and thereby protects against the deleterious effects of endogenous and exogenous agents encountered on a daily basis. Removal of the incorrect or damaged base by a DNA glycosylase (e.g. N-methylpurine DNA glycosylase; MPG) comprises the first step of the BER pathway (Figure 16.1). MPG repairs not only the major alkylated cytotoxic lesion, 3-methyladenine (3-meA) of DNA, but also functions to cleave the major product of all alkylated DNA N7-methylguanine [1], as well as that related to oxidative DNA damage such as

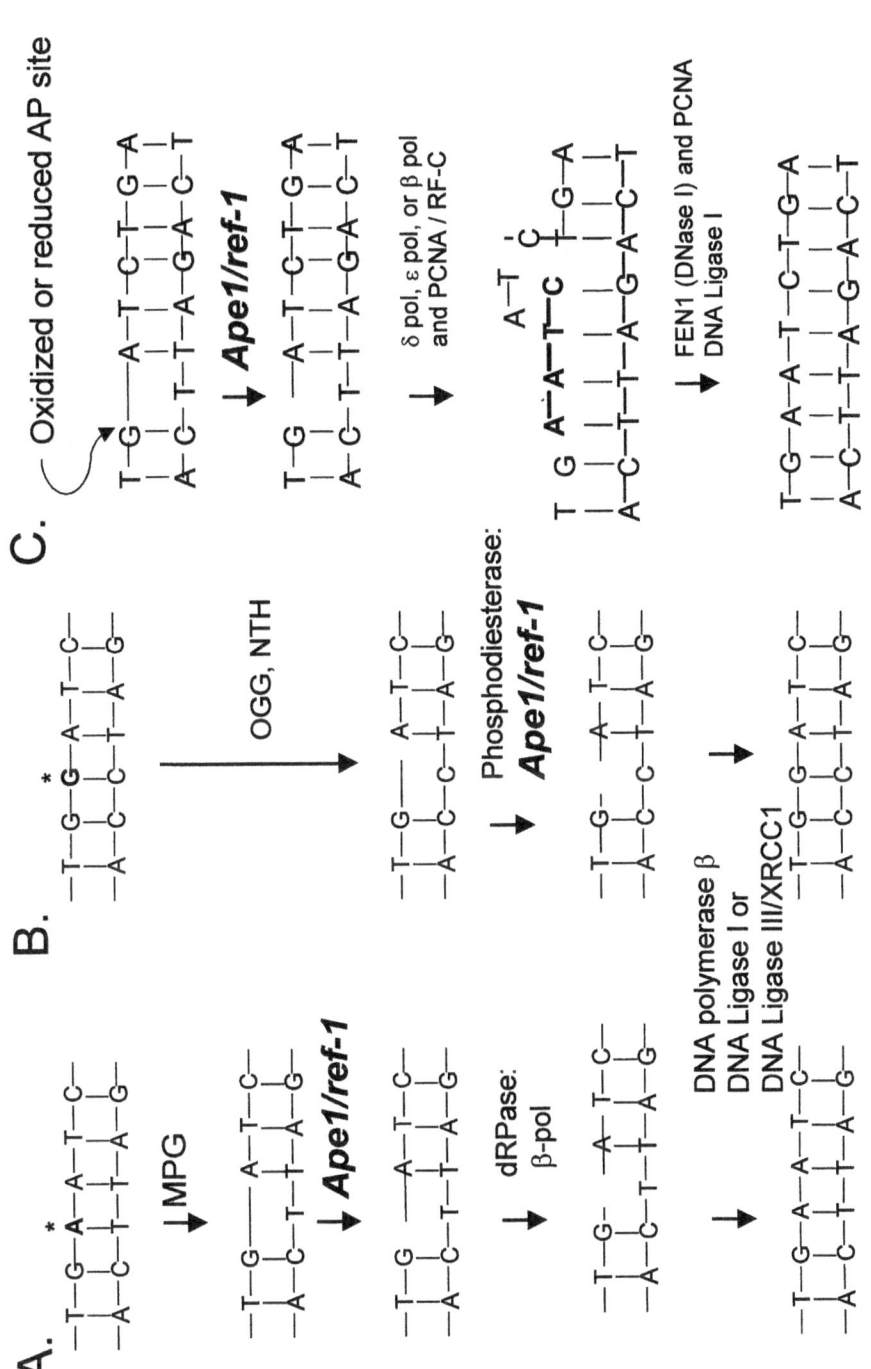

Figure 16.1: DNA base excision repair (BER) pathways and crucial role of Ape1 in these pathways.

N^6ethenoadenine. Although it has been proposed that N^7-methylguanine is relatively innocuous, data suggests that this lesion can rearrange to form both cytotoxic and mutagenic lesions [1].

The second enzyme in the BER pathway, Ape1, is the focus of these studies. Ape1 hydrolyzes the phosphodiester backbone immediately 5' to an AP site, which is generated following chemotherapeutic or ionizing radiation (IR) treatment (Figure 16.1, 16.2). This incision generates a normal 3'-hydroxyl group and an abasic deoxyribose–5–phosphate, which is processed by subsequent enzymes of the BER pathway. AP sites are generated from spontaneous and chemically initiated hydrolysis, IR, UV irradiation, oxidative stress, oxidizing agents, and removal of altered (such as alkylated) bases by DNA glycosylases [2, 3]. For instance, direct alkylation of the base by electrophilic chemotherapeutic agents can result in AP sites as the alkylated base may be excised by specific DNA glycosylases (Figure 16.2) [4–7]. The persistence of AP sites in DNA results in a block to DNA replication, cytotoxic mutations, and genetic instability [3]. Furthermore, AP sites are stimulators of topoisomerase II (topoII) cleavage and function in a manner comparable to topoII poisons such as etoposide [8, 9].

Reactive oxygen species and free radicals are capable of oxidizing the deoxyribose moiety producing 1' and 4' oxidized AP sites along with the 3¢-phosphate (3'-P) and phosphoglycolate species (3'-PG) noted above. Ape1 also contains repair activity for 3'-terminal oxidative lesions, such as those formed by IR and bleomycin (Figure 16.1) [2, 10–14]. By hydrolyzing 3'-blocking fragments from oxidized DNA, Ape1 produces normal 3'-hydroxyl nucleotide termini necessary for DNA repair synthesis and ligation at single or double strand breaks.

Bacteria, yeast or human cells lacking AP endonuclease repair activity are hypersensitive to agents (e.g. alkylating or oxidizing) that induce the formation of AP sites [2]. Moreover, targeted reduction of Ape1 protein by specific anti-sense RNA expression renders mammalian cells hypersensitive to alkylating and oxidizing agents, and bleomycin [15]. Recent studies have shown that the radiosensitivity of cervical cancers is directly correlated to the levels of Ape1 activity, thus validating Ape1 as a target for sensitization or protection schemes in anti-cancer treatments [16–18]. Ape1 levels have also been found to be elevated in a number of other malignancies such as ovarian, cervical and prostate cancer, rhabdomyosarcomas and GCT [19–24].

Ape1 is a multifunctional protein and, in addition to its role in DNA repair, also functions as a redox factor maintaining transcription factors in an active reduced state [25]. As a result of this alternative function, Ape1 was given the name redox effector factor 1 (ref-1) and appears in the literature under this name as well as APE/ref-1, hAPE, HAP1 and others [15]. Ape1 has been shown to stimulate the DNA binding activity of numerous transcription factors that are involved in cancer promotion and progression such as Fos, Jun, NFkB, PAX, HIF–1a, HLF and p53 [15] (Figure 16.3). The redox and repair domains are fairly distinct and alterations to one domain can have little or no effect on the function of the other domain (Figure 16.4).

Given the multifaceted role of Ape1 in DNA repair and redox regulation of transcription factors, and our previous findings that Ape1 is elevated in a variety of GCTs, we wanted to determine if the expression of Ape1 was related to the response of GCTs to front or second line therapy, particularly comparing those patients that relapse to those that remain disease-free. Toward this goal, we have continued to analyze GCTs for Ape1 expression using our monoclonal antibody and

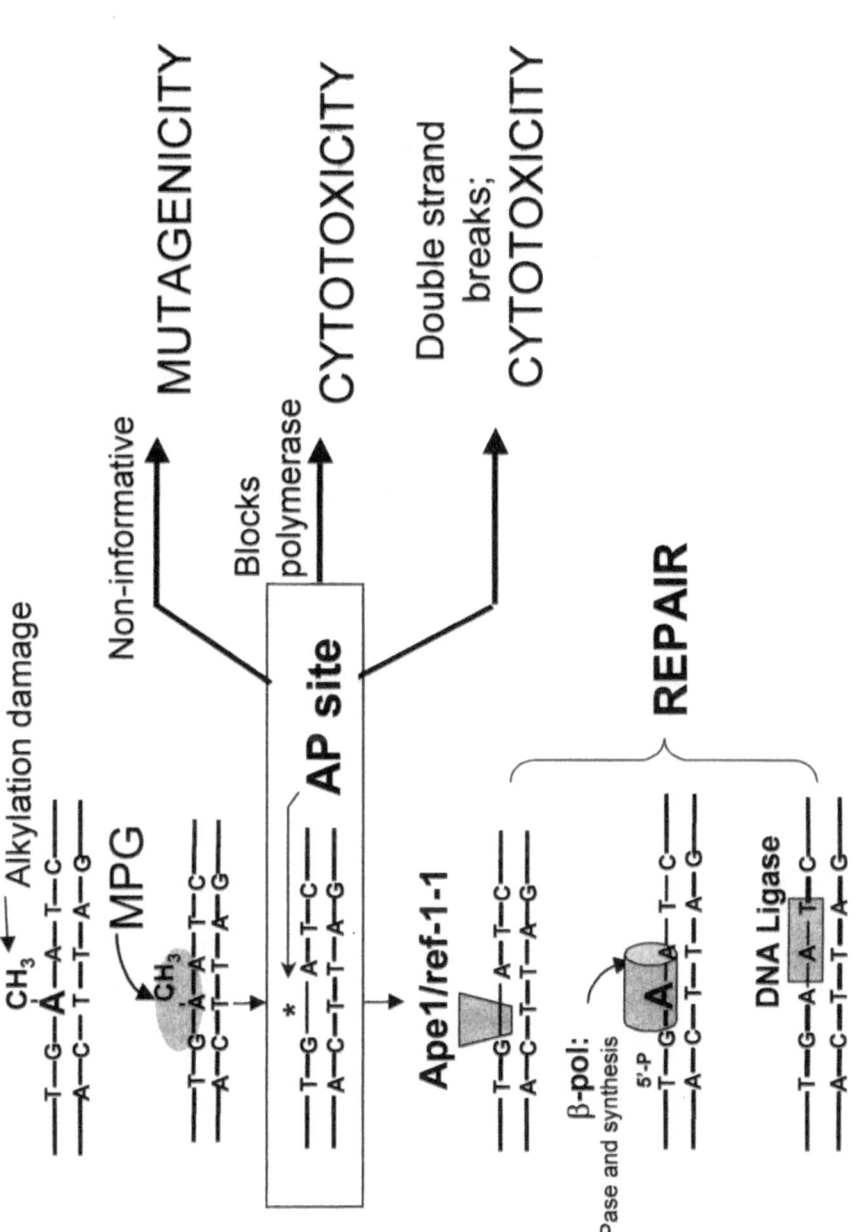

Figure 16.2: DNA BER and the consequences of AP sites.

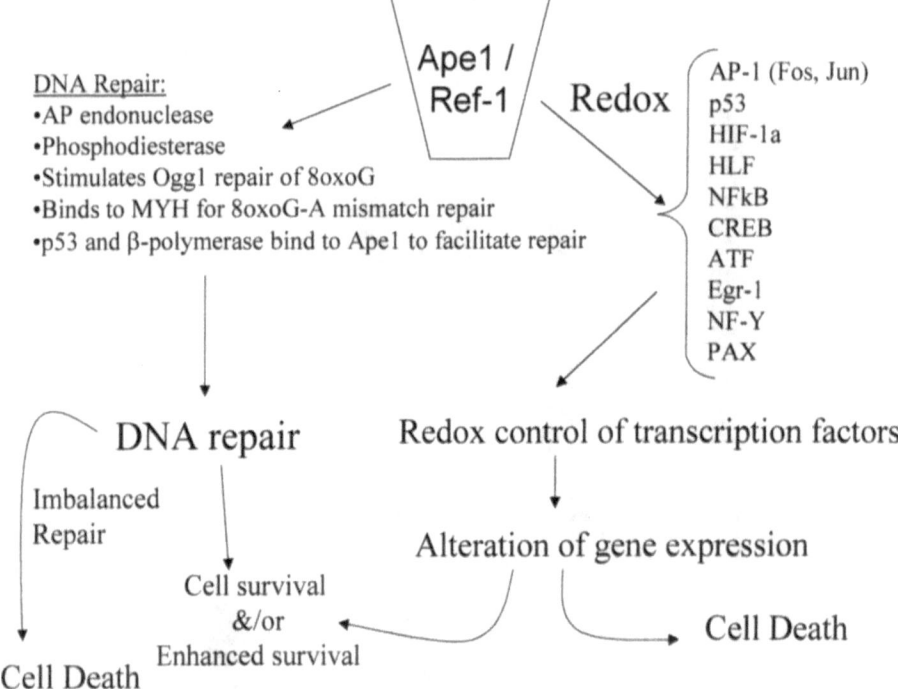

Figure 16.3: Multifunctional role of Ape1 in repair, redox regulation of transcription factors and its relationship to cell death, cell survival and cell cycle (p53) control.

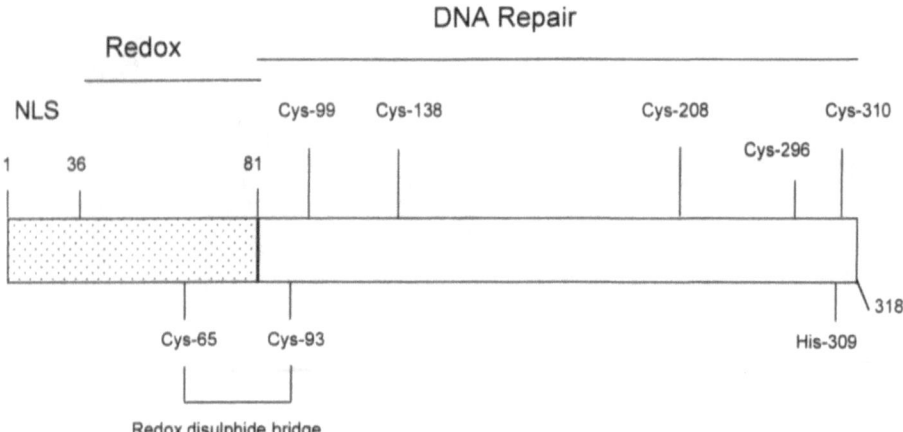

Figure 16.4: Domains of Ape1. The redox domain includes approximately the first 81 amino acids while the DNA repair domain is at the carboxyl end of the protein. The cysteines at amino acids 65 and 93 have been presumed to form a disulphide bridge and are involved in the redox function of Ape1. The histidine at amino acid 309 is in the heart of the DNA repair active site [26–28].

immunohistochemistry (IHC). The preliminary results of our ongoing studies are presented here.

Methods

Patients and Samples

Tissue sections of biopsy material from patients with disseminated GCTs were obtained from the Indiana University Medical Center, University Hospital under an Indiana University Institutional Review Board approved protocol; IU Study No. 9908–47) as 4 per cent buffered formaldehyde fixed tissues embedded in paraffin blocks. These blocks were sectioned at three microns and fixed onto slides. The diagnosis was made from morphological examination of haematoxylin and eosin stained sections of biopsy material.

Immunohistochemistry (IHC)

Tissue sections were stained for Ape1/ref–1 expression using an anti-Ape1 monoclonal antibody, which has been extensively characterized [19–23] and is available commercially (Novus Biologicals, Littleton, CO). The staining process used was identical to that previously described [19–23]. The sections were analysed for the percent of cells that were Ape1 positive, nuclei percent positive, or cytoplasm percent positive, as well as nuclear intensity (+, ++ or +++) or cytoplasmic intensity. Also, stromal cells were scored for percent cells positive. This grading scheme has been previously used by us in a number of studies and is described in more detail in these studies [19–21, 23, 24].

Statistical Analyses

The Wilcox rank sum test with 5 per cent two-sided significance level was used to compare recurrent and non-recurrent patient groups. The mean follow-up is 6.4 years for front line therapy and 5.8 years for second line therapy.

Results and Discussion

In our early analysis, we partitioned the initial 94 cases for which outcome was available. The subdivision of GCTs by pathology is listed in Table 16.1. The only group for which there were adequate numbers of patients for analysis in both the disease-free and relapse groups at this time was the malignant teratoma (teratoma differentiated) group. With additional scoring, we will eventually have enough patients in the other groups to perform a similar comparison. Upon comparing disease-free patients with those with relapse, the best p-values were seen in the "percent cells positive for Ape1 in the cytoplasm" (Table 16.2). There was a trend toward significance in some of the other groups and clearly no significance when looking at the surrounding stromal cells. When the data for "percent cells positive in the cytoplasm" is plotted, there is a clear difference in the disease free versus relapse

Table 16.1: Initial Partitioning of Germ Cell Tumours by Pathology for Ape1 IHC

	Chorio	Embryonal	Seminoma	Yolk	Terat	Sarcoma	PNET	Non-GCT	Total
1st Line Chemo									
Yes	4	8	5	24	10	6	4	6	64
No	0	1	0	1	5	1	0	0	8
2nd Line Chemo									
Yes	4	7	3	21	8	6	4	3	56
No	0	1	2	0	5	1	0	0	9

Chorio = choriocarcinoma
Embryonal = embryonal carcinoma
YST = yolk sac tumour
Terat = teratoma
PNET = primitive neuroendocrine tumour

Table 16.2: Malignant Teratomas and Ape1/ref-1 Expression p-Values Comparing Disease-free vs. Relapse

	Ape1 % Cells Positive	Nuclei % Positive	Cytoplasm % Positive	Nuclear Intensity	Cytoplasm Intensity	Stroma % Cells Positive
1st Line Chemo						
p-value	0.1728	0.2944	0.0770	0.3515	0.2037	0.6601
2nd Line Chemo						
p-value	0.1573	0.3008	0.0594	0.5271	0.0591	0.8807

groups, both after front line therapy (Figure 16.5) and for those that went on to second line therapy (Figure 16.6).

Again, this is the first evaluation at this accumulating data set, which includes retrospective (67 per cent) and prospective cases (33 per cent). We will continue to evaluate the cases we have accumulated, now totaling over 150, and will also compare different sites of disease (mediastinal versus abdominal) and response to specific agents as well as other parameters.

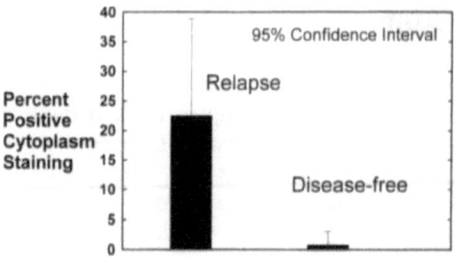

Figure 16.5: Ape1 IHC staining and response to front line therapy of malignant teratomas. The percentage of positive cytoplasmic staining Ape1 cells from relapsed or disease-free patients was plotted and statistical analysis was performed as described in Methods. There is a significant difference at the 95% confidence level of differences in cytoplasmic staining between these two populations.

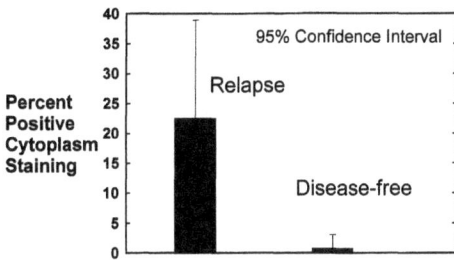

Figure 16.6: Ape1 IHC staining and response to second line therapy of malignant teratomas. The same analysis was performed as in Figure 5, but with patients who were treated with second line therapy.

Conclusion

We have established that Ape1 is elevated in both adult and paediatric GCTs, as previously reported [20, 22]. However, in our ongoing studies with Ape1 in GCT, it is increasingly clear that the level of Ape1 in the cytoplasm is elevated, particularly in those patients that relapse compared to those that remain disease-free. Cytoplasmic localization of Ape1 may be a marker for patients who may not be responsive to standard GCT treatments or act as a predictor of relapse with current therapeutic regimens, particularly for teratomas. The function of Ape1 in the cytoplasm is unknown a this time and is a focus of our continuing studies.

Acknowledgements

National Institutes of Health grants CA76643 (KAR, MRK), NS38506 (MRK), P01–CA75426 (MRK) and a P30 DK49218 Center Grant (MRK) supported this work. The Riley Memorial Association also supported it.

References

1. Friedberg EC, Walker GC, Siede W. *DNA Repair and Mutagenesis.* Washington, D. C.: ASM Press;1995
2. Demple B, Harrison L. Repair of oxidative damage to DNA: Enzymology and Biology. *Ann Rev Biochem* 1994;63:915–948
3. Loeb LA, Preston BD. Mutagenesis by apurinic/apyrimidinic sites. *Ann Rev Genet* 1986;20:201–230
4. Barzilay G, Walker LJ, Robson CN, Hickson ID. Site-directed mutagenesis of the human DNA repair enzyme HAP1: identification of residues important for AP endonuclease and RNase H activity. *Nucl Acids Res* 1995;23:1544–1550
5. Barzilay G, Mol CD, Robson CN, et al. Identification of critical active-site residues in the multifunctional human DNA repair enzyme HAP1. *Nat Struct Biol* 1995;2:561–568
6. Barzilay G, Hickson ID. Structure and function of apurinic/apyrimidinic endonucleases. *Bioessays* 1995;17:713–719
7. Wood RD. DNA repair in eukaryotes. *Annu Rev Biochem* 1996;65:135–167
8. Kingma PS, Osheroff N. Apurinic sites are position-specific topoisomerase II poisons. *J Biol Chem* 1997;272:1148–1155
9. Kingma PS, Osheroff N, Kingma PS, et al. Spontaneous DNA damage stimulates topoisomerase II–mediated DNA cleavage. *J Biol Chem* 1997;272:7488–7493
10. Ramotar D, Popoff SC, Gralla EB, Demple B. Cellular role of yeast Apn1 apurinic endonuclease/3'-diesterase: repair of oxidative and alkylation DNA damage and control of spontaneous mutation. *Mol Cell Biol* 1991;11:4537–44

11. Ramotar D. The apurinic-apyrimidinic endonuclease IV family of DNA repair enzymes. *Biochem Cell Biol* 1997;75:327
12. Suh D, Wilson DM, Povirk LF. 3'-Phosphodiesterase activity of human apurinic/apyrimidinic endonuclease at DNA double-strand break ends. *Nucl Acids Res* 1997;25:2495–2500
13. Mitra S, Hazra TK, Roy R, et al. Complexities of DNA base excision repair in mammalian cells. *Mol Cells* 1997;7:305–312
14. Doetsch PW, Cunningham RP. The enzymology of apurinic/apyrimidinic endonucleases. *Mutat Res* 1990;236:173–201
15. Evans AR, Limp-Foster M, Kelley MR. Going APE over ref-1. *Mutat Res* 2000;461:83–108
16. Ono Y, Furuta T, Ohmoto T, Akiyama K, Seki S. Stable expression in rat glioma cells of sense and antisense nucleic acids to a human multifunctional DNA repair enzyme, APEX nuclease. *Mutat Res* 1994;315:55–63
17. Walker LJ, Craig RB, Harris AL, Hickson ID. A role for the human DNA repair enzyme HAP1 in cellular protection against DNA damaging agents and hypoxic stress. *Nucl Acids Res* 1994;22:4884–4889
18. Herring CJ, West CM, Wilks DP, et al. Levels of the DNA repair enzyme human apurinic/apyrimidinic endonuclease (APE1, APEX, Ref-1) are associated with the intrinsic radiosensitivity of cervical cancers. *Br J Cancer* 1998;78:1128–1133
19. Thomson B, Tritt R, Davis M, Kelley MR. Histology-Specific Expression of a DNA Repair Protein in Pediatric Rhabdomyosarcomas. *Am J Pediatr Hematol Oncol* 2001;23:234–239
20. Robertson KA, Bullock +HA, Xu Y, et al. Altered expression of Ape1/ref-1 in germ cell tumours and overexpression in NT2 cells confers resistance to bleomycin and radiation. *Cancer Res* 2001;61:2220–2225
21. Kelley MR, Cheng L, Foster R, et al. Elevated and altered expression of the multifunctional DNA base excision repair and redox enzyme Ape1/ref-1 in prostate cancer. *Clin Cancer Res* 2001;7:824–830
22. Thomson BG, Tritt R, Davis M, Perlman EJ, Kelley MR. Apurinic/apyrimidinic endonuclease expression in pediatric yolk sac tumours. *Anticancer Res* 2000;20:4153–4157
23. Moore DH, Michael H, Tritt R, Parsons SH, Kelley MR. Alterations in the expression of the DNA repair/redox enzyme APE/ref-1 in epithelial ovarian cancers. *Clin Cancer Res* 2000;6:602–609
24. Xu Y, Moore DH, Broshears J, Liu LF, Wilson TM, Kelley MR. The apurinic/apyrimidinic endonuclease (APE/ref-1) DNA repair enzyme is elevated in premalignant and malignant cervical cancer. *Anticancer Res* 1997;17:3713–3719
25. Xanthoudakis S, Miao G, Wang F, Pan YC, Curran T. Redox activation of Fos-Jun DNA binding activity is mediated by a DNA repair enzyme. *EMBO J* 1992;11:3323–3335
26. Rothwell DG, Barzilay G, Gorman M, Morera S, Freemont P, Hickson ID. The structure and functions of the HAP1/Ref-1 protein. *Oncol Res* 1997;9:275–280
27. Wilson DM, 3rd, Takeshita M, Demple B. Abasic site binding by the human apurinic endonuclease, Ape, and determination of the DNA contact sites. *Nucleic Acids Res* 1997;25:933–939
28. Erzberger JP, Barsky D, Scharer OD, Colvin ME, Wilson DM, III. Elements in abasic site recognition by the major human and Escherichia coli apurinic/apyrimidinic endonucleases. *Nucl Acid Res* 1998;26:2771–2778

17. Translational Implications of Ape1 in Germ Cell Tumours: Ape1 as a Therapeutic Target

M.R. Kelley[1,2], M. Luo[1], Y. Xu[1], E. Zimmerman[1], D.M. Wilson III[3], K.A. Robertson[1]

1. Department of Pediatrics, Section of Hematology/Oncology, Herman B Wells Center for Pediatric Research, 2. Department of Biochemistry and Molecular Biology, Indiana University School of Medicine, 702 Barnhill Dr., Indianapolis, IN 46077, 3. Lawrence Livermore National Lab, Biology & Biotechnology Research Program, POB 808, L-452, 7000 East Avenue, Livermore, CA 94551, United States of America

Summary

The second enzyme in the DNA base excision repair (BER) pathway, Ape1, hydrolyzes the phosphodiester backbone immediately 5' to an apurinic site (AP) site. AP sites are generated from spontaneous and chemically initiated hydrolysis, ionizing radiation, UV irradiation, oxidative stress, oxidizing agents, and removal of altered (such as alkylated) bases by DNA glycosylases. In the latter case, this incision generates a normal 3'-hydroxyl group and an abasic deoxyribose-5-phosphate, which is processed by subsequent enzymes of the BER pathway. AP sites are the most common form of DNA damage with some 20–50,000 sites produced in every cell each day under normal physiological conditions. The persistence of AP sites in DNA results in a block to DNA replication, cytotoxic mutations, and genetic instability. However, Ape1 is a multifunctional protein that is not only responsible for repair of AP sites, but also functions as a redox factor maintaining transcription factors in an active reduced state. Ape1 has been shown to stimulate the DNA binding activity of numerous transcription factors that are involved in cancer promotion and progression such as Fos, Jun, NFkB, PAX, HIF–1a, HLF, p53 and others in an ever expanding list. Given the multiple roles of Ape1, both as a DNA repair enzyme and as a major redox-regulating factor, Ape1 is clearly a good target for therapeutic inhibition. We will discuss our initial incursion into three areas that Ape1 could be used as either a target or as a gene therapy approach to tumour cell therapeutics. These include, but are not limited to; 1) inhibition of Ape1 DNA repair activity via the small molecule agent lucanthone, 2) dominant-negative Ape1 mutants that effectively bind to AP sites, but do not cleave the phosphodiester backbone and, 3) cells with elevated levels of Ape1 appear to respond to retinoic acid (RA) resulting in an increased level of cell death compared to those cells with lower amounts of Ape1. These studies are all part of an ongoing series of experiments surrounding the hypothesis that unbalancing DNA repair pathways, particularly BER, can be used in a clinical setting.

Introduction

As previously discussed in an earlier chapter, the DNA Base Excision Repair (BER) pathway is responsible for the repair of alkylation and oxidative DNA damage and its action results in protection against the deleterious effects of endogenous and exogenous agents encountered on a daily basis. In this chapter, we will discuss our rationale for using Ape1 as a therapeutic target, not only for germ cell tumours (GCT), but also for tumour cells in general.

Given its multiple roles, both as a DNA repair enzyme and as a major redox-regulating factor, Ape1 is clearly a good target for inhibition. For example, previous studies, and work performed in our laboratories, have demonstrated that decreased levels of Ape1 lead to the sensitization of cells to alkylating agents, oxidative DNA damaging agents and ionizing radiation (IR) [1–3]. These studies have been conducted in a variety of cell lines such as human lung carcinoma, HeLa and rat glioma cells [1–3]. When transfected with antisense Ape1, these cell lines became hypersensitive to killing by methyl methanesulfonate (MMS), H_2O_2, menadione and paraquat [1], as well as ionizing radiation [2, 3]. However, it is not yet known whether the enhanced sensitivity of cells to these agents results from a loss of the DNA repair function of Ape1 or its redox activity.

We will discuss our initial forays into three areas where Ape1 could be used as either a target or as a gene therapy approach to tumour cell therapeutics. These include, but are not limited to; 1) inhibition of Ape1 DNA repair activity via the small molecule agent lucanthone, 2) dominant-negative Ape1 mutants that effectively bind to AP sites, but do not cleave the phosphodiester backbone and 3) cells with elevated

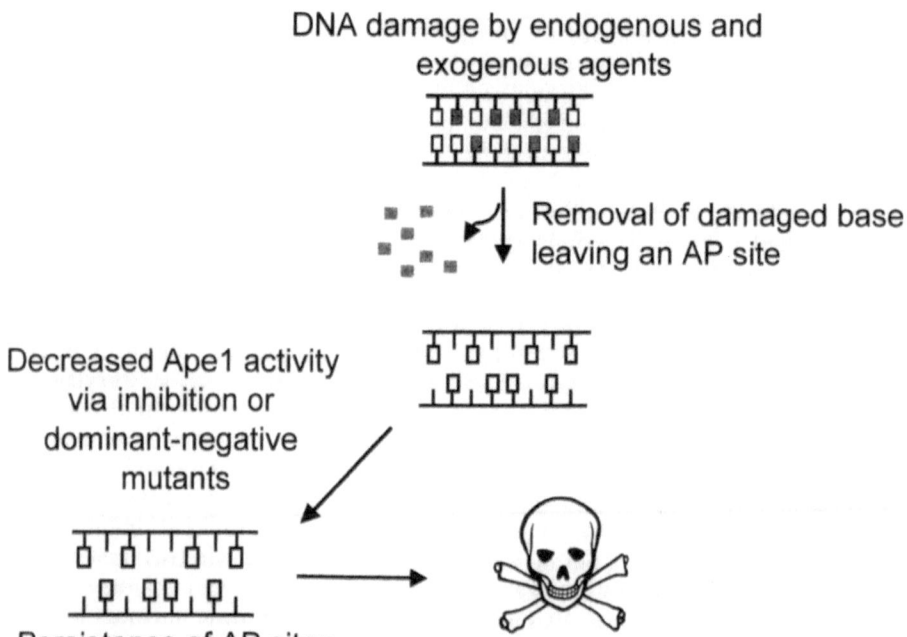

Figure 17.1: Outcomes of imbalanced DNA repair.

levels of Ape1 appear to respond to retinoic acid (RA) resulting in an increased level of cell death compared to those cells with lower amounts of Ape1. This latter finding may be of great interest in those tumours with elevated levels of Ape1 and are not currently treated with RA. These include cancers such as GCT, ovarian, cervical and prostate cancer, and sarcomas [4–9]. Other approaches that we are pursuing but are not discussed here include the use of antisense Ape1 morpholinos, RNA interference [10, 11] and direct administration of dominant-negative Ape1 mutant protein using transactivating transduction (TAT) fusion proteins [12].

These studies are all part of a vigorous series of experiments surrounding the hypothesis that unbalancing DNA repair pathways, particularly BER, can be used in a clinical setting. A cartoon of how the unbalancing of the BER pathway is predicted to mechanistically perform is shown in Figure 17.1.

Methods

Cell Lines and Reagents

Chemicals and enzymes were purchased from Fisher Scientific (Pittsburgh, PA), Sigma (St. Louis, MO), and New England Biolabs (Beverly, MA). The MDA-MB231 cell line was kindly provided by Dr. Martin Smith (Department of Microbiology, Indiana University School of Medicine). MDA-MB231 cells were maintained in RPMI media (GibcoBRL Life Technologies, Gaithersburg, MD), supplemented with 10 per cent Fetal Bovine Serum (Hyclone Laboratories, Logan, UT) and 1 per cent Penicillin/Streptomycin (GibcoBRL Life Technologies, Gaithersburg, MD) in 5 per cent CO_2 at 37°C. HL60 myeloid leukemia cells were cultured as previously described [13]. All-trans retinoic acid (Sigma) stock solutions were made up fresh under amber light the day of use as a 4 mM solution in ethanol and diluted into cultures to the desired concentration. Hl–60 cells were induced to differentiate down the granulocytic pathway with retinoic acid (10^{-5} M) and stained with propidium iodide. The samples were analyzed by flow cytometry. Hey cells were grown as previously described [6]. The wild-type and mutant Ape1 constructs will be described elsewhere (manuscript in preparation). The double mutant, ED, consisted of a change of the glutamic amino acid (E) at position 96 to a glutamine (Q) and the aspartic amino acid (D) at 210 to asparagines (N). This mutant Ape1 (ED) has binding activity equivalent to wild-type Ape1, but no endonuclease activity (DMW, personal communication). HaCaT cells were obtained from Dr. Jeff Travers (Dept of Dermatology, IU School of Medicine) and were grown as described [14].

The pSF91-RE bicistronic retroviral vector has been previously used by us [15] and contains the IRES-EGFP for co-expression of proteins. Viral supernatant was produced from phoenix-AMPHO cells and phoenix-ECO cells by transfection. Viral supernatants from phoenix-AMPHO were used to infect the HaCaT or Hey cells, and infected cells were analyzed for GFP expression using a FACSCalibur (Becton Dickinson, Mountain View, CA) [15].

Ape1 Endonuclease Repair Activity Assay

The Ape1 repair assay was performed as has previously been described using our recently published alteration to the technique [16]. Oligonucleotides for measurement of Ape1 activity were custom synthesized by The Midland Certified Reagent Co. (Midland,

TX) and contained a tetrahydrofuran (THF) lesion, with a 5'-hexachloro-fluorescein phosphoramidite (HEX) molecule. The fluorometric HEX molecule was incorporated into the 5'-end of the lesioned strand during synthesis [16]. The 26 bp oligonucleotide substrate containing a single THF residue in the middle yielded a HEX-labeled 13mer fragment upon endonuclease activity of Ape1. Ape1 activity was measured by incubating 0.2 pmol HEX-labeled (2 pmol/ml) excess oligo substrate with recombinant Ape1 protein in a total volume of 20 µl of assay buffer (50 mM HEPES, 50 mM KCl, 10 mM MgCl$_2$, 1 per cent BSA, 0.05 per cent Triton X–100, pH 7.5) at 37°C for 15 min. [16]. Reactions were terminated by adding formamide loading buffer (10 µl), without dye to each sample and heating each sample at 95°C for 5 min to denature the oligos. Electrophoresis was carried out as previously described [16]. Fluorometric HEX-labeled oligonucleotides were detected and quantitated using the Hitachi FMBio II Fluorescence Imaging System (Hitachi Genetic Systems, South San Francisco, CA). The HEX fluorophore is excited by a solid-state laser at 532 nm (Perkin-Elmer) and emits a fluorescent light signal at 560 nm, which is then isolated using a 585 nm filter. Fluorescence intensity units were quantitated using FMBio software (Hitachi Genetic Systems).

For experiments analysing the inhibiting effect of lucanthone on Ape1, the Ape1 protein was first incubated with lucanthone for 30 or 60 minutes followed by addition of the HEX-oligonucleotide substrate. The reaction was allowed to proceed for 10 minutes before termination with loading dye.

Statistical Analyses

P values for the cell survival data was generated using the one-way Analysis of variance (ANOVA) test with Sigma Stat software (Jandel Scientific, Erkrath, Germany).

Results and Discussion

A previous report had claimed that Ape1 endonuclease (repair) activity could be inhibited by lucanthone, a small molecule that has been reported to be a radiosensitizer and stimulator of topoisomerase II activity [17–19]. However, these studies were not performed with the more sensitive oligonucleotide AP endonuclease activity assay, but rather by the "nicked plasmid" method [17]. Therefore, we repeated these studies and demonstrated that Ape1 is indeed inhibited by lucanthone, regardless of whether Ape1 was incubated with lucanthone for 30 or 60 minutes (Figure 17.2). With these results and given the role of Ape1 in repairing damage due to alkylating agents, we predicted that lucanthone, by inhibiting Ape1, should increase the sensitivity of tumour cell lines, in this case a breast cancer cell line MDA-MB231, to alkylating agents. As shown in Figure 17.3, the addition of 4 µM lucanthone enhances the killing effect of the simple alkylating agent MMS. While these results do not conclusively prove that the effect of lucanthone is due to the inhibition of Ape1 repair activity, the results do support that hypothesis. Additional work that is not presented demonstrated that lucanthone is specific for Ape1 repair function and increases the sensitivity of numerous cell lines to alkylating agents, including more relevant clinical alkylating agents (Luo and Kelley, manuscript in preparation). Therefore, lucanthone, or other small molecule inhibitors of Ape1, are worthy of consideration and research into more effective means of therapeutic intervention with Ape1 as a target.

Another approach using gene therapy and dominant-negative mutants of Ape1 is being tested in ovarian and GCT cell lines. Using retroviral vectors containing either

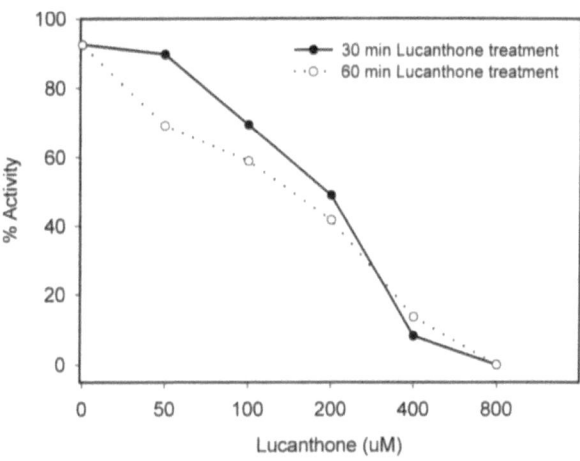

Figure 17.2: Inhibition of Ape 1 endonuclease activity by lucanthone: results of three independent experiments.

the wild-type or double Ape1 mutant (ED] (Figure 17.4], we infected the ovarian cancer cell line, Hey, and measured cell survival (Figure 17.5]. We determined that the wild-type infected cells did not show any decrease in cell survival. However, the Hey cells transfected with the Ape1-ED mutant, which has the binding activity of Ape1 but no endonuclease activity, were all dead by 10 days following infection (Figure 17.5]. This killing effect by the Ape1-ED mutant is observed without the addition of any exogenous agents. We conclude from these initial data that there is sufficient spontaneous depurination occurring in growing cells to cause cell death in the absence of DNA repair and that the ED mutant binds, in a dominant-negative fashion, to the existing AP sites and prevents the endogenous Ape1 entry to the AP site, thereby preventing the completion of the BER pathway. We are repeating these

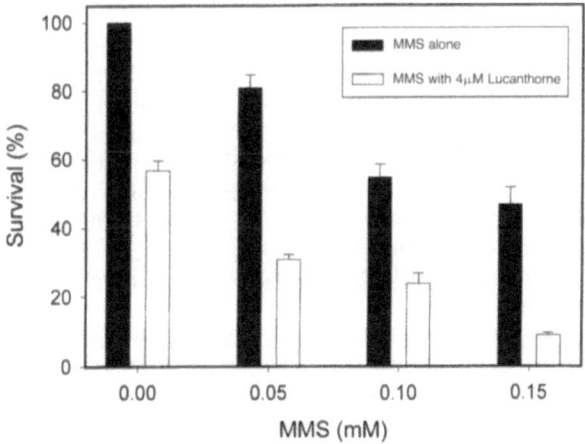

Figure 17.3: Effect of lucanthone on breast cancer cells treated with the alkylating agent MMS: results of three independent experiments show highly significant differences at all doses p ≤ 0.01).

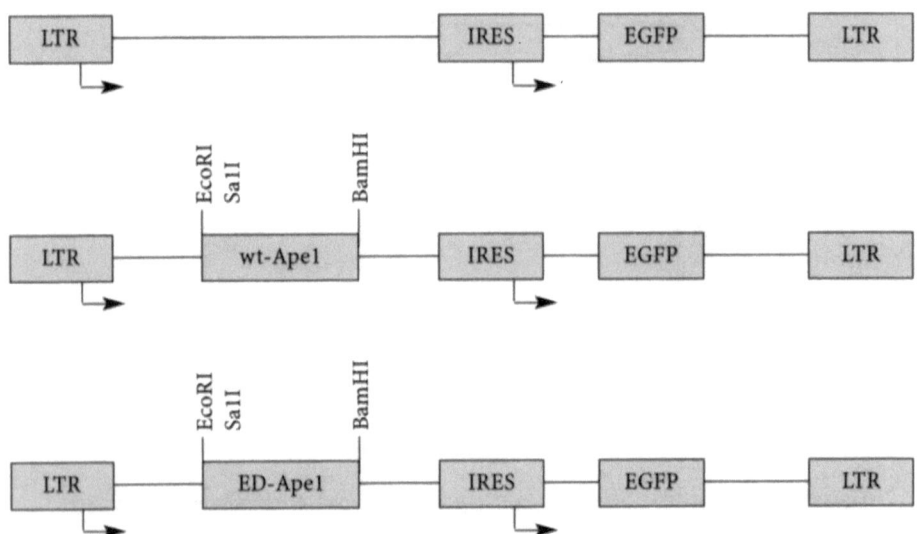

Figure 17.4: pSF91.1 retroviral vector and constructs of wild-type (wt) Ape1 and double Ape1 mutant (ED-Ape1). This vector contains an IRES-EGFP region such that wt-Ape1 or ED-Ape1 can be co-expressed with the EGFP protein to allow flow cytometry sorting of infected cells prior to experiments.

studies with both inducible and retroviral vector systems, in both ovarian and GCT cell lines.

The data resulting from these first two approaches centers on either inhibiting Ape1 repair activity or expressing dominant-negative repair Ape1 mutants in tumour cells. The third method takes advantage of the redox function of Ape1 and the elevated levels of Ape1 found in a variety of tumour cells, including GCT. In this series of experiments, we overexpressed Ape1 in the myeloid leukemia cell line HL60 and then challenged the cells with either vehicle alone (EtOH] or RA. As shown in Table 17.1, 67 per cent or 87 per cent of cells overexpressing Ape1 were undergoing apoptosis as determined by the PI staining and flow cytometry method, whereas 31 per cent of HL60 cells containing the vector backbone and 22 per cent of those with no vector were undergoing apoptosis (Table 17.1). This represents a 2–4 fold increase in apoptosis in the Ape1 overexpressing cells. This was confirmed by morphological examination of these cells with 8.5 per cent and 12.5 per cent of the HL60 cells containing either the vector alone or no vector undergoing apoptosis, while the cells overexpressing Ape1 showed apoptosis levels of 24 and 40 per cent (Table 17.1). Again, a 2–5 fold increase in apoptosis levels. Clearly, the RA cytotoxic effect was enhanced in the cells overexpressing Ape1.

We sought to confirm the RA effect and to determine whether it was a general phenomenon, and to establish whether the effect of Ape1 was related to its redox domain and not to its repair domain. We therefore infected a human keratinocyte cell line, HaCaT, with the pSF91.1 retroviral vector containing either the wild-type or C65A Ape1 mutant. This mutant has a site-directed change from the cysteine at position 65 to an alanine. The cysteine at position 65 has been implicated in the redox activity of the Ape1 protein, forming a disulphide bridge with cysteine at position 93

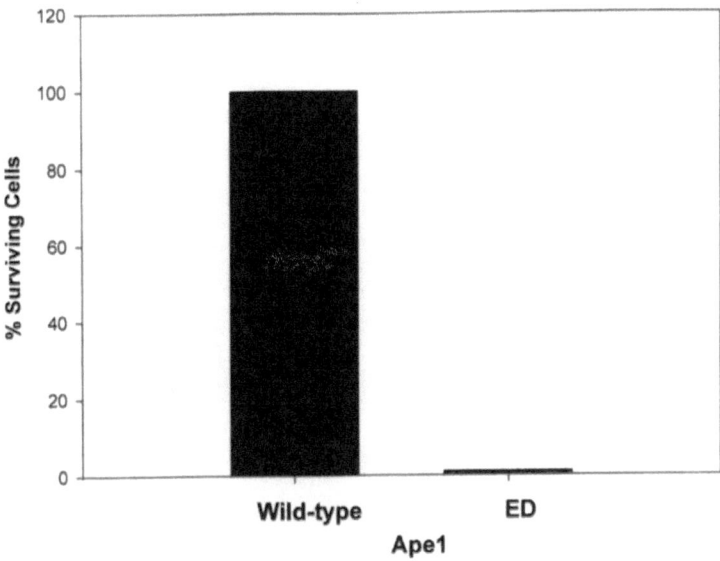

Figure 17.5: Effects of expressing either wt-Ape1 or ED-Ape1 in ovarian cancer cells. Cell survival analyzed as in Figure 17.3.

when oxidized [20–22]. If the enhanced cytotoxic effect of RA in cells overexpressing Ape1 was due to the ability of Ape1 to increase the reduction state of the RA receptor, we predicted that there would be no increase in the cytotoxicity of RA in cells infected with the C65A Ape1 mutant. HaCaT cells were infected with the pSF91.1 vector, or vector containing either the wild-type Ape1 or C65A mutant, and were sorted for green fluorescent protein (GFP) expression since GFP is co-expressed in this vector. The cells were then plated and treated with increasing doses of RA. After three weeks, the cells were analyzed for colony formation and cell survival. We observed an increase in the killing of the HaCaT cells with the wild-type Ape1 retrovirus compared to the vector control (Figure 17.6), which was similar to the results we observed with the HL60 cell line. In addition however, this effect was not seen in the HaCaT cells carrying the C65A Ape1 mutant (Figure 17.6). This latter observation allows us to begin to determine the mechanism by which Ape1 enhances the RA cytotoxic effect and supports our hypothesis that Ape1 is involved in the redox regulation of the RA receptor. Clearly more work needs to be done to confirm these

Table 17.1: Overexpression of Ape1 augments retinoic acid induced apoptosis in HL-60 cells.

Cell Type	Day 5 Apoptosis-Propidium Iodide	Day 5 Apoptosis-Morphology
HL-60 + EtOH	0.7%	1%
HL-60 + RA	22%	12.5%
HL-60-LXSN + RA (vector control)	31%	8.5%
HL-60-HA-Ape1 #1 + RA	67%	24%
HL-60-HA-APE#6 + RA	87%	40%

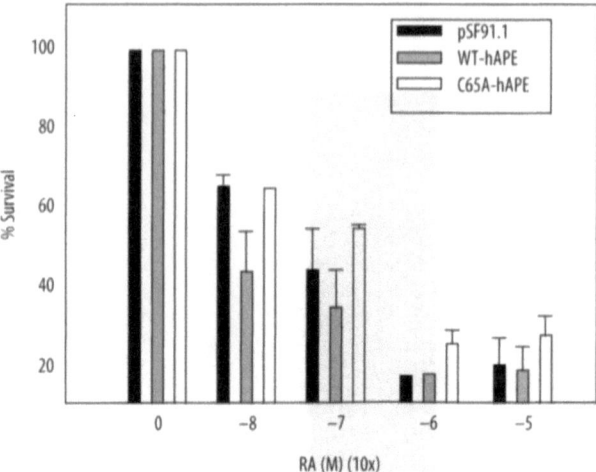

Figure 17.6: Human keratinocyte HaCaT cells overexpressing wt-Ape1 or the redox Ape1 mutant C65A, treated with RA at varying doses for three weeks (experiments in triplicate, repeated twice). There was a significant difference between cells containing the pSF91.1 vector and those overexpressing Ape1 ($p < 0.05$) but not the C65A redox Ape1 mutant.

initial results, but our findings were consistent in two completely different cell lines, and the C65A Ape1 mutant analysis supports our hypothesis that the RA receptor (RAR) functions under redox control and that Ape1 plays a role in this post-translational regulation. It should also be noted that the RA effect was lost at the higher doses of RA, presumably due to either another mechanism or the overwhelming of the cells with such high RA doses.

Conclusions

The data presented in this chapter describe our early experiments aimed at manipulating and exploiting the expression of Ape1 in tumour cells in order to facilitate the therapeutic effectiveness of chemotherapeutic, IR or other agents such as RA. We postulate that Ape1 is an important and valid target given that previous studies have shown that decreased Ape1 levels lead to increased sensitivity to alkylators, oxidizing DNA damaging agents and IR. Furthermore, Ape1 has at least two domains, one of which is involved in its redox function, while the other is the DNA repair domain. Recent reports have indicated another role for Ape1 in the removal of beta-1-dioxolane-cytidine (l-OddC, BCH–4556, Troxacitabine), which is an unnatural stereochemical nucleoside [23]. The inhibition of Ape1 and its impact on this new function is also currently under investigation. Inhibitors of the DNA repair activity of Ape1, such as lucanthone, should sensitize tumour cells to chemotherapeutic agents as well as IR. In contrast, the inhibition of the redox function of Ape1 could cause a decrease in the reduction state of transcription factors, such as Fos, Jun, p53, HIF–1a, NFkB. If this results in decreased DNA binding of these factors to their target DNA, there could be a decrease in cellular proliferation as well as other growth deterrent effects. A similar effect may be occurring through the interaction of Ape1 with the RAR. Additionally, inhibitors to both Ape1 redox and repair functions may lead to decreased tumour proliferation and growth and increased sensitivity to chemotherapeutic and IR treatments. Finally, the preliminary finding that Ape1 may modulate the effect of RA, possibly through redox modification of the RA receptor, opens the door for further studies into exploiting the over- or elevated expression of Ape1 in certain tumour cells types, such as GCT, to induce enhanced apoptosis using RA in combination with other current therapies.

Acknowledgements

This work was supported by National Institutes of Health grants CA76643 (KAR, MRK), NS38506 (MRK), P01-CA75426 (MRK) and a P30 DK49218 Center Grant (MRK). It was also supported by the Riley Memorial Association.

References

1. Walker LJ, Craig RB, Harris AL, Hickson ID. A role for the human DNA repair enzyme HAP1 in cellular protection against DNA damaging agents and hypoxic stress. Nucl Acids Res 1994;22:4884–4889
2. Chen DS, Olkowski ZL. Biological responses of human apurinic endonuclease to radiation-induced DNA damage. Ann N Y Acad Sci 1994;726:306–308
3. Ono Y, Furuta T, Ohmoto T, Akiyama K, Seki S. Stable expression in rat glioma cells of sense and antisense nucleic acids to a human multifunctional DNA repair enzyme, APEX nuclease. Mutat Res 1994;315(1):55–63
4. Kelley MR, Xu Y, Tritt R, Robertson KA. The multifunctional DNA base excision repair and redox protein, AP endonuclease (APE/ref-1), and its role in germ cell tumors. In: W.G. Jones I. Appleyard, P. Harnden, J.K. Joffe, editor. Germ Cell Tumors IV. London, UK: John Libbey & Co.; 1998. p. 81–86
5. Xu Y, Moore DH, Broshears J, Liu LF, Wilson TM, Kelley MR. The apurinic/apyrimidinic endonuclease (APE/ref-1) DNA repair enzyme is elevated in premalignant and malignant cervical cancer. Anticancer Res 1997;17:3713–3719
6. Moore DH, Michael H, Tritt R, Parsons SH, Kelley MR. Alterations in the expression of the DNA repair/redox enzyme APE/ref-1 in epithelial ovarian cancers. Clin Cancer Res 2000;6:602–609
7. Thomson BG, Tritt R, Davis M, Perlman EJ, Kelley MR. Apurinic/apyrimidinic endonuclease expression in pediatric yolk sac tumors. Anticancer Res 2000;20:4153–4157
8. Kelley MR, Cheng L, Foster R, et al. Elevated and altered expression of the multifunctional DNA base excision repair and redox enzyme Ape1/ref-1 in prostate cancer. Clin Cancer Res 2001;7:824–830
9. Robertson KA, Bullock HA, Xu Y, et al. Altered expression of Ape1/ref-1 in germ cell tumors and overexpression in NT2 cells confers resistance to bleomycin and radiation. Cancer Res 2001;61(5):2220–2225
10. Sharp PA. RNA interference – 2001. Genes Dev 2001;15:485–490
11. Zamore PD. RNA interference: listening to the sound of silence. Nat Struct Biol 2001;8:746–750
12. Snyder EL, Dowdy SF. Protein/peptide transduction domains: potential to deliver large DNA molecules into cells. Curr Opin Mol Ther 2001;3:147–152
13. Robertson KA, Hill DP, Xu Y, et al. Downregulation of AP endonuclease expression is associated with the induction of apoptosis in differentiating myeloid leukemia cells. Cell Growth Different 1997;8:443–449
14. Chen WC, Sass JO, Seltmann H, Nau H, Orfanos CE, Zouboulis CC. Biological effects and metabolism of 9-cis-retinoic acid and its metabolite 9,13-di-cis-retinoic acid in HaCaT keratinocytes in vitro: comparison with all-trans-retinoic acid. Arch Dermatol Res 2000;292:612–620
15. Kobune M, Xu Y, Baum C, Kelley MR, Williams DA. Retrovirus-mediated expression of the base excision repair proteins, formamidopyrimidine DNA glycosylase or human oxoguanine DNA glycosylase, protects hematopoietic cells from N,N',N''-triethylenethiophosphoramide (thioTEPA)-induced toxicity in vitro and in vivo. Cancer Res 2001;61:5116–5125
16. Kreklau EL, Limp-Foster M, Liu N, Xu Y, Kelley MR, Erickson LC. A novel fluorometric oligonucleotide assay to measure O(6)-methylguanine DNA methyltransferase, methylpurine DNA glycosylase, 8-oxoguanine DNA glycosylase and abasic endonuclease activities: DNA repair status in human breast carcinoma cells overexpressing methylpurine DNA glycosylase. Nucleic Acids Res 2001;29:2558–66

17. Del Rowe JD, Bello J, Mitnick R, et al. Accelerated regression of brain metastases in patients receiving whole brain radiation and the topoisomerase II inhibitor, lucanthone. Int J Radiat Oncol Biol Phys 1999;43:89–93
18. Dassonneville L, Bailly C. Stimulation of topoisomerase II-mediated DNA cleavage by an indazole analogue of lucanthone. Biochem Pharmacol 1999;58:1307–1312
19. Bases RE, Mendez F. Topoisomerase inhibition by lucanthone, an adjuvant in radiation therapy. Int J Radiat Oncol Biol Phys 1997;37:1133–1137
20. Barzilay G, Hickson ID. Structure and function of apurinic/apyrimidinic endonucleases. Bioessays 1995;17:713–719
21. Barzilay G, Mol CD, Robson CN, et al. Identification of critical active-site residues in the multifunctional human DNA repair enzyme HAP1. Nat Struct Biol 1995;2:561–568
22. Rothwell DG, Barzilay G, Gorman M, Morera S, Freemont P, Hickson ID. The structure and functions of the HAP1/Ref-1 protein. Oncol Res 1997;9:275–280
23. Chou KM, Kukhanova M, Cheng YC. A novel action of human apurinic/apyrimidinic endonuclease: excision of L-configuration deoxyribonucleoside analogs from the 3' termini of DNA. J Biol Chem 2000;275:31009–31015

18. Current Clinical Trials in Germ Cell Tumours in the United States

Craig R. Nichols

Oregon Health & Science University, 3181 SW Sam Jackson, Park Road, OP28, Portland, OR 97201, USA

Introduction

The astonishing success of systemic chemotherapy in patients with disseminated germ cell tumours is largely a result of logical application of clinical trial principles and foresight in asking and answering clinically meaningful questions.

Since the 1970s, large institutional pilot trials have lead to randomized clinical trials that have refined therapy for patients with disseminated germ cell tumours. Over the last twenty years the largest advances have been in defining lower limits of chemotherapy dose and duration in good risk disease and finding better tolerated therapies for advanced disease. The success of therapy in disseminated disease has lead to the application of systemic chemotherapy in localized disease and as a surgical adjuvant.

An additional key to successful management of germ cell tumours has been successful integration of surgery with chemotherapy. As such, careful anatomical studies review of patterns of relapse and prognostic variables in early stage disease has lead to more refined surgery that yields very few local failures and has markedly diminished the morbid consequences of surgery such as infertility, vascular injury and prolonged recovery. Herein, we will review current clinical trials in both these arenas as well as planned clinical trials and potential future directions in clinical and scientific investigations of disseminated germ cell tumours.

Clinical Trials in Good Risk Disseminated Disease

In the United States there are currently no therapeutic trials in good risk disseminated disease nor are any planned. The prevailing opinion is that the near uniform success of brief chemotherapy (3 cycles of BEP or 4 cycles of EP) makes any therapeutic advance in good risk disease difficult to detect without extremely large clinical trials. The current consequences of such chemotherapy appear minimal as the effects are largely short term and manageable.

Such patients certainly are eligible for clinical trials looking at issues of survivorship, health services research, resource utilization and biological studies. It is reasonable to consider careful biological and molecular analysis of the rare failures of systemic chemotherapy in this subset to identify molecular markers of poor outcomes. Such studies are planned, but currently not available.

Intermediate and Poor Risk Germ Cell Tumours

The intergroup trial of PVB versus BEP reported in 1987 by Williams and colleagues was the first randomized trial to show both therapeutic advances and toxicity reductions in poor risk disease[1]. Unfortunately, this is also the last trial that has shown a therapeutic advance in poor risk disease. Subsequent trials were appropriately focused on improving therapeutic outcome in this group of patients accepting enhanced toxicities in an effort to effect cure in these biologically aggressive settings. Unfortunately, both in the US and Europe, no randomized trials shown superiority to 4 cycles of BEP [2–6]. The current US intergroup effort for intermediate and poor risk germ cell tumours compares randomly standard therapy with 4 cycles of BEP versus 2 cycles of BEP followed by two high dose cycles with carboplatin, etoposide and cyclophosphamide. To date, 183 of the approximately 280 patients required for this study have been accrued. Preliminary reports show 5 early deaths in each arm, almost all deaths with the first cycle of conventional BEP. A formal interim analysis has been conducted and the trial continues. The projected completion date is late 2002. The results of this trial are eagerly awaited. Subsequent trials will likely require either new biological understanding or new therapeutic compounds to justify the effort and expense of a large intergroup effort in this relatively rare subset of germ cell tumours.

Early Stage Disease

The current investigative effort in early stage disease is concentrating on improving on predictors of outcome in order to select patients for a lesser therapy after orchiectomy and also identify patients at high risk of dissemination. The current Eastern Cooperative Oncology Group trial seeks to validate a predictive model of outcome for patients with early stage non-seminomatous germ cell tumours. In the original Indiana model, patients underwent careful histopathological and immunohistochemical assessment of the primary testis tumour along with quantitative radiological assessment in an attempt to identify patients with very low risk of dissemination of clinical stage A non-seminoma [7]. In the initial Indiana study, a very significant subset (40 per cent) of patients was identified with a very low chance of recurrence after orchiectomy (5 per cent); a group for which surveillance and perhaps even surveillance at less intense intervals would be appropriate. If these results are confirmed in a multicentre study, a significant fraction of patients with early stage non-seminoma could benefit in terms of reduction of morbidity (e.g. retroperitoneal lymph node dissection) and minimize the burden of close surveillance. This trial requires 315 clinical stage A patients and will provide a 90 per cent power to detect a hazard ratio of 2.0 in the multifactorial model.

Biological Studies in Disseminated Disease

Shipp and colleagues presented a landmark study at plenary session of The American Society of Hematology in which they used gene expression to identify subsets of poor risk patients amongst groups of clinically homogenous presentations of diffuse large cell lymphoma. Investigators have begun to extend this concept to other diseases and Mazumder and colleagues at Memorial Sloan Kettering have begun to use biological end points to predict outcome of disseminated germ cell tumours. While the gene expression analysis is still pending, these results are eagerly awaited and will hopefully set the stage for more rational prognostic systems based on molecular and genetic analysis in the near future.

Salvage Therapies

The investigative study of salvage study of therapy for germ cell tumours in the United States has largely consisted of serial phase II trials conducted at single institutions. The current standard of therapy is VIP with or without stem cell transplantation [8]. Several investigative efforts are underway to identify new combinations of active single agents. For patients with good risk recurrent germ cell tumours, e.g. testis primary, cisplatin sensitive and prior favorable response, the investigators at Memorial Sloan Kettering are exploring the use of paclitaxil, ifosfamide and cisplatin. For those patients with poor risk recurrence, Memorial is using paclitaxil, ifosfamide induction followed by carboplatin, etoposide plus stem cell transplantation (carboplatin AUC = 24). In patients with multiply recurrent germ cell tumours, Oregon Health & Science University and SWOG are exploring the use of arsenic trioxide. In the same category of patients Memorial Sloan Kettering is looking at Temozolomide. The results of all of these phase II trials are pending.

There is an effort at molecularly directed therapies as well. STI-571 is being investigated in germ cell tumour patients who are C-KIT positive. This trial is being spearheaded by Indiana University. Oregon Health and Sciences University, The National Cancer Institute, Memorial Sloan Kettering and CALGB are using STI-571 in C-kit positive seminomas. This particular trial is based on prior work from Oregon that demonstrated that C-KIT mutations in human tumours are spread across several different exons. In each case the reading frame is maintained and results in mutant isoforms that show evidence of constitutive activation. The successful use of enzyme inhibitors in gastrointestinal stromal tumours stems from enzyme phosphorylation (activation) that can be demonstrated in tumour extracts [9]. This supports the hypothesis that altered signaling through KIT pathway supports the development of these tumours. Previously Tian et al demonstrated that 2/23 C-KIT mutations in patients with seminoma had alterations in exon 17, no mutations were demonstrated in 10 non-seminomas [10]. However, the Tian study was limited to exons 11 and 17. Michael Heinrich and Chris Corless along with other colleagues at Oregon Health & Science University have repeated this effort with more modern techniques and demonstrated 7/35 (20 per cent) mutations in exon 17 including novel mutations. Screening for mutations in exon 8, 9, 10, 11 and 13 continues. The finding of a modest level of potentially activating mutations in seminomas raises the prospect of effective therapies with STI-571. This trial will be coordinated across a number of cooperative groups in the US.

Conclusions

The progress of clinical trials in germ cell tumours has lead to extremely effective therapy for good risk disseminated disease and lowered the toxicity in patients with poor risk disseminated disease. We are however at a crossroads in terms of clinical trials and clinical advancement in patients with germ cell tumours. The effort to increase biological understanding and molecularly driven approaches is certainly appropriate. It is unlikely that additional combinations of existing nonspecific antineoplastics will result in significant advances in germ cell tumours and further breakthroughs await improved biological predictors and development in investigations of molecular targets.

References

1. Williams SD, Birch R, Einhorn LH et al., Treatment of Disseminated Germ-Cell Tumors with Cisplatin, Bleomycin and either Vinblastine or Etoposide. *N Engl J Med* 1987;316:1435–40
2. Nichols Cr, Williams S, Loehrer P et al., Randomized study of cisplatin dose intensity in advanced germ cell tumors: A Southeastern Cancer Study Group and Southwest Oncology Group protocol. *J Clin Oncol* 1991;9:1163–1172
3. Droz, J., et al., Preliminary results of a randomized trial comparing bleomycin, etoposide, cisplatin(BEP) and cyclophosphamide, doxorubicin, cisplatin/vinblastine.bleomycin (CISCA/VB for patients(Pts) with intermediate and poor risk metastatic nonseminomatous germ cell tumors (NSGCT). *Proc Am Soc Clin Oncol* 2001;20: 173a
4. Droz J, Pico J et al., No evidence of a benefit of early intensified chemotherapy (HDCT) with autologous bone marrow transplantation (ABMT) in first line treatment of poor risk non seminomatous germ cell tumors. *Proc Am Soc Clin Oncol* 1992;11: 197
5. Nichols CR, Catalano PJ, Crawford ED, Vogelzang NJ, Einhorn LH, Loehrer PJ. Randomized Comparison of Cisplatin and Etoposide and Either Bleomycin of Ifosfamide in Treatment of Advanced Disseminated Germ Cell Tumors: An Eastern Cooperative Oncology Group, Southwest Oncology Group, and Cancer and Leukemia Group B Study. *J Clin Oncol* 1998;16:1287–1293
6. Kaye SB, Mead GM, Cullen M et al., Intensive-induction sequential chemotherapy with BOP/VIP-B compared with treatment with BEP/EP for poor prognosis metastatic nonseminomatous germ cell tumor: a randomized Medical Research Council/European Organization for Research and Treatment of Cancer study. *J Clin Oncol* 1998;16:692–701
7. Leibovitch, I, et al., Characterization of an extremely low risk cohort of clinical stage A nonseminomatous testicular cancer (NSGCT): Quantitative immunohistochemistry, histopathology and radiology. *Proc Am Soc Clin Oncol* 1996;14
8. Bhatia, S, et al., High dose chemotherapy with peripheral stem cell or autologous bone marrow transplant as initial salvage chemotherapy for testicular cancer. *Proc Am Soc Clin Oncol*, 1998;17: 321A, #1239
9 Tuveson DA, Willis NA, Jacks T et al. STI–571 inactivation of the gastrointestinal stromal tumor c-KIT oncoprotein: biological and clinical implications. *Oncogene* 2001;20:5054–8
10. Tian Q, Frierson HF Jr, Krystal GW, Moskaluk CA. Activating c-kit gene mutations in human germ cell tumors. *Am J Pathol* 1999;154:1643–7

19. Topoisomerase I and II in Germ Cell Cancer as Indicators of Possible Drug Selection for Salvage Chemotherapy Studies

D.M. Berney[1], J. Shamash[2], J. Gaffney[2], R.T.D. Oliver[2]

*Departments of 1. Histopathology and 2. Medical Oncology, St Bartholomew's Hospital,
St Bartholomew's and The Royal London School of Medicine and Dentistry*

Introduction

DNA Topoisomerase I (Topo I) is the target of the camptothecins, topotecan and irinotecan, which show activity against several solid cancers. DNA topoisomerase II (Topo II) is the target of etoposide, which is active against some testicular tumours. The immunohistochemistry of these molecular targets has not been investigated in non-seminomatous germ cell tumours.

Materials and Methods

Samples of testicular germ cell tumours (GCTs) and retro-peritoneal lymph node dissections (RPLND) were collected from the Bart's and the London Medical oncology database. Twenty-seven post-chemotherapy RPLND were investigated, 14 of which had matching orchidectomy samples. Thirteen primary seminomas were also tested for comparison. 3mm formalin fixed, paraffin embedded tissue sections were cut from the selected tissue blocks. Antigen retrieval was used for all of the antibodies used. Protocols for assessment were followed according to those used for the topoisomerases in previous studies.

Topo I expression was assessed on a subjective scale of 0 to 3+, and Topo II by calculating the number of positive cells out of 500.

Results

All the antibodies used showed nuclear staining. There was a negative correlation between the expression of Topo I and Topo II.

Topo I was significantly more strongly expressed in post-chemotherapy teratoma differentiated (TD) ($p < 0.015$) and in yolk sac tumour (YST) ($p < 0.001$) than in seminomas. There was no significant difference between embryonal carcinoma (EC) and seminoma.

There was a significant correlation between the two anti-Topo II antibodies used. Topo II was most strongly positive in EC ($p < 0.05$) and there was no significant difference between the other groups.

Conclusions

Anti-Topo I drugs may be of use in the salvage chemotherapy of selected GCTs. They are likely to be most effective in tumours with a high proliferative fraction, which are generally tumours with a high Topo II index. Tumours expressing both high Topo I and Topo II include primary EC and seminomas. In relapsed GCTs, both TD and YST are uniformly positive. However, TD has a low proliferation index and is unlikely to be sensitive to anti-Topo I drugs but recurrent YSTs are a possible target. Late recurrences of YSTs are well reported and may be resistant to standard germ cell chemotherapy. Recurrent EC, unlike primary EC, is predominantly negative for Topo I and is unlikely to be responsive to these agents. Therefore, anti-Topo I agents may be of use in salvage chemotherapy, but only in selected tumours.

Section 3

Non-testicular Germ Cell Tumours

20. Overview of Female Germ Cell Tumours

S.A. Tjulandin

The Russian Cancer Research Center, Moscow

Introduction

Ovarian germ cell tumours (OGCT) are a rare (2–3 per cent of all ovarian cancers) but potentially curable group of malignancies that usually affect adolescent girls and young women with median age between 16 to 20 years and range from 6 to 46 years [1]. Like testicular germ cell tumours (GCTs), malignant OGCTs demonstrate an aggressive nature with a very high growth rate and early spread to the adjacent organs and regional lymph nodes. As a result of surgical treatment followed by cisplatin-based chemotherapy most women with this disease will survive with little long-term treatment related morbidity. As a person who has been involved for a long time in the management of male GCTs, I will critically review the current status of the diagnosis, staging and treatment of OGCT.

Pathology

Like testicular cancer, all ovarian GCTs are divided into two clinically and histologically distinct entities: dysgerminoma and tumours other that dysgerminomas [2]. Dysgerminoma is the female equivalent of seminoma with a similar morphological picture and high sensitivity to radiotherapy. Dysgerminomas account for almost half of malignant OGCTs. Non-dysgerminomas include endodermal sinus (yolk sac) tumour, embryonal cell carcinoma, choriocarcinoma, polyembryoma and combinations of all these types, which have a very aggressive nature with a high risk of disease progression after surgical treatment. Immature teratomas are the third most common OGCT and are graded by the degree of immaturity [3]. Mature cystic teratoma is a benign tumour and often contains such cell types as cartilage, neural tissue, and mucinous and nonmucinous glands. On occasion, somatic cell types in mature teratoma undergo malignant transformation with the development, for example, of a squamous cell carcinoma or primitive neuroendocrine tumour. Histologically solid immature teratomas have a mixture of immature and mature tissue. Their prognosis worsens with the increasing proportion of immature tissues present and if one of the components is truly carcinomatous or sarcomatous.

Cytogenetic Abnormalities

GCTs derive from totipotential germ cells. The cause of OGCTs is not known, as the molecular mechanism of the germ cell transformation is poorly understood. Several cytogenetic studies have examined the genetic changes associated with OGCT development. Ploidy measurements have revealed that most dysgerminomas and yolk sac tumours (endodermal sinus tumours) have cell populations in the triploid to tetraploid range [4]. By contrast, immature teratomas are usually diploid, although aneuploidy has been detected in some grade 3 lesions [4,5]. An isochromosome for short arm of chromosome 12 is very common in primary testicular GCTs, and several authors reported the occurrence of an i(12p) in patients with dysgerminomas (four of four tumours), yolk sac tumour (one of two tumours) and mixed GCTs (four of 10 tumours), but not in any of the three pure immature teratomas [7-9]. Also, gain of chromosome 12 or 12p sequences was found in the majority of dysgerminomas and yolk sac tumours, indicating that the changes of the short arm of chromosome 12 are a very common event in patients with OGCTs [9]. Comparative genomic hybridisation studies in OGCTs have also revealed recurrent gains of all or parts of chromosomes and chromosome arms 1q, 7, 8, and 21 as well as losses from 13q [8, 9]. The target genes affected by these changes remain unknown.

The inactivation of tumour suppressor genes plays a central role on the development and progression of human cancers. Several studies reported the frequent deletions at 3q27-3q28, 5q31, 5q34-q35, 9p22-p21, 11p15.5, 11p13, 11q13, 12q22, 17p13, and 18q21.1 in male GCTs [10-12]. A similar frequency of chromosomal loss in the same regions was found in all histological subtypes of malignant OGCTs [13]. The most striking losses were observed in the chromosomal regions located at 3q27-q28, 5q31, 5q34-q35, 9p21-p22, and 12q22. These chromosome regions may contain tumour suppressor genes that are important in the initiation and progression of both malignant ovarian and testicular GCTs. The presence of i(12p) in both female and male GCTs and the similarities in other, presumably secondary, chromosomal abnormalities, and ploidy indicate that these tumours evolve through some of the same pathogenetic mechanisms in both sexes. On the other hand, immature teratomas show fewer DNA changes (no gain of 12p, diploid), indicating that they arise via different pathogenetic mechanisms [9].

Tumour Markers

GCTs, including ovarian, have a unique property to secrete tumour-associated antigens that can be detected in serum. This has allowed accurate diagnosis, comprehensive monitoring during treatment and detection of recurrence. Both human chorionic gonadotropin (hCG) and alpha-fetoprotein (AFP) have been identified as sensitive markers in most patients with OGCTs [14]. AFP is most often elevated in yolk sac tumours but also has been detected in immature teratomas and embryonal carcinomas. HCG is often elevated in choriocarcinomas, embryonal carcinomas, and polyembryomas. Clusters of syncytiotrophoblastic cells in dysgerminoma can result in a measurable hCG level. Lactate dehydrogenase (LDH) is not specific for GCTs but when raised, it can be useful in monitoring treatment of OGCTs negative for hCG and AFP, especially in dysgerminomas [15]. Macrophage colony-stimulating factors (M-CSF), neurone-specific enolase and CA-125 have also been identified in the serum of patients with OGCTs, but their clinical roles are not well defined [16-18].

Staging

The staging system used for OGCTs is identical to that used for epithelial ovarian cancer. In contrast to epithelial tumours, approximately 60 per cent to 70 per cent of OGCTs are stage I at diagnosis [19]. Stage II and stage IV are relatively uncommon, and stage III accounts for approximately 25 per cent to 30 per cent of tumours. Primary OGCTs can be very large and often are greater than 10 cm in diameter. The contralateral ovary is involved by a synchronous tumour in 10 per cent of dysgerminoma patients but only rarely in tumours other than dysgerminoma. Spread beyond the ovaries occurs most commonly to the peritoneal surface and paraaortic lymph nodes. In spite of peritoneal surface involvement, ascites is infrequent. Distant metastases, mainly to liver and lung, occur occasionally but is less common than in testicular cancer.

Surgical Management

Surgery is the initial approach for both diagnosis and treatment of a patient suspected of having a malignant OGCT. Before the initial surgical procedure, every effort should be made to diagnose OGCT in adolescent and young women presenting with an ovarian tumour, and this includes markers determination. Also a frozen section facility is necessary to confirm the presence of OGCT and to plan the extent of the primary surgery. As a result of the curative potential of modern chemotherapy, one of the goals of the initial surgical procedure is to preserve fertility.

The principles of surgical staging of OGCT are similar to those described for epithelial tumours [20]. After the vertical midline incision, the entire peritoneal cavity should be carefully inspected. Ascitic fluid or a peritoneal washing with normal saline should be submitted for cytological examination. Any suspicious areas should be biopsied and, if none are present, random biopsies should be performed. The retroperitoneal nodes should be carefully palpated and suspicious areas biopsied; otherwise random biopsies should be performed.

The type of primary surgery depends on the extent of disease and tumour histology. Bilateral ovarian involvement with tumour is rare except in cases of pure dysgerminoma. Therefore, unilateral salpingo-oophorectomy with preservation of the contralateral ovary and the uterus can be performed in most patients, thus preserving the potential for fertility. Results from several studies clearly demonstrate similar cure rates in patients treated with conservative unilateral salpingo-oophorectomy compared with patients who had bilateral salpingo-oophorectomy with or without abdominal hysterectomy [21]. If the contralateral ovary appears grossly normal on careful inspection, it should be left undisturbed, as biopsy may result in future infertility due to peritoneal adhesions or ovarian failure. If frozen section of the ovarian tumour confirms the presence of pure dysgerminoma however, careful examination and biopsy of the contralateral ovary is necessary to exclude bilateral tumour involvement. If the contralateral ovary appears abnormally enlarged, a biopsy or ovarian cystectomy should be performed. If frozen section analysis reveals malignant disease or a dysgenetic gonad, then bilateral salpingo-oophorectomy is indicated. If a benign cystic teratoma is found (5 per cent to 10 per cent of cases), then only ovarian cystectomy with preservation of as much normal ovarian tissue as possible is recommended. In spite of the fact that all malignant GCTs have a propensity for lymphatic spread, the risk of lymph node involvement in OGCTs is low. Thus routine lymph node dissection is not necessary, although enlarged paraaortic and pelvic lymph nodes should be resected.

If metastatic disease is found at initial surgery, cytoreductive surgery is essential to achieve maximal resection and minimal residual disease. The GOG study showed that 91 of 93 patients remained disease free following complete surgical excision and adjuvant chemotherapy [22]. The cure rate dropped 60–80 per cent in patients with incompletely resected tumour, indicating that all reasonable efforts should be applied to achieve a complete tumour removal [23, 24]. GCTs, especially dysgerminomas, are generally very chemosensitive, and, in selected patients with advanced disease, preservation of reproductive function remains an option as long as the uterus and contralateral ovary are not grossly involved with tumour [25, 26].

Postsurgical Management of Dysgerminomas

Dysgerminomas are the most common ovarian germ cell malignancy, accounting for 50 per cent of all cases [19]. They are likely to be localized to the ovary at the time of diagnosis. The contralateral ovary is involved by a synchronous tumour in 10 per cent and by microscopic spread from the primary tumour in another 5 per cent of cases. Spread beyond the ovaries occurs in 25 per cent of patients, most commonly to the paraaortic lymph nodes. The diagnosis of dysgerminoma requires a normal AFP value; however, an elevation of hCG is not inconsistent with this diagnosis. An elevated level of LDH is a sensitive though non-specific marker, and the degree of elevation has been correlated with the size of the tumour.

With precise staging, approximately 60 per cent to 70 per cent of patients are diagnosed with stage I disease. Patients with stage IA dysgerminomas may be observed closely without adjuvant treatment [19, 27]. Patients should be monitored at 4–6 week intervals with measurements of tumour markers (AFP, hCG, LDH) followed by pelvic ultrasound. An abdominal CT scan is advisable every 3–4 months. The overall 10-year survival rate for these patients approaches 100 per cent. The relapse rate varies from 15 per cent to 25 per cent in different studies, but all relapses can be retreated successfully with a high likelihood of cure. Dysgerminomas are highly radiosensitive, but even with shielding there is considerable scatter of radiation to the uterus and contralateral ovary, leading to ovarian failure and loss of reproductive function. Therefore, radiation therapy for dysgerminomas has been replaced by effective and less toxic chemotherapy regimens.

Patients with more advanced disease and completely resected tumour should receive adjuvant chemotherapy. Three courses of BEP (cisplatin, etoposide and bleomycin) will nearly always prevent a recurrence [19, 27].

All patients with residual tumour masses after surgery or disease recurrence are candidates for chemotherapy. Based on the results obtained in the treatment of testicular GCTs, BEP has replaced previously used combinations, such as VAC (vincristine, actinomycin-D, cyclophosphamide) and PVB (cisplatin, vinblastine, bleomycin) [19]. Limited experience with BEP chemotherapy in dysgerminoma has shown excellent results. Gershenson et al. treated nine patients with advanced and recurrent disease and all of them were free of disease with a median follow up of 23 months [28]. The same results were reported by GOG and the M.D.Anderson Cancer Center [29, 30]. These studies led to the recommendation of 4 cycles of BEP as a standard regimen for advanced or recurrent dysgerminoma.

Post-surgical Management of Non-dysgerminomas

The non-dysgerminomatous tumours include yolk sac tumours, immature and mature teratomas, mixed GCTs, choriocarcinomas, embryonal carcinomas, and polyembryomas [2]. Yolk sac tumours are the second most common GCTs after dysgerminomas, comprising 25 per cent of all cases. They secrete AFP as a tumour marker. They are very rapidly growing tumours, although 70 per cent of patients present with stage IA disease, with 6 per cent falling into stage II and 23 per cent into stage III. Contralateral ovary involvement is reported in 5 per cent of patients.

Immature teratomas are the third most common GCT and 5 per cent of contralateral ovaries contain a benign cystic teratoma. Immature teratomas are graded from 1 to 3 based on the amount of primitive neuroectodermal tissue present [3]. The grade has been correlated with prognosis and dictates the mode of therapy. Mixed primitive GCTs account for about 19 per cent of all OGCTs. Dysgerminomas and yolk sac tumours are the most common combination encountered. Embryonal carcinomas, choriocarcinomas, and polyembryomas are extremely rare in pure forms and are most likely to be seen as components of mixed primitive GCTs.

Patients with completely resected OGCTs have a risk of recurrence that ranges from 25 per cent in grade 1 immature teratomas to nearly 100 per cent in yolk sac and mixed tumours [30]. These patients are routinely treated with adjuvant chemotherapy. GOG reported the results of adjuvant chemotherapy in 93 non-dysgerminomatous patients with stage I–III who were disease-free after initial surgery [22]. All of them received 3 cycles of classical BEP. With a median follow up of 39 months, four patients developed recurrences, two of which had immature teratoma and were salvaged by surgery alone. Thus, 91 of 93 patients were free of disease, and one died of disease progression. Several studies confirmed the effectiveness of cisplatin-based chemotherapy given as a short course of the BEP regimen in completely resected GCTs [23, 31].

The role of adjuvant chemotherapy in grade I immature teratoma is still controversial. Norris et al. showed that only one of 14 patients with stage I, grade 1, immature teratoma developed a recurrence [32]. However, recurrence was observed in nine of 20 patients with grade 2 and in four of six with grade 3. Based on these data, in patients with stage I grade 1 immature teratoma, no adjuvant chemotherapy is recommended. On the other hand, three groups have presented their results of surveillance in patients with stage I resected immature teratoma. The Pediatric Oncology group followed 31 patients with immature teratoma of any grade and 30 of them remained continuously disease-free with a median follow up of 33 months [33]. Investigators from the UK observed one recurrence in nine patients with grade 2–3 immature teratomas [34]. Italian investigators reported that one of nine patients with grade 2–3 immature teratoma developed recurrence and all are currently free of disease with follow up ranges from 11 to 138 months [35]. These results questioned the prognosis of stage I, grade 2–3 teratoma and the role of the adjuvant chemotherapy. Although these three studies combined 49 patients with pure immature teratomas and only three recurrences were documented, the results are too premature to draw definitive conclusions. Further study is needed before we can recommend omission of adjuvant chemotherapy in these patients. Patients with stage II or III immature teratoma should receive adjuvant chemotherapy irrespective of tumour grade. Of the 42 patients with resected grade 2–3 immature teratoma who received three cycles of adjuvant BEP in the GOG study, 39 have been-continuously disease-free [22].

All patients with incompletely resected tumours, metastatic or recurrent non-dysgerminomas should be considered for platinum-based chemotherapy. The results of several studies concluded that platinum-based therapy was effective for non-dysgerminomatous OGCTs [23, 27, 28, 36]. PVB, POMB-ACE (cisplatin, vincristine, methotrexate, bleomycin, actinomycin-D, cyclophosphamide, etoposide), and BEP are among the most popular regimens. These regimens have shown that about 60 per cent to 80 per cent of patients will be long-term survivors. Based upon data from randomized trials in testicular cancer, BEP is a standard therapy. The recommended duration of chemotherapy is now four cycles. For patients with elevated tumour markers, the usual practice is to administer two cycles beyond the time of achieving marker negativity. However, in the advanced disease, results with this regimen were less favourable than in the testicular cancer group, and it was thought that further improvement is possible.

Postchemotherapy Surgery

Several studies have been performed to assess the role of second-look laparotomy in patients with an initial complete resection, who received adjuvant cisplatin-based chemotherapy. In the GOG study, 45 surgical procedures were performed in patients who received three courses of BEP after initial complete tumour resection [37]. No tumour or mature teratoma was found in 43, and immature teratoma was found in two patients. Both these patients and 44 of the total are disease free. In a series from the M. D. Anderson Cancer Centre, findings were negative in 52 of 53 patients, who underwent this procedure [38]. These data indicate that second-look laparotomy is not necessary to document a disease-free status in patients with initial complete tumour resection.

In the GOG study, 72 patients with incompletely resected tumour underwent surgery after three cycle of BEP [37]. Forty-eight of these patients did not have teratoma elements in their primary tumour. At surgery 45 patients had no tumour, and three had persistent yolk sac tumour or embryonal carcinoma. All three patients progressed and died despite further treatment. Twenty-four patients had teratoma elements in their primary tumour. At surgery 16 had mature teratoma, which in seven was bulky or progressive. Fourteen of the 16 remain disease free after surgery. These data show that patients with incomplete tumour resection but without teratoma do not need second-look surgery. However, patients with teratoma elements in the primary tumour often presented after chemotherapy with marker negative mature teratoma, which should be resected. The role of postchemotherapy surgery in patients with persistent marker negative or even marker positive non-dysgerminoma should be further clarified despite the negative GOG study.

Second-line Chemotherapy

The prognosis of patients who progress during or shortly after cisplatin-based chemotherapy is very poor. There is little information regarding the efficacy of salvage chemotherapy for recurrent and persistent OGCTs after initial BEP chemotherapy. Based on the testicular cancer experience it is logical to offer VeIP (cisplatin, ifosfamide and vinblastine) in case of recurrent cisplatin-sensitive disease. If we are dealing with cisplatin–refractory disease there are no reasonable therapeutic options, except an investigational chemotherapy. Patients who had been initially treated with PVP might benefit from BEP or EMA-CO (etoposide, methotrexate, actinomycin-D, cyclophosphamide and vincristine) [30].

Fertility Issues

Because OGCTs occur in young women of reproductive age and are now potentially curable, fertility issues are of great concern. Effective chemotherapy allows the consideration of fertility sparing surgery in the most of patients. Modern chemotherapy like BEP might cause ovarian dysfunction or even failure, but the majority of survivors can anticipate normal menstrual and reproductive function. Most of the data suggest that 60 per cent to 80 per cent of patients who underwent unilateral salpingo-oophorectomy and 3–4 cycles of cisplatin-based chemotherapy returned to their normal prechemotherapy menstrual pattern, and many of them had successful pregnancies followed by the delivery of healthy children [23, 39, 40]. Factors such as older age at initiation of therapy, extent of the primary surgery, greater cumulative dose of anticancer agents, and longer duration of chemotherapy have an adverse affect on future gonadal function. But one of the first priorities for fertility preservation is to exclude the unnecessary bilateral salpingo-oophorectomy and hysterectomy in young women with OGCT, which is still a standard approach in many general hospitals and gynaecology departments.

Prognostic Factors

In male GCT patients, in order to achieve the best treatment results, we plan our treatment strategy based on clinically proved prognostic classification, such as the IGCCCT prognostic classification. No such classification has been developed for OGCTs. Currently treatment strategy is based on tumour histology and the FIGO or WHO staging systems, which do not consider the extent of disease, the presence or absence of tumour after initial surgery, and tumour markers. Several groups retrospectively determined the most important prognostic factors in OGCTs. Mitchell et al. found in multivariate analysis that relapse after surgery and chemotherapy was generally seen in patients with yolk sac tumours who had an AFP over 1000 U/l, as well as patients who received nonplatinum-based chemotherapy [40]. Univariate analysis also showed a non-significant trend to more frequent relapse with tumour diameter over 2 cm prior to chemotherapy. Couline S. et al. analysed the treatment results of 102 OGCT patients. On univariate analysis, the presence of residual disease after initial surgery and elevated hCG attained significant prognostic value but neither the initial FIGO stage (I versus II–IV), elevated AFP nor the histological type were significant [23]. Only the presence of residual disease after initial surgery retained significant prognostic value in the multivariate analysis. Newlands et al. treated 95 patients with OGCTs with POMB-ACE chemotherapy and determined that age over 30 negatively affected survival [36]. Neither FIGO stage at diagnosis nor initial tumour marker concentrations influenced survival. These studies clearly demonstrate that tumour histology (dysgerminoma versus non-dysgerminoma) and the FIGO staging system do not predict the treatment outcomes of OGCT patients. Obviously, the development of a prognostic classification for OGCTs is one of the first priorities.

Conclusion

Twenty years ago the prognosis of OGCT patients was dismal. Development of effective cisplatin-based chemotherapy and conservative surgery has made cure probable and and retention of fertility possible for most patients. In spite of significant success in the treatment of OGCTs we are far from understanding the cause of the disease, mechanisms of tumour development, and optimal surgical and chemotherapy strategy. Prospective randomised trials in subgroups of patients with different prognoses should allow the development of more effective treatment and minimize toxicity. Given the rarity of the disease, every effort should be made to start an international collaboration in this area.

References

1. Creasman WT, Soper JT. Assessment of the contemporary management of germ cell malignancies of the ovary. *Am J Obstet Gynecol* 1985;153: 828–835
2. Scully RE, Sobin LN. Histological typing of ovarian tumors. In: *World Health Organization International Classification of Tumors*, 2nd ed. Berlin: Springer-Verlag, pp 28–36, 1999
3. Norris HJ, Zirkin HJ, Benson WL: Immature (malignant) teratoma of the ovary. *Cancer* 1976;37: 2359–2372
4. Baker BA, Frickey L, Yu IT, Hawkins EP, Cushing B, Perlman EJ. DNA content of ovarian immature teratomas and malignant germ cell tumors. *Gynecol Oncol* 1998;71:14–18
5. Silver SA, Wiley JM, Perlman EJ. DNA ploidy analysis of pediatric germ cell tumors. *Mod Pathol* 1994;7: 951–956
6. Atkin NB, Baker MC. Abnormal chromosomes including small metacentrics in 14 ovarian cancers. *Cancer Genet Cytogenet* 1987;26:355–361
7. Jenkin DJ, McCartney AJ. A chromosome study of three ovarian tumors. *Cancer Genet Cytogenet* 1987;26:327–337
8. Riopel MA, Spellerberg A, Griffin CA, Perlman EJ. Genetic analysis of ovarian germ cell tumors by comparative genomic hybridization. *Cancer Res* 1998;58:3105–3110
9. Kraggerud SM, Szymanska J, Abeler VM, et al. DNA copy number in malignant ovarian germ cell tumors. *Cancer Res* 2000;60:3025–3030
10. Faulkner SW, Leigh DA, Oosteerhuis JW, Roelofs H, Looijenga LHJ, Friedlander ML. LOH analysis of small regions of testicular germ cell tumor microdissected from paraffin-embedded tissue. *Proc. ASCO* 1998;17:2169 [abstract]
11. Murty VVVS, Bosl GJ, Houldsworth J, et al. Allelic loss and somatic differentiation in human male germ cell tumors. *Oncogene* 1994;9:2245–2251
12. Peng H-Q, Bailey D, Bronson D, Goss PE, Hogg D. Loss of heterozygosity of tumor suppressor genes in testis cancer. *Cancer Res* 1995;55:2871–2875
13. Faulkner SW, Friedlander ML. Molecular genetic analysis of malignant ovarian germ cell tumors. *Cynecil Oncol* 2000;77:283–288
14. Kawai M, Kano T, Kikkawa F, et al. Seven tumor markers in benign and malignant germ cell tumors of the ovary. *Gynecol Oncol* 1992;45:248–253
15. Schwartz PE, Morris JM. Serum lactic dehydrogenase: a tumor marker for dysgerminoma. *Obstet Gynecol* 1988;72:511–515
16. Suzuki M, Kobayashi H, Ohwanda M, et al. Macrophage colony-stimulating factor as a marker for malignant germ cell tumors of the ovary. *Gynecol Oncol* 1998;68:35–37
17. Kawata M, Sekiya S, Hatadeyama R, Takamizawa H. Neuron-specific enolase as a serum marker for immature teratoma and dysgerminoma. *Gynecol Oncol* 1989;32:191–197
18. Altaras MM, Goldberg GL, Levin W, et al. The value of cancer antigen-125 as a tumor marker in malignant germ cell tumors of the ovary. *Gynecol Oncol* 1986;25:150–159
19. Hurteau JA, Williams SJ. Ovarian germ cell tumours. In: Rubin SC, Sutton GP (eds). *Ovarian Cancer*, 2nd edn. Philadelphia: Lippincott Williams & Wilkins, pp 373–382, 2001
20. Trimbos JB, Bolis G. Guidelines for surgical staging of ovarian cancer. *Obstet Gynecol Surv* 1994;49: 814–820
21. Williams S, Wong LC, Ngan HYS. Management of ovarian germ cell tumors. In: Gershenson DM, McGuire WP (eds). *Ovarian Cancer: Controversies in management.* New York: Churchill Livingstone, pp 399–416, 1998

22. Williams SD, Blessing JA, Liao S-Y, et al. Adjuvant therapy of ovarian germ cell tumors with cisplatin, etoposide and bleomycin: a trial of the Gynecologic Oncology Group. *J Clin Oncol* 1994;12:701–706
23. Culine S, Lhomme C, Kattan J, Michel G, Duvillard P, Droz JP. Cisplatin-based chemotherapy in the management of germ cell tumors of the ovary: The Institute Gustave Roussy Experience. *Gynecol Oncol* 1997;64:160–165
24. Schwartz PE, Chambers SK, Chambers JT, et al. Ovarian germ cell malignancies: the Yale University experience. *Gynecol Oncol* 1992;45:26–31
25. Wu P, Huang R, Lang J, et al. Treatment of malignant ovarian germ cell tumors with preservation of fertility: a report of 28 cases. *Gynecol Oncol* 1991;40:2–6
26. Thomas GM, Dembo AJ, Hacker NF, et al: Current. therapy for dysgerminoma of the ovary. *Obstetr Gynecol* 1987;70:268–275
27. Williams SD, Blessing JA, Moore DH, et al. Cisplatin, vinblastine, and bleomycin in advanced recurrent ovarian germ-cell tumors. *Ann Intern Med* 1989;111:22 –27
28. Gershenson DM, Morris M, Cangir A, et al. Treatment of malignant germ cell tumors of the ovary with bleomycin, etoposide, and cisplatin (BEP). *J Clin Oncol* 1990;8:715–720
29. Williams SD, Blessing JA, Hatch KD, Homesley HD. Chemotherapy of advanced dysgerminoma: trials of the Gynecologic Oncology Group. *J Clin Oncol* 1991;9:1950–1955
30. Gershenson DM. Update on malignant ovarian germ cell tumors. *Cancer Suppl* 1993;71:1581–1590
31. Segelov E, Campbell J, Ng M, et al. Cisplatin-based chemotherapy for ovarian germ cell malignancies: the Australian experience. *J Clin Oncol* 1994;12:378–384
32. Norris HJ, Zirkin HJ, Benson WL. Immature (malignant) teratoma of the ovary. *Cancer* 1976;37: 2359–2372
33. Marina NM, Cushing B, Giller R, et al. Complete surgical excision is effective treatment for children with immature teratomas with or without malignant elements: a Pediatric Oncology Group/Children's Cancer Group intergroup study. *J Clin Oncol* 1999;17:2137–2143
34. Dark CG, Bower M, Newlands ES, et al. Surveillance policy for stage I ovarian germ cell tumors. *J Clin Oncol* 1997;15:620–624
35. Bonazzi C, Peccatori F, Columbo N, et al. Pure ovarian immature teratoma, a unique and curable disease: 10 year's experience of 32 prospectively treated patients. *Obstet Gynecol* 1994;84:598–604
36. Newlands ES, Bower M, Holden L, Rustin GJ, Paradinas FJ, Dark GG. Management of Stage I and metastatic ovarian germ cell tumors (OGCT).). *Proc ASCO* 1996;15: A774 (abstr)
37. Williams SD, Blessing JA, DiSaia PJ, et al. Second-look laparotomy in ovarian germ cell tumors: the Gynecologic Oncology Group experience. *Gynecol Oncol* 1994;52:287–291
38. Gershenson DM, Copeland LJ, Del Junco G: Second-look laparotomy in the management of malignant germ cell tumors of the ovary. *Obstetr Gynecol* 1986;67:789–794
39. Brewer M. Gershenson DM, Herzog CE, et al. Outcome and reproduction function after chemotherapy for ovarian dysgerminoma. *J Clin Oncol* 1999;17:2670–2675
40. Mitchell PL, Al-Nasiri N, A'Hern R, et al. Treatment of nondysgerminomatous ovarian germ cell tumors: an analysis of 69 cases. *Cancer* 1999;85:2232–2244

21. Germ Cell Tumours of the Ovary: a Clinicopathological Study of 121 Cases from Nepal

S.P. Sah[1], D. Upreti[2], M. Lakhey[1], S. Rani[1]

Departments of 1. Pathology, and 2. Obstetrics & Gynaecology, B.P. Koirala Institute of Health Sciences (BPKIHS), Dharan, NEPAL

Background

Germ cell tumours (GCTs) of the ovary occur more frequently than epithelial tumours in Orientals and Africans [1]. Although much has been published about ovarian GCTs from the Western countries, there has been no such documentation from Nepal. This retrospective study aimed to report the clinicopathological profile of ovarian GCTs reported at BPKIHS, Dharan, Nepal.

Methods

We identified 121 histopathologically proven ovarian GCTs reported at our institute from November 1995 to April 2001 (5 and half years). The clinical data, histopathological findings and complications were recorded. The GCTs and other tumours of the ovary were distributed in different caste/ethnic populations of Nepal e.g., Terai caste, Hill caste and Hill native [2].

Results

The prevalence of GCTs was 43.36 per cent (121/279) of all ovarian neoplasms. The ages of the patients varied from 8 to 65 (mean 31) years. The largest number of cases was found in patients between the age of 21 and 40 years. Only 8 out of 121 (6.61 per cent) cases were malignant and the rest (93.39 per cent) were mature teratomas. The prevalence of GCTs seemed to correlate with the ethnic background, representing 60.41 per cent, 42.85 per cent and 18.75 per cent of all ovarian neoplasms in the Hill native, Hill caste and Terai caste respectively (Chi square 14.63, DF 2, p = 0.0006). Pain and abdominal fullness were the common symptoms noted in 85.95 per cent and 79.31 per cent of patients respectively. Seventeen (14 per cent) asymptomatic cases were found either on routine physical examination (12 cases) or during pregnancy (5 cases). The left ovary was involved in 39.7 per cent and the right in 35.5 per cent of patients, with bilateral involvement in 24.8 per cent. Torsion was noted in 20.66 per cent and was the most common complication. Only 6.61 per cent of GCTs were solid on gross appearance, and 93.39 per cent were cystic. Of the 118 cases of teratoma, 110 cases were benign mature teratomas (solid or cystic) and four cases were immature, three cases were mature monodermal teratomas and one case showed squamous cell carcinoma arising in mature teratoma. There were three cases of malignant GCTs (one yolk sac tumour and two dysgerminomas). Six cases of mature cystic teratoma were associated with mucinous cystadenoma (four cases), serous cystadenoma (one case) or yolk sac tumour (one case) in either the same or the contralateral ovary.

Conclusion

Mature teratoma is the most common form of GCT and accounts for 40.50 per cent of all ovarian neoplasms. The high prevalence of GCTs in Hill natives needs to be investigated in a large scale study.

References

1. Bugharara FA. Incidence of the histologic types of ovarian tumours in Benghazi (Libya) and Poland. *Neoplasma* 1983;30:251–254
2. Bal Kumar KC. Social composition of population. In: Population monograph of Nepal. Central Bureau of Statistics, Kathmandu, Nepal, 1995, pp 301–337

22. Serum Lactate Dehydrogenase Isoenzyme 1 in Patients with Testicular and Ovarian Germ Cell Tumours

F.E. von Eyben[1], M.R. Mirza[2], E.L. Madsen[3], O. Blaabjerg[1], P.H. Petersen[1], B. Hølund[4]

1. Department of Clinical Chemistry, 2. Department of Oncology, Odense University Hospital, 3. Department of Oncology, Sønderborg Hospital, 4. Department of Pathology, Odense University Hospital, Denmark

Background

Serum lactate dehydrogenase isoenzyme 1 catalytic concentration (S-LD-1) is raised both in patients with ovarian germ cell tumours (OGCT) and with testicular germ cell tumours (TGCT). This overview combines results from the literature with the experience at a single oncological institution.

Patients

Eleven patients with OGCT and 108 previously reported patients with TGCT treated at Odense University Hospital [1–4] and the previous literature [5] were reviewed.

Methods

At Odense University Hospital, S-LD-1 was measured with an immunochemical method as previously described [1]. S-LD-1 was measured only after the initial salpingo-oophorectomy in patients with OGCT. TGCT patients were monitored mainly from start of treatment after orchiectomy. All patients were followed for 5 years after treatment.

Results

Four of seven patients with metastatic or suspected OGCT had a raised S-LD-1, as did half of the patients with metastatic TGCT, and this normalized following initiation of platinum-based combination chemotherapy. None of the patients with OGCT but 20–30 per cent of those with TGCT stage I treated by surveillance relapsed. A quarter of these patients had a raised S-LD-1 up to six months before clinical evidence of relapse [6].

S-LD-1 remained normal during pregnancy. However, some patients with OGCT and TGCT had a transient increase in S-LD-1 with values up to 1.4 upper limit of reference values. Raised S-LD-1 was not predictive of poor prognosis for patients with metastatic OGCT but was a highly significant for patients with metastatic TGCT [7].

A raised S-LD-1 has been demonstratedin 35 of 40 patients with OGCT (88 per cent, 95 per cent CI 73-96) and in 423 of 696 patients with TGCT (61 per cent) [5]. Raised S-LD-1 is therefore more common in patients with OGCT than TGCT (p = 0.0006, Fisher's exact test).

Neither S-LD-1, serum alpha fetoprotein (S-AFP), or serum human chorionic gonadotropin (S-hCG) levels were predictive of prognosis in patients with OGCT unlike their importance in TGCT [8, 9]. Some studies indicate that S-LD-1 might be a better prognostic predictor for patients with metastatic TGCT compared with S-LD [2, 7, 10]. S-LD-1 reflects the high copy number of chromosome 12p in TGCT with the gene locus *LDHB* [4, 11]. LD-1 is a homotetramer of the LD-B sub-unit that is produced by *LDHB*. OGCT also have isochrome (12p) but the relation between the tumour copy number of 12p and level of S-LD-1 has not been studied yet.

Conclusion

OGCT is rarer than TGCT, and the experience with S-LD-1 for OGCT patients is limited. S-LD-1 may be more often raised in OGCT patients with active disease compared to TGCT patients. However in general, tumour markers have a larger role in the monitoring of patients with TGCT than OGCT. Pregnancy can induce a raised S-AFP and S-hCG in OGCT patients so S-LD-1 has an advantage. Larger series of OGCT and TGCT patients monitored with S-LD-1 are required.

References

1. von Eyben FE, Blaabjerg O, Petersen PH et al. Serum lactate dehydrogenase isoenzyme 1 as a marker of testicular germ cell tumor. *J Urol* 1988;140:986–90
2. von Eyben FE, Blaabjerg O, Madsen EL, Petersen PH, Smith-Sivertsen C, Gullberg B. Serum lactate dehydrogenase isoenzyme 1 and tumour volume are indicators of response to treatment and predictors of prognosis in metastatic testicular germ cell tumours. *Eur J Cancer* 1992;238:410–5
3. von Eyben FE, Madsen EL, Blaabjerg O, Petersen PH. Serum lactate dehydrogenase isoenzyme 1 as an early indicator of relapse in patients with testicular germ cell tumors. *Acta Oncol* 1995;34:925–9
4. von Eyben FE, Blaabjerg O, Petersen PH et al. Lactate dehydrogenase isoenzyme 1 in testicular germ cell tumors. In: Oosterhuis JW, Walt H, Damjanov I (eds). *Pathobiology of human germ cell neoplasia*. Berlin: Springer Verlag;pp 85–92, 1991
5. von Eyben FE. A systematic review of lactate dehydrogenase isoenzyme 1and germ cell tumors. *Clin Biochem* 2001;in press
6. von Eyben FE, Madsen EL. Serum lactate dehydrogenase isoenzyme 1 as predictor of tumor-associated death in patients with testicular germ cell tumours. *Andrologia* 1997;29:137–45
7. von Eyben FE, Madsen EL, Liu F, Amato R, Fritsche H. Serum lactate dehydrogenase isoenzyme 1 as a prognostic predictor for metastatic testicular germ cell tumours. *Br J Cancer* 2000;83:1255–7
8. International Germ Cell Cancer Collaborative Group. International germ cell concensus classification. A prognostic factor-based staging system for metastatic germ cell cancers. *J Clin Oncol* 1997;15:594–603
9. International Union Against Cancer, Sobin LH, Wittekind C. TNM classification of malignant tumours. Fifth edition. New York: Wiley-Liss;1997
10. von Eyben FE, Liu FJ, Amato RJ, Fritsche HA. Lactate dehydrogenase (LD) isoenzyme 1 is the most important LD isoenzyme in patients with testicular germ cell tumor. *Acta Oncol* 2000;39:509–17
11. von Eyben FE, de Graaff W, Marrink J et al. Serum lactate dehydrogenase isoenzyme-1 activity in patients with testicular germ cell tumors correlates with the total number of copies of the short arms of chromosome 12 in the tumor. *Mol Gen Genet* 1992;235:140–6

Section 4

Paediatric Germ Cell Tumours

23. Low Dose Bleomycin Every Three Weeks with Cisplatin and Etoposide Results in Excellent Event Free and Survival Rates for Children and Adolescents with Gonadal Malignant Germ Cell Tumours (MGCT): a POG/CCG Intergroup Report

J.W. Cullen, T.A. Olson*, R.H. Giller, S.J. Lauer, B. Cushing,
P.C. Rogers, W.B. London, A.R. Albin, R.M. Weetman

*Department of Pediatrics, Atlanta, USA

Pediatric Oncology Group (POG) and Children's Cancer Group (CCG) institutions treated 208 patients with gonadal MGCT in studies CCG 8891/8882, POG 9048/9049. There were 17 Stage II, 17 Stage III, and 43 Stage IV testicular primaries, plus 41 Stage I, 16 Stage II, 58 Stage III, and 16 Stage IV ovarian primaries. Stage II testicular and stage I and II ovarian patients were treated with cisplatin 20 mg/m^2/day for 5 days, etoposide 100 mg/m^2/day for 5 days and low dose bleomycin 15 units/m^2 on day 1 of each course. Stages III and IV ovarian and testicular patients received the same etoposide and bleomycin doses, but the dose of cisplatin was randomly assigned to 20 or 40 mg/m^2/day for 5 days (100 mg/m^2 or 200 mg/m^2 per course). Courses were administered every 21 days for a total of four.

Six-year event free survival (EFS) was 93.1 per cent (SE 2.4 per cent) and six-year survival was 95.5 per cent (SE 1.9 per cent) for the entire cohort. The six year EFS for testicular patients was 100 per cent, 94.1 per cent, and 88.3 per cent for stages II, III and IV respectively with corresponding survival rates of 100 per cent, 100 per cent, and 90.6 per cent. The six-year EFS for ovarian patients was 95.1 per cent, 87.5 per cent, 96.6 per cent, and 87.5 per cent for stages I, II, III and IV and the survival was 95.1 per cent, 93.8 per cent, 98.3 per cent, and 93.3 per cent respectively. There was no statistically significant difference in EFS rates (p = 0.191) or survival rates (p = 0.410) between the different cisplatin arms for the randomized Stage III and IV gonadal patients.

Studies of adult testicular GCT patients use bleomycin at a dose of 30 U weekly irrespective of body surface area. Total bleomycin doses for 4 cycles would be 360 U and for 3 cycles, 270 U [1]. The total paediatric bleomycin dose in this study was 60 U/m^2. Theoretically, a large adolescent (2.0 m^2) could receive 120 U of bleomycin. The total paediatric bleomycin dose was 25 per cent to 33 per cent of the dose administered in the standard adult MGCT treatment.

We conclude that in children and adolescents with gonadal MGCT, low dose bleomycin in combination with cisplatin and etoposide maintains excellent efficacy while limiting the cumulative dose of bleomycin, with the potential for a decrease in late pulmonary toxicity. Treatment by four courses of PEB is curative for more than 90 per cent of children with Stage I-IV gonadal GCT. The next Children's Oncology Group (merging POG and CCG) study will decrease the number of cycles from four to three, thus, decreasing the total bleomycin dose by another 25 per cent.

Reference

1. De Wit R, Roberts JT, Wilkinson PM et al. Equivalence of three or four cycles of bleomycin, etoposide, and cisplatin chemotherapy and of a 3-or 5-day schedule in good-prognosis germ cell cancer: A randomized study of the European Organization for Research and Treatment of Cancer Genitourinary Tract Cancer Cooperative Group and the Medical Research Council. *J Clin Oncol* 2001;19:1629–40

24. Treatment Strategy for Childhood Extracranial Secreting Germ Cell Tumours Based on Alphafoetoprotein (AFP) Level: Protocol TGM95 of the Société Française d'Oncologie Pédiatrique (SFOP)

C. Patte*, E. Quintana, D. Frappaz, P. Lutz, G. Leverger, C. Behar,
F. Millot, J.L. Stephan, E. Sariban, M.C. Baranzelli, on behalf of the SFOP

* IGR, Villejuif, France

The previous SFOP TGM85 and TGM90 studies showed that carboplatin (400 mg/m^2) was less efficient that cisplatin (100 mg/m^2), that patients with AFP levels over 15000 ng/ml had a worse outcome, and that the VIP regimen (VP16, Ifosfamide, cisplatin) was an efficient salvage therapy [1–3]. Based on these results, the SFOP developed the TGM95 protocol, a cisplatin-based chemotherapy adapted to initial resection, serum AFP and presence of metastases. Patients are stratified into three risk groups with the following guidelines: low risk (LR) patients with complete resection of a localized tumour (pS1): "watch and wait" with chemotherapy only in cases of tumour marker increase; median risk (MR) patients: non metastatic incompletely resected or unresectable tumour with AFP less than 15000: VBP (Vinblastine, Bleomycine, cisplatin) regimen; high risk (HR) patients: AFP 15000 or more, and/or metastasis: VIP regimen. In both groups, patients received two additional courses of chemotherapy after normalization of tumour markers. The residual tumour or the organ initially involved (if not previously done) were excised after normalization of tumour markers.

Results

From January 1995 to December 1998, 90 patients were registered: 27 LR, 26 MR and 37 HR (19 metastatic). Ages ranged from 2 months to 17 years. There were 17 testicular, 34 ovarian, 18 sacrococcygeal and 11 "other site" tumours. Sixty-six patients had AFP secretion, five HCG, 10 both and three none (but with a yolk sac or embryonal carcinoma component in their tumour). Nineteen patients were treated with surgery alone. There were eight events: six relapses followed by death in three cases, one death after an accident, one toxic death after allograft for AML of a patient with concomitant pS1 ovarian tumour and AML with iso12p. With a follow-up of 44 months, the overall (OS) and event free (EFS) survivals are 94 per cent (95 per cent CI: 87–98 per cent) and 90 per cent (81–94 per cent), without any difference between the therapeutic groups and the AFP levels. The OS and EFS are 94 per cent (73–99 per cent) and 84 per cent (61–84 per cent) in metastatic patients.

Conclusion

With this strategy, the outcome of secreting germ cell tumours was greatly improved compared to our previous studies, and the importance of the previously recognized prognostic factors, such as high AFP level or advanced stage, disappeared.

References

1. Baranzelli MC, Flamant,F, De Lumley L et al. Treatment of non-metastatic, non-seminomatous malignant germ-cell tumours in childhood: experience of the "Societe Francaise d'Oncologie Pediatrique" MGCT 1985–1989 study. *Med. Pediatr. Oncol.* 1993;21:395–401
2. Patte C, Baranzelli MC, Quintana E et al. Carboplatin is less efficient than Cis-platinum in childhood nonmetastatic non seminomatous germ cell tumor treated in SFOP TGM 85 and TGM 90 protocols. *J.Clin.Oncol.* 1995;14, 438
3. Baranzelli MC, Kramar A, Bouffet E et al. Prognostic factors in children with localized malignant nonseminomatous germ cell tumors. *J. Clin. Oncol.* 1999;17:1212

25. Risk Factors in Malignant Extracranial Germ Cell Tumours (MGCTs) of Childhood: Analysis of UKCCSG's GCII Study

J.R. Mann[1], F. Raafat[1], K. Robinson[2], J. Imeson[2], J. Hale[3], E. Bouffet[4], A. Oakhill[5]

1. The Children's Hospital, Steelhouse Lane, Birmingham B4 6NH, 2. UKCCSG Data Centre, Leicester, 3. Royal Victoria Infirmary, Newcastle upon Tyne, 4. Hospital for Sick Children, Toronto, Canada, 5. Royal Hospital for Sick Children, Bristol

Introduction

Most groups now obtain high cure rates in paediatric extracranial MGCTs, mostly using cisplatin-based chemotherapy [1-4]. In Britain, a carboplatin-based regimen (carboplatin, etoposide and bleomycin – JEB) is preferred because it is less oto– and nephrotoxic [5]. An analysis of the UKCCSG's second study (GCII) aimed to define risk groups in order to refine therapy.

Patients and Methods

Children aged 0–16 years with histologically verified extracranial MGCTs were treated by excision of the tumour if this was feasible without major morbidity, or were biopsied. Chemotherapy with JEB [5] was given if excision was incomplete or if tumour recurred. Uni- and multivariate analyses of survival were performed [5].

Results

From 1989 to 1997, 192 patients were registered. Eight were excluded (no histology: three; non-protocol chemotherapy: five). The remaining 184 had germinoma (20), malignant teratoma (55), embryonal carcinoma (one), yolk sac tumour (107) or choriocarcinoma (one). Surgery cured 47 patients (40 testicular, six ovarian, one thoracic) and 137 required JEB. Overall five-year survival (OS) was 93.2 per cent. For the 137 JEB-treated patients OS was 90.9 per cent and five-year event-free survival (EFS) was 87.8 per cent.

Univariate analysis of the JEB-treated patients showed five-year EFS per cent by site: testis 100, ovary 91, vagina/uterus 80, sacrococcygeal 87, thorax 75, other 73 ($p = 0.011$); age: 0-4: 87.4, 5-9: 87.5, 10-16: 88.9 ($p = 0.93$); stage I: 100, II: 94, III: 85, IV: 78 ($p = 0.07$); histology germinoma: 100, malignant teratoma: 87, yolk sac tumour: 86 ($p = 0.32$); AFP $< 10,000$: 95, $\geq 10,000$: 77 ($p = 0.014$). Multivariate analysis on 124

JEB-treated patients aged > 1 year confirmed AFP to be the strongest prognostic factor, followed by stage and site.

Three risk groups were defined among the entire 184 patients: low (45 per cent of cases, treatment surgery, JEB if recurrence) had four year OS of 100 per cent, intermediate (19 per cent, all given JEB) had OS of 97 per cent and high (32 per cent, all given JEB) had OS of 82 per cent.

Conclusions

The confirmed prognostic significance of AFP, stage and site [3] has been used to modify the British protocol, giving fewer courses of chemotherapy for low and intermediate risk disease and a cisplatin-based protocol for high risk cases who develop relapse.

References

1. Haas RJ, Schmidt P, Göbel U, Harms D. Testicular germ cell tumors, an update. Results of the German Co-operative studies 1982-1997. *Klin Pädiatr* 1999;211:300–305
2. Göbel U, Schneider DT, Calaminus G et al. Multimodal treatment of malignant sacrococcygeal germ cell tumors: a prospective analysis of 66 patients of the German cooperative protocols MAKEI 83/86 and 89. *J Clin Oncol* 2001;19:1943–1950
3. Baranzelli MC, Kramer A, Bouffet E et al. Prognostic factors in children with localized malignant nonseminomatous germ cell tumors. *J Clin Oncol* 1999;17:1212–1218
4. Rescorla F, Billmire D, Stolar C et al. The effect of cisplatin dose an surgical resection in children with malignant germ cell tumors at the sacrococcygeal region: a Pediatric Intergroup Trial (POG 9049/CCG 8882). *J Ped Surg* 2001;36:12–17
5. Mann JR, Raafat F, Robinson K et al. The United Kingdom Children's Cancer Study Group's second germ cell tumor study: carboplatin, etoposide, and bleomycin are effective treatment for children with malignant extracranial germ cell tumors, with acceptable toxicity. *J Clin Oncol* 2000;22:3809–3818

26. A Watch-and-Wait-Strategy Is a Safe Procedure in Children and Adolescents with Malignant Non-testicular Germ Cell Tumours (GCTs): Results of the German Consecutive MAKEI 83/86/89 and 96 Protocols

U. Göbel[1], G. Calaminus[1], J. Engert[2], D. Harms[3] for the MAKEI Study Group

1. University of Düsseldorf, 2. Department of Pediatric Surgery, Herne, 3. University of Kiel, Germany

Purpose

The watch-and-wait-strategy (w/w) is already established in children with testicular tumours [1]. In young men this treatment approach is not a standard as insufficient compliance during follow-up increases the risk of late diagnosis of relapse [2]. To determine the value of w/w in non-testicular GCTs, we assessed the group of patients with malignant seminomatous and non-seminomatous GCTs treated in three consecutive German protocols.

Patients and Methods

In the consecutive studies for non-testicular malignant GCTs (MAKEI 83/86 and 89 protocols), patients with ovarian germinoma stage Ia were operated on and then went on to w/w. In MAKEI 96, w/w was introduced into the management of microscopically resected non-germinomatous malignant tumours of any localisation. After surgery, a follow-up programme was mandatory, which included clinical examination, serum tumour markers and imaging at short intervals, in the first year every month, in the second year every 2 months, and during the third to fifth every 3 months. Sixty-five patients were treated as watch-and-wait patients. Patients were divided into three groups. Group A: Patients who received w/w according to protocol, Group B: Non-protocol patients who received w/w, Group C: Patients who had relapsed and who had received w/w as first line treatment.

Results

Group A (n = 41): All patients had ovarian tumours, 14/41 with non-germinomatous histology. Ten progressions occured, one was diagnosed with advanced stage. Group B (n = 16): 13 had non-germinomatous histology, five were microscopically incompletely resected and seven were extragonadal primaries. Three progressions occured, two of which had bulky disease and one died of disease. Group C (n = 8): three were initially microscopically incompletely resected, one was an extragonadal tumour. Three of eight were diagnosed with advanced stage disease, two died of disease. A common characteristics of all patients who progressed was that follow-up was not done at the suggested intervals. All patients who progressed in Groups B and C did not have complete resections. All of the progressing patients of Group A were salvaged by additional treatment (overall survival 100 per cent), unlike patients in Groups B (overall survival 92 per cent) and C (overall survival 75 per cent).

Conclusions

Patients with microscopically incomplete resections need adjuvant chemotherapy. Patients with no or insufficient follow-up are frequently diagnosed with an advanced tumour stage resulting in decreased survival. In children and young women, w/w is possible and safe in case of stage I microscopically completely resected tumours with close follow-up.

Supported by Deutsche Krebshilfe

References

1. Haas RJ, Schmidt P, Göbel U, Harms D. Treatment of malignant testicular tumors in childhood: results of the German National Study 1982-1992. *Med Pediatr Oncol* 1994;23:400–405
2. Foster RS, Nichols CR. Testicular cancer: what's new in staging, prognosis and therapy. *Oncology* 1999;13: 1689–1703

27. Mediastinal Germ Cell Tumours (MGCT) in Children and Adolescents: Age Correlates with Histological Differentiation, Genetic Profiles and Clinical Outcome

D.T. Schneider*, E.J. Perlman, D. Harms, M.K. Fritsch, G. Calaminus, U. Göbel

*Clinic of Pediatric Hematology and Oncology, Heinrich-Heine-University, Moorenstr. 5, Duesseldorf, Germany

The aim of this study was to evaluate the influence of age on biology and clinical outcome of MGCTs in children and adolescents. Between 1983 and 2000, 67 patients (median age 4 years, range neonate-26 years; 35 male, 32 females) were prospectively enrolled onto the German cooperative protocols of nontesticular GCTs in children and adolescents. Median follow-up was 29 (range 1–166) months. Histological diagnosis was seminoma in three patients, all of whom were older than 10 years. The incidence of teratoma differentiated was highest among neonates; only four of 26 patients were older than 10 years. Of 38 patients with malignant nonseminomatous MGCTs, 17 were adolescents (16 male, 1 female). Two patients had Klinefelter's syndrome. Girls predominated (15 to 6) among infants with secreting MGCTs. During infancy, yolk sac tumour (YST) was the exclusive malignant histology, whereas in adolescence, mixed malignant GCTs with embryonal carcinoma, seminoma and choriocarcinoma components also occurred.

Teratomas were treated with resection and follow-up. We observed no relapse, although resection was microscopically incomplete in six patients. Patients with malignant MGCTs were treated with 4 to 8 cycles of cisplatinum/etoposide-based chemotherapy and resection. One patient was excluded from the analysis, since the parents refused treatment. Event free survival (EFS) for seminoma was 1.0 (3/3). For all patients with malignant nonseminomatous MGCT, EFS was 0.73 ± 0.08, recurrence free survival was 0.75 ± 0.08, and overall survival was 0.84 ± 0.07. Seventeen patients with malignant nonseminomatous MGCTs underwent resection at diagnosis, and this was incomplete in 12 patients. Nine of these patients received complete resection on second look surgery. In 13 of 15 patients who received delayed surgery after preoperative chemotherapy, resection was complete. The final completeness of resection was the strongest prognostic parameter (EFS: 0.94 ± 0.05 versus 0.36 ± 0.16, $p < 0.01$). Patients younger than 10 years showed a trend towards better prognosis compared to older children (EFS 0.82 ± 0.09 versus 0.6 ± 14, $p = 0.19$; overall survival 0.94 ± 0.06 versus 0.70 ± 0.13, $p = 0.07$).

In a collaborative effort, 35 MGCT samples from the US-POG and the German MAKEI study groups were collected and screened for chromosomal imbalances with comparative genomic hybridization (CGH). CGH revealed normal profiles in mature or immature teratomas, and distinguished two genetically distinct groups of malignant nonseminomatous MGCTs by age. Infants and young children showed losses at 1p, 4q and 6q, and gains at 1q, 3 and 20q. Conversely, MGCT of adolescents most commonly showed gain of 12p, 21, X, and loss of 13. Genetic aberrations consistent with Klinefelter's syndrome were restricted to adolescents.

The prognosis of young children with mediastinal malignant MGCTs is comparable to other non-gonadal sites. These tumours are characterized by female predominance and YST histology. In contrast, during adolescence, patients are almost exclusively male, may suffer from Klinefelter's syndrome, show composite histology and are at higher risk. The genetic profiles correspond to gonadal tumours of the respective age groups.

Supported by Deutsche Krebshilfe, Maryland Children's Cancer Foundation, and American Cancer Association.

28. Intracranial Malignant Germ Cell Tumours (CNS GCTs): Interim Results of the SIOP Trial

G. Calamınus[1], M.L. Garré[2], J.R. Mann[3], C. Patte[4], R. Kortmann[5],
J. Nicholson[6], F. Saran[7], U. Riccardi[8], D. Frappaz[9], C. Alapetite[10],
U. Göbel[1] for the SIOP CNS GCT group

*University Children's Hospitals, 1. Düsseldorf, 2. Genua, 3. Birmingham, 4. Institut
Gustave-Roussy, Villejuif, 5. University Tübingen, 6 Cambridge, 7. Sutton, 8. Torino,
9. Lyon, 10. Institut Curie, Paris*

Aims

A European protocol for malignant CNS GCTs was initiated in 1996. The purpose was to compare patients with germinoma treated either with reduced craniospinal irradiation (CSI) (24 Gy craniospinal/16 Gy tumour boost) or with a combined therapy (2 courses Carbo PEI) and focal irradiation (40 Gy). In non-germinomatous malignant tumours (choriocarcinoma, yolk sac tumours, embryonal carcinoma) (sGCTs) the efficacy of intensive preoperative chemotherapy (4 courses PEI) followed by radiotherapy was investigated. Irradiation was either focal (54 Gy) if negative spinal MRI and negative CSF–cytology, or CSI in metastatic patients (30 Gy CSI/24 Gy tumour boost). Measurement of markers was mandatory. Elevated markers in serum or CSF (ß-HCG > 50 IU/l, AFP > 25 ng/ml) together with an intracranial primary suggested the clinical diagnosis of a sGCTs.

Patients

We assessed 96 patients with germinoma and 48 patients with sGCTs diagnosed before 1.1.2000. Intracranial metastases were found in 15 per cent of the germinoma and 18 per cent of the sGCTs patients. Spinal metatastasis were diagnosed in 3 per cent of the germinoma and 8 per cent of the sGCT patients. A positive CSF-cytology was apparent at diagnosis in 15 per cent of germinoma and 20 per cent of sGCT patients. Information on increased markers at diagnosis was available in 80 per cent of the sGCT patients. There was information about markers in the CSF in 60 per cent of the patients with sGCTs. Seventy-four patients with germinoma received CSI, 22 had combined treatment. Seventeen patients with sGCTs received CSI after chemotherapy, 31 were focally irradiated.

Results

4/96 patients with germinoma had a relapse, 3 after CSI and 1 after combined treatment (event free survival (EFS) 95 per cent resp. 96 per cent). Relapses were locoregional. All except one was salvaged by additional treatment. 16/48 patients with sGCTs had a relapse, 4 after CSI and 12 after focal radiotherapy (EFS 74 per cent resp. 44 per cent). Relapses were mainly combined (locoregional and spinal). One recurrence in non-metastatic sGCTs occured 51 months after diagnosis. Only one child with spinal relapse after focal radiotherapy was salvaged by high dose chemotherapy and radiotherapy. Two other patients are on treatment, 13 died of their disease. Long-term side effects were mainly endocrinological in suprasellar primaries, whereas effects on motor, cognitive and psychomotor functions as well as cerebral nerve palsies appeared in pineal tumours.

Conclusions

Germinoma: CSI and chemotherapy + irradiation is equally effective. Non-Germinoma: The combination of intensive chemotherapy and focal radiotherapy does not sufficiently control the locoregional and the spinal area, whereas the combination of chemotherapy and CSI reduces the risk of locoregional and spinal relapse. Long-term effects are strongly related to the primary tumour site.

Supported in part by Deutsche Krebshilfe

29. Treatment of Primary Intracranial Germ Cell Tumours with Carboplatin-based Chemotherapy and Focal Irradiation

C. Patte*, D. Frappaz, M.A. Raquin, E. Bouffet, C. Kalifa*,
M.C. Baranzelli on behalf of the Société Française d'Oncologie
Pédiatrique (SFOP)

* IGR, Villejuif, France

In the SFOP TC-90 and TC-92 protocols, patients with intracranial germinomas and secreting germ cell tumours (sGCT) were treated with a combination of chemotherapy and focal radiotherapy. One chemotherapy cycle included alternating Carboplatin-VP16 and Ifosfamide-VP16. Germinoma patients received two cycles followed by 40 Gy focal radiotherapy, and sGCT three or four cycles followed by focal 55 Gy. Metastatic patients received craniospinal radiotherapy.

One hundred and eighteen patients, median age 13 years, were registered between 1990 and 1999: 80 germinomas (two associated with mature and one with immature teratoma) and 38 sGCT. Twelve tumours were bifocal and 17 metastatic.

Eight patients had protocol deviations, including high dose (HD) chemotherapy without radiotherapy in two metastatic germinomas. All germinomas responded to chemotherapy. All sGCT patients except two (including one early perioperative death), achieved biological remission. Twenty patients underwent surgery for residual masses, which were teratoma or fibrosis. Twenty-two patients relapsed. Eight of them died of tumour progression. Relapses in germinomas were later (median delay 29 months, range 9-56) and in ventricles compared to the sGCT (median 11months, range 6-30, mainly spinal). One sGCT patient died of MDS. Median follow-up is 62 months (5-103). The event-free and overall survivals were 77 per cent (+/-8) and 90 per cent (+/-5) for the whole population, 83 per cent (+/-9) and 98 per cent (+/-3) for germinomas, and 67 per cent (+/-14) and 78 per cent (+/-14) for sGCT.

30. Patterns of Relapse Following Focal Irradiation of Intracranial Germinoma: Critical Review of TGM-TC90 SFOP protocol

C. Alapetite[1], C. Carrie[2], H. Brisse[1], P. Thiesse[2], J-L. Habrand[3], J-C. Cuilliere[4], V. Moncho[5], G. Gaboriaud[1], D. Frappaz[2], M-C. Baranzelli[5], C. Patte[3] on behalf of the French Society for Paediatric Oncology (SFOP)

1.Institut Curie, Paris, 2 C.L.B., Lyon, 3 Institut G. Roussy, Villejuif, 4 C.R.G., Nantes, 5 C.O.L., Lille, France

In the SFOP protocol TGM-TC90 for localised tumours, craniospinal (CS) prophylactic radiotherapy fields were replaced by carboplatin-based chemotherapy together with focal irradiation of the initial tumour volume (40 Gy). Metastatic tumours received CS irradiation and a local boost. In order to refine radiation-treatment volumes, patterns of relapse with respect to radiation technique were documented.

Initial and relapse MR/CT scans and radiation treatment planning were reviewed. Seventy-nine patients were registered between 1990-1999. The median age was 13 yrs (5–24 yrs). At 62 months, overall survival and event free survival were 97 per cent and 82 per cent respectively. Nine of 73 patients treated according to the protocol relapsed : 8/62 (13 per cent) of the initially localised disease and 1/11 of the metastatic patients. Median time to relapse was 29 months (10–56m). Six relapses occurred in the supratentorial ventricular system (combined with tumour bed in 2, positive CSF in 1, posterior fossa in 1). These relapses were all partly or exclusively outside the radiation field. In 2 cases, distant leptomeningeal relapses occurred (bulbo-medullary junction and medullary axis). The metastatic patient who received 36 Gy CS radiation and 45 Gy to the primary site relapsed at the primary site only. No extra-CNS relapses were observed. Treatment of relapses included high dose chemotherapy and re-irradiation in 6/9 patients.

Conclusions

Subependymal infiltration relapses were observed in 6/9 cases. Expected benefits of both approaches for prophylaxis – chemotherapy (and focal irradiation) or large volume irradiation – should be balanced against their respective toxicities. Enlargement of prophylactic radiation volume to the ventricles should be considered, particularly in older patients.

31. Impact of Residual Lesions in Intracranial Germinoma – Interim Results from the SIOP CNS GCT 96 Study

S. Eisert[1], J. Nicholson[2], F. Saran[3], M. L. Garré[4], D. Frappaz[5], U. Göbel[1], G. Calaminus[1], for the study group

Children's University Hospitals: 1 Düsseldorf, 2 Cambridge, 3 Sutton, 4 Genova, 5 Lyon

Aims

The significance of residual lesions after therapy for intracranial germinomas remains a controversial issue [1]. We therefore assessed: a) the frequency of residual tumour after surgery, b) the frequency of residual abnormalities after radiotherapy (RT) and during follow-up and c) the impact of residual lesions on patient outcome.

Patients and Methods

One hundred and sixteen patients enrolled in the SIOP CNS GCT 96 Study for the treatment of an intracranial germinoma were studied. Sufficient information about residual lesions was available in 82 (median age 12 years). Tumour location was: 34 pineal region, 29 suprasellar region, 19 bifocal. Eighteen patients had metastatic disease (9 with cranial metastases, 2 with spinal metastases and 9 with positive CSF cytology). Fifty patients underwent open surgery: 11 had complete and 39 only partial tumour resection. In 31 patients, the histological diagnosis was made by stereotactic biopsy.

Sixty patients were treated according to option A of the study protocol. They received RT only (24 Gy craniospinal irradiation + 16 Gy tumour boost). The other 22 underwent combined treatment (option B) consisting of 2 courses of CarboPEI chemotherapy (CT) + 40 Gy focal RT. Follow-up ranged from 5-85 months. The incidence of residual lesions was evaluated after surgery, 3-6 months after RT, and during follow-up.

Results

We found residual tumour after surgery in 70/82 patients (85 per cent). In 19 (23 per cent), there was still some radiographic abnormality after RT. The size of these lesions ranged from 0.3 to 2 cm. In 8/19 patients the lesion resolved spontaneously between 10 and 35 months. In 9/19 patients, the size of the lesion remained stable or decreased. Tumour site, metastatic disease and treatment option did not affect the incidence of residual lesions after therapy. Surgical management such as partial resection vs. stereotactic biopsy did not influence the frequency of residual abnormalities. No patient with residual abnormality after RT underwent surgery or received any additional therapy. None of these patients developed progressive disease (mean follow-up 28 months) whereas 5 (8 per cent) without a residual lesion after surgery and/or RT had a relapse.

Conclusion

Residual lesions after therapy are common in intracranial germinomas. They are not apparently associated with a risk of early relapse. Therefore, a watch and wait strategy seems appropriate, at least in patients with residual lesions of less than 2 cm after RT. Residual lesions will be routinely assessed in germinomatous and non-germinomatous GCTs in the SIOP CNS GCT 2002 study to further evaluate the risk.

Supported in part by Deutsche Krebshilfe

Reference

1. Weiner HL, Finlay JL. Surgery in the management of primary intracranial germ cell tumors. *Childs Nerv Syst.* 1999;15:770–3

32. Failure of Treatment in Childhood Extracranial and Extratesticular Malignant Germ Cell Tumours (MGCT)

M. Lo Curto*, P. D'Angelo, G. Turdo, P. Dall'Igna, I. Mazzarino, M. Conte, A. Sandri, G. Bernini, T. De Laurentis, A. Di Cataldo, M.G. Fugardi, F. Siracusa, G. Cecchetto, for AIEOP TCG Cooperative Study

*Dipartimenta Materno Infantile, Palermo, Italy

Platinum based chemotherapy improves the cure rate of patients with MGCT [1, 2] to over 80 per cent, but tumour recurrence is associated with an unfavourable prognosis. We sought to identify factors predictive of poor outcome following relapse.

Methods

We investigated the clinical features at first presentation and at relapse in 21 patients, seven of whom remained in second remission after treatment and 14 with poor outcome.

Results

The parameters at first presentation and at relapse of the 21 patients (16 females, 5 males) are shown in tables 32.1 and 32.2. Levels of AFP, HCG and LDH were not predictive of progression. The features more commonly associated with progression following relapse were: extragonadal site of the primary tumour, stage IV, incomplete resection and incomplete response to primary treatment. All patients had local

Table 32.1

Pt	Site	Histology	Stage	Primary surgery	Subsequent surgery	Treatment	Remission (months)
1	Ovary	YST	IIIb	P	P	CT+RT	52
2	Ovary	G	II	C	–	RT	15
12	SC	YST	IIIc	B	C	CT+RT	36
15	SC	YST	IV	B	C	CT+RT	24
18	Ovary	YST	IIIb	P	C	CT	12
20	Ovary	M+T	I	C	–	CT	6
21	SC	YST+EC	IIIc	B	C	CT	6

Table 32.2

Pt	Site	Histology	Stage	Primary surgery	Subsequent surgery	Treatment	Death (months)
3	SC	YST	IV	B	–	CT	8
4	SC	YST	IV	B	P	CT	10
5	Other	YST	IIIc	B	–	CT	5
6	SC	M+T	IIIc	B	P	CT	14
7	SC	M+T	IIIb	P	P	CT+RT	20
8	Ovary	G	IV	B	P	CT	20
9	SC	YST	IV	B	C	CT+RT	37
10	SC	YST	IV	P	–	CT	16
11	Ovary	YST	IIIb	P	–	CT	20
13	SC	YST	IV	B	P	CT	2
14	Other	YST	IV	B	–	CT	16
16	SC	M+T	IIIb	P	–	Nil	23
17	SC	M+T	IIIb	P	P	CT	32
19	Other	YST	IIIc	B	P	Nil	14

SC = sacrococcygeal   YST = yolk sac tumour   P = partial resection
CT = chemotherapy   G = germinoma   C = complete resection
RT = radiotherapy   M = malignant germ cell tumour   B = biopsy
    T = teratoma
    EC = embryonal carcinoma

recurrence and distant metastases developed in eight, one of whom achieved a second remission (patient 15). Cure was only achieved in patients who underwent both surgery and chemotherapy. Radiotherapy appeared to provide additional benefit.

Conclusions

In agreement with recent data [3], complete resection of the recurrent mass appeared to be the major determinant of long-term remission.

References

1. Mann J.R., Raafat F., Robinson K. et al. The U.K. C.C.S.G. Second Germ Cell Tumor Study: Carboplatin, Etoposide and Bleomycin are Effective Treatments for Children with Malignant Extracranial Germ Cell Tumors, with Acceptable Toxicity. *J. Clin. Oncol.* 2000;18:3809–3818
2. Marina M., Fontanesi J., Kun L. et al. Treatment of Childhood Germ Cell Tumors; Review of the St. Jude Experience from 1979 to 1988. *Cancer* 1992;70:2568–2575
3. Schneider D.T., Wessalowski R., Calaminus G. et al. Treatment of Recurrent Malignant Sacrococcygeal Germ Cell Tumors: Analysis of 22 Patients Registered in the German Protocols MAKEI 83/86, 89 and 96. *J. Clin. Oncol.* 2001;19:1951–1960

Section 5

Current Status – Surgery

33. Surgery for Germ Cell Tumours: Current Status in the USA

R.S. Foster, R. Bihrle, J.P. Donohue

Indiana University Medical Center, 535 N. Barnhill Drive, Ste. 420, Indianapolis, Indiana, USA, 46202

No nationwide registry exists for the treatment of testis tumours in the United States. The American Cancer Society estimates that in 2001 there will be 7200 new cases of testicular cancer and 400 deaths attributed to testis cancer [1]. Because testis cancer is a relatively rare tumour, a few referral centers in the United States provide the bulk of surgical care for these patients. As mentioned, because no nationwide registry exists for the treatment of these patients, the material presented herein is based upon abstracts and presentations from referral centers and the experience of the authors from Indiana University.

This presentation will concern the authors' impressions of differences in surgical treatment compared to the previous Germ Cell Tumour Conference IV in Leeds in 1997. We have chosen to categorize this discussion into three basic areas: the treatment of the local tumour when discovered in the testis, evolving concepts in early stage disease and, finally, trends in post chemotherapy surgery.

Primary Local Surgery

Radical inguinal orchiectomy has been the standard treatment for a solid intratesticular mass suspicious for being a germ cell tumour. This remains generally the case in the United States. However, based upon the European experience with partial orchiectomy in highly selected patients with solid intratesticular masses, partial orchiectomy has gained acceptance in the United States. Patients with small second primary tumours are candidates for partial orchiectomy. Patients with a normal contralateral testis are not offered partial orchiectomy and instead undergo radical orchiectomy. Based on the German experience, after partial orchiectomy patients are routinely administered radiotherapy to minimize the chance of a local recurrence [2]. This effectively eliminates spermatogenesis but can over the long term preserve Leydig cell function. Therefore, it is the authors' impression that in this highly selected group of patients partial orchiectomy has gained acceptance in the United States.

Treatment of Early Stage Disease

Retroperitoneal Lymph Node Dissection Versus Surveillance

Formerly in the United States, most patients with clinical stage I non-seminoma were managed with retroperitoneal lymph node dissection (RPLND) and nerve sparing

139

techniques have more recently been introduced. The rationale for RPLND in clinical stage I non-seminoma was that it provided accurate staging and provided a therapeutic benefit for those patients with metastatic disease to retroperitoneal nodes. The staging benefit was important in that accurate pathological staging allowed an earlier definition of appropriate therapy and accelerated the time line for the course of the disease.

With increasing acceptance of surveillance as a management scheme in the United States, the staging benefit of RPLND in low stage disease is less important. Even if its diagnosis is deferred, metastatic disease can be treated effectively with "good risk" chemotherapy and therefore, except for the psychological benefit to some patients of defining the pathological stage, any potential therapeutic benefit of earlier pathological staging has diminished. However, the therapeutic benefit of RPLND remains for those patients with metastatic disease to retroperitoneal nodes as evidenced by cure rates with surgery alone in pathological stage IIA disease of 67 to 90 per cent, and around 50 per cent in pathological stage IIB disease [3, 4, 5]. Even in so called high risk patients who are found to have metastatic disease to the retroperitoneum, 65 to 70 per cent of patients are cured with RPLND alone [3].

It is well documented and recognized, however, that patients who have high risk features such as large amounts of embryonal carcinoma and/or vascular or lymphatic invasion are at slightly increased risk not only for lymphatic metastasis, but also haematogenous spread. In the Indiana University experience, this increased risk of haematogenous metastasis in high risk patients is approximately 5 to 10 per cent compared to low risk patients [3]. Unfortunately, we have no predictors of lymphatic metastasis as compared to haematogenous metastasis. Such a predictive ability would be desirable as patients could be more appropriately assigned to RPLND for lymphatic metastasis and chemotherapy for systemic metastasis. Efforts to improve this predictive ability are warranted. Currently the only strong predictor of haematogenous (systemic) metastasis is elevation of alpha fetoprotein and/or beta HCG in a patient otherwise felt to be clinical stage I [6, 7].

Currently at Indiana University, high risk patients are given the option of nerve sparing RPLND or surveillance as are all other clinical stage I patients. It is well recognized that approximately 50 per cent of high risk patients will have metastatic disease but the converse of this is that 50 per cent will not. In the Medical Research Council large trial of surveillance, patients with so called high risk features did just as well in terms of overall outcomes as did patients with low risk features who recurred and required chemotherapy [8]. Therefore, at Indiana University such high risk features do not mandate assignment to surveillance or nerve sparing RPLND and patients are given the choice of therapy as are all other clinical stage I patients.

Primary Chemotherapy in Early Stage Disease

Primary chemotherapy in high risk clinical stage I patients has not gained widespread acceptance in the United States. The reason for this is that such high risk patients have a 50 per cent chance of not having metastatic disease, and two other extremely effective alternatives (RPLND and surveillance) are available. Certainly special situations may warrant the use of primary chemotherapy, but in the overall population of informed patients who have access to medical care, it is felt that surveillance and nerve sparing RPLND are considered to be equivalent therapies. Historically, patients who underwent retroperitoneal lymph node dissection for low stage disease and who were found to have metastatic disease to retroperitoneal nodes were cured at the 50 to 70 per cent level, depending upon the volume of metastases. Such patients were offered two courses of adjuvant chemotherapy after RPLND, decreasing the risk of recurrence to less than 1 per cent. The rationale for such adjuvant therapy was that three courses of chemotherapy was associated with significantly more morbidity than two courses and therefore it was desirable to avoid a third course of chemotherapy because of marrow suppression, vomiting, etc. With newer anti-emetics and immune stimulants, the morbidity of three courses of chemotherapy is not significantly different from two courses. Therefore, at Indiana University, the current policy is to inform patients that if it is their desire to treat any metastatic disease with chemotherapy (as opposed to RPLND), a surveillance scheme should be undertaken with three courses of chemotherapy administered at relapse. Patients who choose RPLND are informed that the reason for proceeding with RPLND is to treat any metastatic disease surgically. Such patients are observed after RPLND and only those patients who recur are administered three courses of chemotherapy.

Therefore, in terms of clinical stage I non-seminoma, patients are given the choice between nerve sparing RPLND and surveillance regardless of the presence or absence of high risk features. The only strong argument for mandating RPLND is non-germ cell cancerous elements in the orchiectomy specimen. Furthermore, it is felt that staging is less of an issue compared to former times and that the major benefits of nerve sparing RPLND are avoidance of chemotherapy and the psychological benefit of earlier definition of therapy. Patients who choose RPLND are strongly encouraged to undergo surveillance if proven to be pathological stage II. Patients who have no objection to treating any metastatic disease with chemotherapy are advised that surveillance, as opposed to primary chemotherapy, is a very reasonable option.

Laparoscopic Retroperitoneal Lymph Node Dissection

The option of laparoscopic RPLND in order to decrease hospitalization time and hopefully allow an earlier return to full activity exists in the United States as in Europe. It is recognized that there is a learning curve for a surgeon to attain skill at laparoscopic RPLND and therefore if such a procedure is considered, it should be performed in an institution where there is significant prior experience with the procedure.

As currently practiced in the United States, if pathological stage II disease is identified at laparoscopic RPLND, patients are routinely administered postoperative chemotherapy, usually either two or three courses of Bleomycin, Etoposide, and Cisplatin (BEP) [9, 10]. Based upon the published literature from the United States and abstracts presented at national meetings, only a few patients who have refused postoperative chemotherapy have had the possibility of surgical cure with laparoscopy in pathological stage II disease. Therefore, it is impossible to know the therapeutic benefit of removing involved retroperitoneal lymph nodes. Whether or not this will be tested in the future is unclear.

Two series of laparoscopic RPLND in clinical stage I from Europe have presented hospitalization times. The mean hospital times in the series of Rassweiler was 5.3 days [10]; the experience of Januszek et al. showed an average hospitalization of 3.3 days [11]. We recently compiled the mean hospitalization for the most recent 25 cases of primary nerve sparing RPLND at Indiana University and post chemotherapy RPLND at Indiana University. The mean hospitalization time for primary RPLND was 3.3 days; mean hospitalization for post chemotherapy RPLND was six days.

Therefore, it appears there is little difference in hospitalization times between laparoscopic RPLND and open RPLND.

As currently practiced, it appears the only two benefits of laparoscopic RPLND are firstly a different abdominal scar (Trochar insertion marks as opposed to a midline incision), and secondly a probable earlier return to full activity. Data on return to full activity is very difficult to assemble. In a paper from several investigators in the United States, patients returned to "full activity" after a mean of 17 days [9]. If this is substantiated worldwide, laparoscopic RPLND is very likely to offer a quicker return to full activity compared to open RPLND. Currently patients around the world must determine whether or not this putative benefit is important to them, especially if they are treated with a staging procedure (laparoscopic RPLND) and a separate therapeutic procedure (two or three courses of BEP postoperatively). Nevertheless, if laparoscopic RPLND is shown to be therapeutically equivalent to open RPLND and is equivalent in all other measures but allows a more rapid return to full activity it may become the standard. However, since current standard treatment offers a 98 to 99 per cent chance for cure, laparoscopic RPLND must reach this very high standard and any poor outcomes associated with it (surgical misadventures or more significant morbidity from higher dose chemotherapy) should be monitored if the therapeutic capability of laparoscopic RPLND is to be proven.

Treatment of Advanced Disease

Traditionally patients who present with metastatic germ cell cancer have been treated with three or four courses of good risk chemotherapy. Such patients who have normalization of serum markers but who have persistent radiographic tumour undergo post chemotherapy RPLND. Formerly, when post chemotherapy RPLND was performed in such patients, fibrosis was identified pathologically in approximately 45 per cent of residual masses, teratoma in 40 to 45 per cent and other germ cell malignancy in 5 to 10 per cent. At Indiana University, patients with metastatic testis cancer who are treated with good risk chemotherapy and who experience a clinical complete remission are observed. Only around 5 per cent of these patients recur. At some other centers, including Memorial Sloan-Kettering, patients with clinical complete remission undergo post chemotherapy RPLND if the initial retroperitoneal tumour diameter was 3 cm. or greater [12]. This controversy remains in the United States.

Lumpectomy Versus Complete Lymphadenectomy

Another pertinent issue in post chemotherapy RPLND is whether or not lumpectomy is equivalent to full RPLND. Certainly, there are some patients who have only a single focus of teratoma in the retroperitoneum and lumpectomy in this situation is likely to be adequate. On the other hand, in centers around the world where lumpectomy rather than complete clearance is standard practice, there is some evidence to suggest that local recurrence is more frequent, indicating that microscopic foci of unresected disease can remain and grow [13]. The early mapping studies suggested that in patients with reasonably high volume retroperitoneal tumour there is a likelihood of bilateral disease [14]. Currently at Indiana University, post chemotherapy RPLND is a full bilateral dissection with removal of all lymphatic tissue and tumour from ureter to ureter, from crus to bifurcation of iliac arteries. In patients with low volume disease, nerve sparing is usually employed, preserving the emission and ejaculation of these patients. In good risk patients, local recurrence is extremely rare. Therefore, the rationale for full bilateral rather than limited RPLND is that there is no increase in morbidity but there is a potential gain through removal of additional nodes containing microscopic foci of tumour.

Complicated Post Chemotherapy Resections

It is the impression of the authors that referral centers in the United States are also providing care for an increasing number of patients designated as complicated post chemotherapy RPLND. These patients are those who have elevated tumour markers but localized retroperitoneal tumour and have failed all chemotherapy. These patients are described as desperation RPLND patients. Two other categories of complicated post chemotherapy RPLND patients are re-do procedures and patients with late relapse.

Data from Indiana University from 1996 to 2000 has revealed that the number of primary RPLNDs performed on a yearly basis has fallen from 46 per cent to 26 per cent of all RPLNDs. The absolute number of post chemotherapy RPLNDs has risen from 62 in 1996 to 116 in the year 2000. This provides objective evidence that in referral centers, a higher proportion of RPLNDs are post chemotherapy surgeries. Analysis of the pathology of the last 100 post chemotherapy RPLNDs performed at Indiana University, showed fibrosis in 31 per cent of resected retroperitoneal tumours, teratoma in 53 per cent, and other germ cell malignancy in 16 per cent. Of the latter, ten patients had yolk sac tumour, four embryonal carcinoma, and two choriocarcinoma. Also, 10 per cent of patients in this series required resection of the vena cava. Although these figures may represent a referral bias, they provide interesting information as to the increasingly complicated nature of post chemotherapy RPLNDs seen at referral centers in the United States.

Re-do Procedures

The experience with re-do RPLND at Indiana University from 1975 to 1993 has been described [15]. Two hundred and two such patients were presented, of whom 14 were lost to follow up. Pathologically, 40 per cent had mature teratoma in the specimen, 37 per cent had another germ cell malignancy, and 23 per cent necrosis. At the time of analysis, approximately 55 per cent of these patients were disease free.

More recently two other centers reported their experience with re-do RPLND. These presentations were at the American Urological Association National Meeting in 2001. Investigators from M.D. Anderson presented nineteen patients, two of whom required an aortic graft. Fifteen of nineteen had germ cell malignancy in the operative specimen, and at a median of sixty months postoperatively twelve of nineteen (63 per cent) were disease free [16]. Similarly, investigators from Memorial Sloan-Kettering presented fifty cases of re-do RPLNDs [17]. Fifty per cent of these had germ cell malignancy in the specimen or teratoma with somatic malignant transformation. The median follow-up was 6.6 years, and 71 per cent of patients were disease free. The experience of these three centers with re-do RPLND has shown that the procedure is feasible and is associated with acceptable morbidity. Hence, patients who have incompletely resected tumours at original RPLND and have disease restricted to the retroperitoneum should be referred to centers experienced in performing these re-do procedures.

Desperation Procedures

A second category of complicated post chemotherapy RPLND is so called desperation RPLND. These are patients with elevated alpha fetoprotein, beta HCG, and localized retroperitoneal tumour who have failed chemotherapeutic attempts at marker normalization. The Indiana experience with such patients was presented at the American Urological Association National Meeting in 2001 [18]. One hundred and fourteen patients were identified with localized retroperitoneal tumour and elevated alpha fetoprotein, beta HCG, or both. Complete resection was achieved in all but three patients. All patients were followed-up for at least two years. Sixty-one of these 114 patients had germ cell malignancy in the surgical specimen and therefore really were desperation RPLNDs, and the remainder did not. This experience, along with the experience of other investigators from around the world, has shown that not all patients with elevated tumour markers and tumour restricted to the retroperitoneum and who undergo RPLND have germ cell malignancy in the resected specimen.

In the Indiana series of patients with elevated tumour markers and malignancy in the specimen, patients were divided into two groups: either surgery after induction chemotherapy alone or after both induction and salvage chemotherapy. Of 14 patients who underwent RPLND after induction therapy alone, four of nine (44 per cent) with elevated alpha fetoprotein and two of five (40 per cent) with elevated HCG were disease free with at least two years of follow up. Three of eight patients who received postoperative chemotherapy and three of six patients who did not receive postoperative chemotherapy are disease free. This difference is not significant.

The outcomes were similar in 44 patients who had desperation RPLND after induction and salvage chemotherapy. Ten of 23 patients (43 per cent) who had elevated AFP and two of 18 (11 per cent) who had elevated HCG were disease free. None of the three patients who had elevation of both markers were disease free. Considering postoperative chemotherapy in this group, six of 23 (26 per cent) who had postoperative chemotherapy were disease free. Conversely, six of 21 (29 per cent) who did not receive postoperative chemotherapy were disease free. This difference is also not significant. Therefore, overall, 18 of 58 patients (31 per cent) were disease free at the time of analysis. Morbidity was very acceptable in this group of patients. In these complicated patients who have failed attempts at chemotherapeutic cure, roughly 30 per cent of the patients who have germ cell malignancy in the operative specimen can be cured with desperation RPLND.

Late Relapse

Late relapse is defined as recurrence after more than two years following initial successful therapy of testis cancer. Presumably, it is due to indolent cells, which were unresected and reactivate. It is well recognized that most of these patients are not cured with chemotherapy alone and it is similarly well known that around 2 to 5 per cent of all testis cancer patients will experience a late recurrence. Recently the Indiana experience with late relapse has been updated [19]. Originally in 1995, 81 patients were analysed with a median time to late relapse of 6.2 years. Thirty five of 81 (43 per cent) were disease free and but only two following chemotherapy alone. Seventy seven additional patients have been identified who have been treated for late relapse at Indiana University from 1995 to 2000. Median time to late relapse was seven years. Forty three of 77 (56 per cent) are disease free, eight with chemotherapy alone but six of these eight patients had not received chemotherapy prior to late relapse.

Recently at the American Urological Association meeting in 2001 the surgical experience with late relapse at Memorial Sloan-Kettering was presented [20]. These investigators stated that the number of late relapses seen at Memorial Sloan-Kettering has doubled in the last ten years. Furthermore, they stated that over 50 per cent of patients referred for late relapse had retroperitoneal masses after induction chemotherapy, which were observed. Only 24 of 50 late relapses could be completely resected at RPLND.

It therefore appears that patients with late relapse are increasingly being seen at referral centers in the United States. Whether this represents a better recognition of the entity, a referral bias, or a true increase in late relapse is unknown. Late relapse is an intriguing biological phenomenon and should be studied in the basic science laboratory to gain insights as to the mechanisms of chemo-resistance.

Conclusions

With the limitations of not having a national tumour registry for the surgical treatment of testis cancer, it is the authors' opinion that the following issues regarding the surgical treatment of testis cancer has emerged since the previous Germ Cell Conference at Leeds.

1. Partial orchiectomy is accepted in the United States in selected patients.
2. Surveillance and nerve sparing RPLND are seen as equivalent therapeutic modalities.
3. There may be an increase in the number of patients seen at referral centers with more complicated post chemotherapy RPLNDs such as desperation, re-do, and late relapses; however, this simply could represent referral bias.
4. The biology of late relapse needs to be better studied and elucidated.

References

1. Greenlee RT, Hill-Harmon B, Murray T, Thun M. *Cancer statistics*, 2001. CA 2001;51:15.
2. Heidenreich A, Holtl W, Albrecht W, Pont J, Engelmann UH. Testis-preserving surgery in bilateral testicular germ cell tumours. *Brit J Urol* 1997;79:253.
3. Sweeney CJ, Hermans BP, Heilman DK, Foster RS, Donohue JP, Einhorn LH. Results and outcome of retroperitoneal lymph node dissection for clinical stage I embryonal carcinoma – predominant testis cancer. *J Clin Oncol* 2000;18:358.
4. Richie J, Kantoff PW. Is adjuvant chemotherapy necessary for patients with stage B1 testicular cancer? *J Clin Oncol* 1991;9:1393.
5. Rabbani F, Sheinfeld J, Farivar-Mohsen H et al: Low volume nodal metastases detected at retroperitoneal lymphadenectomy for testicular cancer: Pattern and prognostic factors for relapse. *J Clin Oncol* 2001;19:2020.
6. Saxman SB, Nichols CR, Foster RS, Messemer JE, Donohue JP, Einhorn LH. The management of patients with clinical stage I nonseminomatous testicular tumours and persistently elevated serologic markers. *J Urol* 1996;155:587.
7. Davis BE, Herr HW, Fair WR, Bosl GJ. The management of patients with nonseminomatous germ cell tumours of the testis with serologic disease only after orchiectomy. *J Urol* 1994;152:111.
8. Read G, Stenning SP, Cullen MC et al. Medical Research Council Prospective Study of surveillance for stage I testicular teratoma. *J Clin Oncol* 1992;10:1762.
9. Nelson JB, Chen RN, Bishoff JT et al. Laparoscopic retroperitoneal lymph node dissection for clinical stage I nonseminomatous germ cell testicular tumours. *Urology* 1999;54:1064.
10. Rossweiler JJ, Frede T, Lenz E, Seeman O, Alken P. Long term experience with laparoscopic retroperitoneal lymph node dissection in the management of low stage testis cancer. *Eur Urol* 2000;37:251.

11. Janetschek G: Laparoscopic retroperitoneal lymph node dissection. Evolution of a new technique. *World J Urol* 2000;18:267.
12. Toner G, Panicek D, Heelan R et al. Adjunctive surgery after chemotherapy for nonseminomatous germ cell tumours: Recommendation for patient selection. *J Clin Oncol* 1990;8:1683.
13. Horwich A, Norman A, Fisher C, Hendry WF, Nicholls J, Dearnaley DP. Primary chemotherapy for stage II nonseminomatous germ cell tumours of the testis. *J Urol* 1994;151:72.
14. Donohue J, Zachary J, Maynard B. Distribution of nodal metastases in nonseminomatous testicular cancer. *J Urol* 1982;128:315.
15. Donohue JP, Leibovitch I, Foster RS, Baniel J, Tognoni P. Integration of surgery and systemic therapy: Results and principles of integration. *Sem in Urol Oncol* 1998;16:65.
16. Kim R, Sexton WJ, Wood CG, Pisters LL. Repeat retroperitoneal lymph node dissection for metastatic testis cancer. American Urological Association National Meeting 2001; Abstract 628.
17. McKiernan JM, Sheinfeld J, Bacik J, Motzer RJ, Bajorin DF, Bosl GJ. Reoperative RPLND for germ cell tumour: Initial presentation, complications, and outcome. American Urological Association National Meeting 2001;Abstract 627.
18. Beck SD, Foster RS, Bihrle R et al. Post chemotherapy desperation retroperitoneal lymph node dissection for patients with elevated tumour markers. American Urological Association National Meeting 2001;Abstract 632.
19. George D, Foster R, Hromas R et al. Update on late relapse (LR) of germ cell tumours (GCT): A clinical and molecular analysis. *Proc Am Soc Clin Oncol* 2001;20:Abstract 689.
20. Sheinfeld J. Late recurrence of testicular cancer. American Urological Association National Meeting 2001; Plenary Session 2, June 4, 2001.

34. Surgery for Testicular Cancer: UK and European Experience

David Kirk

Urology Department, Gartnavel General Hospital, Glasgow G12 0YN

Introduction

Surgery for metastatic testis cancer is done for several reasons. It gives diagnostic information, especially in staging apparent stage 1 disease, it provides prognostic information by defining the pathological results of chemotherapy, and, most importantly, is done therapeutically, to remove residual viable disease. The purpose of this article is to define European practice, for comparison with that in the USA, as described elsewhere by Foster and colleagues. The author will, of necessity, provide the most detailed information on UK, rather than general European, practice, using data, involving 909 patients (Table 34.1), from a survey carried out of the majority of British centres performing surgery for metastatic testis cancer [1].

Primary Surgery

Staging retroperitoneal lymph node dissection in stage 1 disease is a procedure little practiced in Europe. Primary surgery for low volume disease is generally not considered an option. Most European oncologists consider that such surgery would not obviate the need for subsequent chemotherapy and that chemotherapy alone may be curative in many of these patients. However, there may be a subgroup of patients in whom primary surgery, with subsequent surveillance, would be an option, a topic possibly worthy of a future clinical trial. Despite this, in the UK and Europe, surgery is most commonly performed following chemotherapy, and will be the main concern of this article.

Table 34.1: UK Survey – Case numbers by year (total 909)

Year	Number	Year	Number
1990	80	1994	114
1991	97	1995	125
1992	91	1996	158
1993	108	1997	136

Surgery for Seminoma

Post chemotherapy surgery is normally considered to be most appropriate in non-seminomatous germ cell tumours (NSGCT). The high chemosensitivity of seminoma means that most residual masses will be necrotic. Also, the tumour is typically infiltrative and often poorly defined at surgery, making complete resection difficult. Finally, radiotherapy is available for salvage. However, a recent publication described a group of patients with well defined masses over 3 cm in diameter in whom resection is relatively simple, and in which 55 per cent will demonstrate viable residual tumour [2]. In the author's own practice, patients with seminoma are now considered more critically for surgery. It is also clear that some patients in whom the primary tumour is considered pure seminoma may harbour NSGCT, which manifests itself in a metastatic pattern typical of that tumour type. Each case should be considered on its merits, and emphasises the importance of close and regular contact between surgeon and oncologist, as discussed later. To what extent practice in the surgical management of seminoma generally is changing is unclear – as shown in Table 34.2, very few cases were reported in the survey.

The British Survey

The British survey collected data retrospectively from 1990–1997 on 909 patients from 15 centres (Table 34.1). Individual totals of cases varied from 4 to 211. During the period surveyed, only two surgeons had operated on over100 patients, (with four between 50 and 99), although taking into account operations performed outside the study period, there were four surgeons with personal series of over 100 cases. Five operated on more than 10 patients per year. As this was a retrospective study, in many cases the data were incomplete in some respects, accounting for apparent discrepancies in numbers reported below.

Indications for Surgery Post Chemotherapy

Response to chemotherapy is monitored by measurement of tumour markers and by serial CT scans. In most centres, it is the patient in whom there is still a detectable mass on the post chemotherapy CT who is considered for surgery. However, a small proportion of patients with complete resolution on CT will have undetected residual disease [3], and the majority of these will relapse. Is there a case for routine surgery

Table 34.2: UK Survey – Pathology (n = 860)

Pathology	Number	Percentage	Range
Necrosis	249	29	10–60
Differentiated teratoma	395	46	30–63
Other NSGCT	205	24	10–33
Seminoma	4	1	
Adenocarcinoma or sarcoma developing from teratoma differentiated	7		

in all patients to detect these few? The consensus would be that this proportion is too small to justify routine surgery when in more than 90 per cent it will prove to have been unnecessary, and when careful surveillance will enable those who do relapse to be successfully salvaged [4]. However, Fosså and her colleagues consider that routine post chemotherapy surgery in all patients is justified since in their practice they find 20 per cent of residual masses of 2cms or less will contain mature teratoma/residual germ cell malignancy. Operating on all these patients reduces the need for follow-up CTs, and is particularly advantageous where follow-up takes place in non-cancer centres [5]. However, this position is under review, as more effective modern chemotherapy may well reduce the percentage of patients with residual malignancy (Fosså, personal communication).

As reported elsewhere in this volume, models are being developed to predict the pathology of residual masses, based on a number of factors including histology of the primary tumour, the pre-chemotherapy markers, the response to treatment and the size of residual mass. The aim is mainly to avoid unnecessary operations where complete necrosis has occurred [6]. These models do not appear yet to be in general routine use, and management decisions are usually based on the size of any residual disease mass. In the British survey, four centres operated on residual masses of any size, two on masses greater than 1.5cm and five only on masses greater than 2cm. The remaining centres did not apply rigid rules.

Outcome

Pathological data was available on 611 patients in the survey (Table 34.2). Although the overall distribution of necrosis, differentiated teratoma and germ cell malignancy is similar to that in the literature [7], there is considerable variation from centre to centre. Whether this reflects differences in chemotherapy regimes, different selection criteria for surgery, or is merely a statistical quirk in centres with small numbers is not clear. Survival data were available for 703 patients. Ninety percent were alive, 83 per cent disease free and 7 per cent with tumour. Death was due to GCT (54 patients), treatment (10 patients), other tumour (4 patients) or unrelated causes (1 patient).

Surgical Strategies

There is general agreement that the ideal management of metastatic NSGT is to operate following chemotherapy, when tumour markers have returned to normal, and to completely excise the residual disease. In Glasgow we would describe this as *elective* surgery. However, this ideal is not always achievable. Sometimes, as judged by tumour markers, poor response occurs, and here we consider *interventional* surgery, in the hope that removing the tumour, and then completing the chemotherapy, will bring disease under control. Where either elective surgery has not been done because of complete remission, or relapse occurs after previous surgery, we would perform *salvage* surgery [8]. In general (Table 34.3) we have found interventional surgery successful with disease at one rather than multiple sites, in agreement with others [9]. In the British survey, seven respondents stated that they only operated if the markers had normalised, while eight would on occasion perform interventional surgery in poor responders.

Table 34.3: Outcome of interventional survery (Glasgow data)

	Disease free	Alive with disease	Dead	Total
RP disease only	5	1	0	6
RP and lung	0	1(?)	0	1
RP and pelvic	1	0	1	2
RP and liver	0	0	1	1
RP and mediastinal	0	1	2	3
Total	6	3	4	13

RP: Retroperitoneum

Other Surgical Issues

There remains discussion and disagreement about a number of issues relating to the surgical procedure itself.

Surgical Approach

The opinion in Britain concerning the best surgical approach is divided. In 11 centres the preferred incision was a mid-line, transabdominal approach. Two favoured a thoraco-abdominal approach and two used a chevron incision. Probably most surgeons will vary their approach depending on the technical problems posed by the disease process in each case.

"Lumpectomy" or Complete Retroperitoneal Dissection

There are those who simply excise the residual lump, probably in an attempt to reduce morbidity. Others will prefer in all cases to do a complete dissection fearing that para-aortic recurrence may lead to a more difficult second operation. While most UK surgeons adopt the former policy (12/15 in the survey), this may be partly a matter of semantics. The author will perform a complete dissection on the side of the tumour in most cases, but reserve bilateral dissection for those with bilateral disease. Perhaps the debate is more about the merits unilateral or bilateral dissection in disease apparently confined to one side.

Nerve Sparing Lymphadenectomy

The surgeon who only operates on post-chemotherapy cases is at a disadvantage here. It is in the staging lymphadenectomy for stage 1 disease, or primary surgery for early metastases that nerve sparing techniques are most easily learnt. Following chemotherapy, when only a proportion of cases are suitable, and some have substantial disease modified by chemotherapy, the scope for nerve sparing is reduced and opportunities to acquire the skill limited. Although only one of the survey respondents indicated that he does not attempt to preserve nerves, no information was available on success rates of the remainder.

Strategy for Dealing with Multiple Metastatic Sites

When there is disease in both abdomen and chest, should the urologist and the thoracic surgeon perform a joint operation, or should abdominal and thoracic disease be dealt with at separate sessions? The author and his thoracic surgical colleague have a pragmatic approach to the latter. Depending on the extent of the disease at each site, if a thoraco-abdominal incision gives adequate access to both disease sites, a joint approach is sensible, while when two, separate, long procedures are necessary, little is gained from a joint session. In the survey five respondents elected to operate on the abdomen first with the thoracic disease being dealt with at a separate operation. Four usually did a combined operation with a thoracic surgical colleague and with three the policy varied. One urologist removed pulmonary metastases himself.

Relapsed Disease

The final issue is the role of surgery in relapsed disease. There is little objective data on individual practice here, and further research and study of this difficult area is needed. However, surgery has a pivotal role in management of relapsed disease, and in late relapse, likely to be due to differentiated teratoma, it is probably the immediate choice. Where chemotherapy is used in early relapse, particularly in cases where surgery has not already been used, elective surgery, planned to coincide with the end of chemotherapy may be appropriate. In patients whose disease progresses on surveillance without previous chemotherapy, in suitable cases, for example cystic disease, a shortened course of chemotherapy with early surgery might be considered.

Surgery for Metastatic Testis Cancer – Who Should Do It?

It is generally recognised that a minimum caseload is necessary to achieve and maintain surgical expertise in complicated cancer surgery. Equally important is the communication and contact between oncologist and surgeon, resulting from joint clinics and/or conferences, made possible where both work in a Cancer Centre. In the survey, 11 respondents had either joint clinics or a review meeting (or both). The environment in which these cases are dealt with is critical, and more than just the expertise of the surgeon is essential for the best results. Peri-operative care is dependent on dedicated anaesthetic, theatre and ward staff. Flexible operating facilities to enable prompt attention in special circumstances (e.g. interventional operations), thoracic (and vascular) surgical support in complicated disease, appropriate ITU/HDU facilities, including epidural anaesthesia, and familiarity with the particular problems created by chemotherapy, particularly its chest complications, are all required.

As will be seen from Figure 34.1, the average number of cases operated per year in many centres per year in Britain is small. Indeed by the standards of the USA and large European centres, it could be argued that only one surgeon was doing enough cases. This in turn reflects the populations served by the various oncology services managing testicular cancer in the UK. If, in the interests of increasing case numbers, surgery alone were centralised, this would be at the expense of communication with the referring oncologist. The majority of the author's patients come through a joint clinic and he becomes involved at an early stage in their management. However, some patients are referred by oncologists from other areas, when communication, and opportunities to see the patient at an early stage are limited. As a result, the management of these patients can be more difficult.

The National Cancer Guidance Group and National Institute for Clinical Effectiveness are about to issue a framework for cancer services in England and

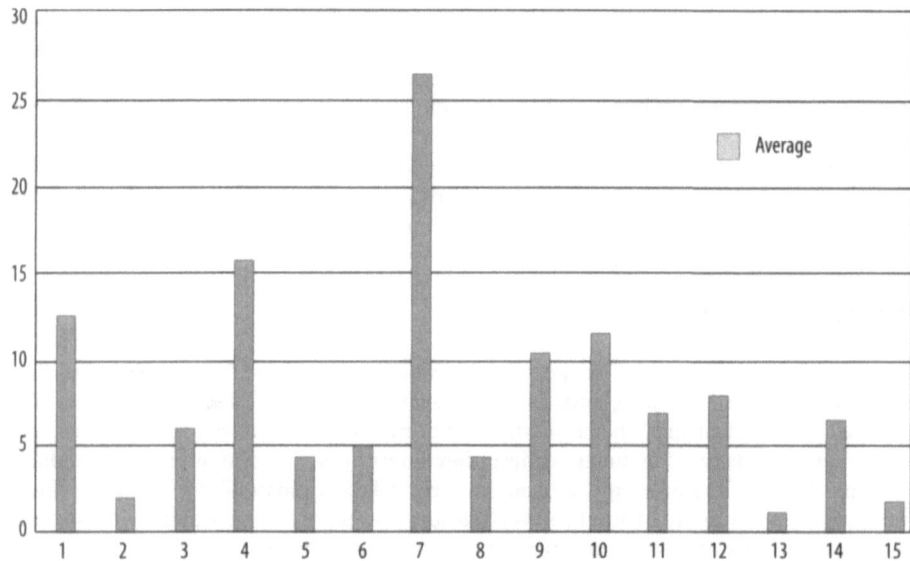

Figure 34.1: British survey of surgery for metastatic germ cell tumour. Average number of cases per year, by centre.

Wales. This recommends that testicular cancer be managed by a centralised service, combining small and medium networks to create a population base of 2 to 4,000,000 per centre, which would be expected to produce 50 to 100 new patients with testicular cancer per year. It is further recommended that surgical centres doing less than 10 operations per year – "should consider whether they have the necessary expertise to continue". On the basis of 1997 figures, only a minority of surgical centres fulfil this criterion. In practice, some of those doing less than 10 cases do have the expertise and should be given the opportunity to increase their numbers, but the process of selecting those who will pass their patients over to achieve this will require careful and diplomatic handling.

Conclusions

Surgery for NSGCT masses is now a routine part of their management. Selection of cases for surgery is appropriate but improvements are needed in the identification of those for whom surgery is needed. Although surgery will continue to have a smaller role in the management of seminoma, it should be considered for some patients.

While elective surgery after normalisation of tumour markers is ideal, interventional surgery may be appropriate in selected cases, but the outcome is poor when there are multiple sites of disease.

In elective cases, dealing with multiple disease sites requires a pragmatic approach. Surgery has central role in managing relapsed disease.

Testis cancer in UK should be managed in bigger centres. This will enable surgery to be concentrated in the hands of surgeons with a sufficient case load who have appropriate support and facilities, and yet maintain the close co-operation between surgeon and oncologist which is essential in the management of this challenging condition.

References

1. Kirk D, Fordham MVP, Wallace DM et al. Surgery for metastatic germ cell tumours: a survey of practice in Britain. *UroOncology* 2001;1:123–129
2. Ravi R, Ong J, Oliver RTD, Badenoch DF, Fowler CG, Hendry WF. The management of residual masses after chemotherapy in metastatic seminoma. *BJU Int* 1999;83:649–53.
3. Wood DP, Herr HW, Heller G et al. Distribution of retroperitoneal metastases after chemotherapy in patients with nonseminomatous germ cell tumors. *J Urol* 1992;148:1812–5
4. Donohue JP. Editorial comment on "Distribution of peritoneal metastases after chemotherapy in patients with nonseminomatous germ cell tumours." *J Urol* 1992;148;1815–1817
5. Fossa S, Qvist H, Stenwig AE, Lien HH, Ous S, Giercksky KE. Is post-chemotherapy retroperintoneal surgery necessary in patients with non-seminomatous testicular cancer and minimal residual tumour masses. *J Clin Oncol* 1990;10;569–573
6. Steyerberg E, Keizer H, Fossa S et al. Prediction of residual retroperitoneal mass histology after chemotherapy for metastatic nonseminomatous germ cell tumour: multivariate analysis of individual patient data from six study groups. *J Clin Oncol* 1995;13:1177–1187
7. Steyerberg EW, Keizer JH, Messemer JE et al. Residual pulmonary masses after chemotherapy for metastatic nonseminomatous germ cell tumour. *Cancer* 1997;79:345–355.
8. Hollins GW, Thomas S, Lanigan DJ et al. Retroperitoneal surgery: its wider role in the management of malignant teratoma. *Br J Urol* 1996;77:571–576
9. Eastham JA, Wilson TG, Russell C, Ahlering TE, Skinner DG. Surgical resection in patients with nonseminomatous germ cell tumour who fail to normalize serum tumour markers after chemotherapy. *Urology* 1994;43:74–80

35. Resection of Residual Masses: a Decade of Research with Jan Keizer

E.W. Steyerberg

Centre for Clinical Decision Sciences, Dept of Public Health, Erasmus University, P.O. Box 1738, 3000 DR Rotterdam, The Netherlands

Background

Surgical resection is a generally accepted treatment to remove remnants of metastases in patients who were treated with cisplatin-based chemotherapy for metastatic non-seminomatous testicular cancer. A wide variation is however noted in the selection of patients for resection by country and by centre. As a tribute to the recently deceased clinical oncologist Dr H. Jan Keizer, a review was performed of 10 of his co-authored papers that were devoted to residual mass resection.

Prognosis After Resection

The prognosis after resection may be positively influenced by resection. First, surgery prevents growth and metastases from residual tumour. Second, additional chemotherapy is valuable after resection of viable cancer, especially in patients at intermediate risk [1]. We found that incomplete resection and pre-chemotherapy HCG level were prognostically important [2]. Patients with residual viable cancer had a favourable prognosis, which may be attributed to the fact that post-resection chemotherapy was different to the original regimen. Unfortunately, the optimum choice of post-resection chemotherapy has not yet been clarified [1].

Prediction of the Residual Histology

Resection may be beneficial for patients with residual tumour but is unnecessary when the histology is benign (necrosis/fibrosis). Preoperative identification of patients with benign histology has been attempted in several studies. In a meta-analysis, we showed that the primary histology, pre-chemotherapy tumour markers, residual mass size and reduction in size were important predictors, but insufficient to confidently identify a clear subgroup without residual tumour [3]. Viable cancer, including teratoma differentiated, was also found in some small masses (10–19mm) or 'normal' nodes (0–9mm). Better predictors need to be identified. Although PET scanning has gained attention in recent years, analyses of PET for residual masses in non-seminoma are thus far based on a limited series of patients, and do not correct for readily available predictive characteristics [4, 5].

We have subsequently combined these predictors in multivariate statistical models. A model for retroperitoneal lymph nodes was developed in 544 patients [6], and subsequently externally validated [7,8]. For very small residual masses, the model predicts a substantial risk of tumour in some patients [9]. For example, when the mass was normal in size post-chemotherapy (2mm) and 30mm pre-chemotherapy, the model predicts a probability of residual tumour of 50 per cent (95 per cent confidence interval 38–62 per cent) when pre-chemotherapy AFP and HCG were elevated, LDH at the upper limit of normal and the primary tumour contained teratoma differentiated. We further analysed the histology of residual lung metastases [10] and showed that necrosis in the abdomen was highly predictive: 48 out of 54 patients (89 per cent) had necrosis only in the lung. When the primary tumour was teratoma-negative, the probability was further increased to 93 per cent [11]. In contrast, necrosis in the lung did not sufficiently predict necrosis in the retroperitoneum. Hence, if sequential resection procedures are required, the retroperitoneal resection should be performed first. Some authors have recommended an aggressive approach to residual masses at multiple sites [12]. The supporting analyses were unfortunately inadequate, e.g. a study of the agreement between all residual histologies instead of only those with necrosis in the retroperitoneum.

Resection Policies

We compared alternative resection policies in two papers, which also included simplified versions of the prediction model for retroperitoneal histology [13,14]. Policies based on the prediction model could achieve an improvement in sensitivity without increasing the number of resections. On the other hand, the only rule that guarantees that residual tumour is not missed is to perform resection in all patients, irrespective of residual mass size or any other characteristic. A formal decision analysis supported the view that the probability of benign tissue should exceed 70 per cent or 80 per cent to decide against resection [15]. This would imply that many patients with masses less than 10mm would be benefit from post-chemotherapy retroperitoneal lymph node resection.

Discussion

The 10 papers reviewed here have received considerable attention in the medical literature, with over 150 citations by September 2001. Contributing to this success are the substantial numbers of patients in the analyses, which increases the statistical precision, as well as the international collaboration, which increases the generalisability of results. The clinical impact of the prediction models has however been more modest. Prediction models are relatively new in the medical field, and practical experience in individual patients is limited yet. For further research, histological findings in resected masses may be used to validate the prediction models further. Especially relevant is their validity for small masses. Follow-up of unresected masses may allow comparison of relapse rates and survival between groups with different predicted probabilities of tumour and might further clarify the benefit of resection.

References

1. Fizazi K, Tjulandin S, Salvioni R et al. Viable malignant cells after primary chemotherapy for disseminated nonseminomatous germ cell tumors: prognostic factors and role of postsurgery chemotherapy – results from an international study group. *J Clin Oncol* 2001;19:2647–57.
2. Steyerberg EW, Keizer HJ, Zwartendijk J et al. Prognosis after resection of residual masses following chemotherapy for metastatic nonseminomatous testicular cancer: a multivariate analysis. *Br J Cancer* 1993;68:195–200.
3. Steyerberg EW, Keizer HJ, Stoter G, Habbema JD. Predictors of residual mass histology following chemotherapy for metastatic non-seminomatous testicular cancer: a quantitative overview of 996 resections. *Eur J Cancer* 1994;30A:1231–9.
4. Stephens AW, Gonin R, Hutchins GD, Einhorn LH. Positron emission tomography evaluation of residual radiographic abnormalities in postchemotherapy germ cell tumor patients. *J Clin Oncol* 1996;14:1637–41.
5. Cremerius U, Effert PJ, Adam G et al. FDG PET for detection and therapy control of metastatic germ cell tumor. *J Nucl Med* 1998;39:815–22.
6. Steyerberg EW, Keizer HJ, Fossa SD et al. Prediction of residual retroperitoneal mass histology after chemotherapy for metastatic nonseminomatous germ cell tumor: multivariate analysis of individual patient data from six study groups. *J Clin Oncol* 1995;13:1177–87.
7. Steyerberg EW, Gerl A, Fossa SD et al. Validity of predictions of residual retroperitoneal mass histology in nonseminomatous testicular cancer. *J Clin Oncol* 1998;16:269–74.
8. Vergouwe Y, Steyerberg EW, Foster RS, Habbema JD, Donohue JP. Validation of a prediction model and its predictors for the histology of residual masses in nonseminomatous testicular cancer. *J Urol* 2001;165:84–8.
9. Steyerberg EW, Keizer HJ, Sleijfer DT et al. Retroperitoneal metastases in testicular cancer: role of CT measurements of residual masses in decision making for resection after chemotherapy. *Radiology* 2000;215:437–44.
10. Steyerberg EW, Keizer HJ, Messemer JE, Toner GC, Schraffordt Koops H, Fossa SD, et al. Residual pulmonary masses after chemotherapy for metastatic nonseminomatous germ cell tumor: prediction of histology. *Cancer* 1997;79:345–55.
11. Steyerberg EW, Donohue JP, Gerl A et al. Residual masses after chemotherapy for metastatic testicular cancer: the clinical implications of the association between retroperitoneal and pulmonary histology. *J Urol* 1997;158:474–8.
12. Gels ME, Hoekstra HJ, Sleijfer DT et al. Thoracotomy for postchemotherapy resection of pulmonary residual tumor mass in patients with nonseminomatous testicular germ cell tumors: aggressive surgical resection is justified. *Chest* 1997;112:967–73.
13. Steyerberg EW, Keizer HJ, Fossa SD et al. Resection of residual retroperitoneal masses in testicular cancer: evaluation and improvement of selection criteria. *Br J Cancer* 1996;74:1492–8.
14 Steyerberg EW, Keizer HJ, Habbema JD. Prediction models for the histology of residual masses after chemotherapy for metastatic testicular cancer. *Int J Cancer* 1999;83:856–9.
15. Steyerberg EW, Marshall PB, Keizer HJ, Habbema JD. Resection of small, residual retroperitoneal masses after chemotherapy for nonseminomatous testicular cancer: a decision analysis. *Cancer* 1999;85:1331–41.

36. Predictive Factors for Residual Teratoma after Chemotherapy for Non-seminomatous Germ Cell Tumours (NSGCT)

L.H. Larsen, H. von der Maase

Department of Oncology, Aarhus University Hospital, Denmark

Background

About 25 per cent of patients with NSGCT receiving chemotherapy will have a residual tumour after the completion of treatment. These residual tumours may harbour malignant cells or only necrosis and/or fibrosis. Resection of residual tumours is of the utmost importance in case of viable tumour whereas one obviously should try to avoid operating on patients with only necrosis/fibrosis. However, the criteria for the selection of patients that should be offered resection of a residual tumour are controversial. We have therefore investigated potential predictive factors for residual malignancy.

Patients

All patients with NSGCT diagnosed between January 1990 and December 2000, who had received chemotherapy (BEP) at Aarhus University Hospital and subsequently had resection of one or more residual masses were included in the study. Two criteria for resection were used, residual mass over 2 cm or cystic residual mass regardless of size.

Methods

A total of 60 patients fulfilled the inclusion criteria. Data concerning the histology of the primary and residual tumour, tumour size and appearance prior to and after chemotherapy, tumour markers, response to treatment, relapse and survival were registered. Potential predictive factors for residual viable tumour were analysed in univariate analyses, and subsequently by multivariate analysis to test for independent importance.

Results

Thirty-five patients (58 per cent) had teratoma differentiated in the residual mass, no other germ cell malignancy was found. Twenty-five patients had necrosis or fibrosis only. After surgery, four patients had a relapse, two with teratoma differentiated and two with other germ cell malignancy, and both these patients have died. One patient died of a non-cancer related cause. Overall, 95 per cent of patients were alive with no evidence of disease after a median follow-up time of 47 months.

Teratoma in the primary tumour, a cystic residual tumour and progressive disease (PD) without marker elevation during or immediately after chemotherapy were all independent predictive factors for residual teratoma. All 14 patients with PD had teratoma in their residual mass and represented all the patients who progressed without marker elevation during the study period. Tumour size before or after chemotherapy and elevated AFP or HCG prior to treatment were not associated with a residual teratoma.

Discussion

We used the three significant factors, primary teratoma, cystic residual tumour and PD, to construct a predictive index for a residual teratoma. Using this index, 77 per cent of all our patients would have been offered an operation, detecting residual teratoma in 74 per cent of these cases. The index would have identified 97 per cent of all patients with residual teratoma, missing one patient. Whether this index may be useful in the selection of patients for surgery should be confirmed in larger patient population.

37. Orchidectomy Following Chemotherapy for Patients with Metastatic Testicular Germ Cell Cancer

T. Geldart

Medical Oncology, Wessex Medical Oncology Unit, Southampton, UK

Patients with testicular germ cell tumours (GCT) may present with advanced or life threatening metastatic disease, requiring urgent treatment with primary chemotherapy with consideration given to subsequent orchidectomy. However, the value of routine post-chemotherapy orchidectomy remains controversial.

A retrospective review of patients with metastatic testicular GCT undergoing primary chemotherapy followed by orchidectomy between 1985 and 2000 was undertaken. Sixty patients were identified. The median age of patients was 32 years and median follow-up 4.3 years.

Only 23 of 60 patients (38 per cent) had testicular symptoms or signs at presentation although 55 (92 per cent) had an abnormal testicular ultrasound. Forty-four patients (73 per cent) underwent a diagnostic biopsy. All but one patient had elevated tumour markers. Forty-one patients (68 per cent) had non-seminomatous (NSGCT) or mixed GCT with 5 per cent, 37 per cent and 58 per cent falling into the good, intermediate and poor prognosis groups respectively. Eighteen patients (30 per cent) had seminoma (SEM) with 94 per cent and 6 per cent falling into the good and intermediate prognosis group respectively. One patient's disease could not be sub-classified.

Following systemic chemotherapy, tumour markers normalised prior to orchidectomy in 68 per cent of patients. For those with abnormal markers prior to surgery, tumour markers were falling in all but three patients. In 56 of 60 patients (93 per cent) markers normalised following surgery. Fifty-seven patients (95 per cent) underwent orchidectomy at a median of 7 weeks following chemotherapy, and three patients during primary chemotherapy. Out of 41 patients with NSGCT or mixed GCT, 34 (83 per cent) required additional surgical resection of residual post chemotherapy masses.

The orchidectomy specimens of 24 patients (40 per cent) revealed the presence of GCT (three SEM and 21 NSGCT, including 18 teratoma differentiated) or intratubular germ cell neoplasia (five specimens). The remaining specimens contained fibrous scarring or necrosis. In the 34 per cent of patients who underwent additional post chemotherapy surgery, 65 per cent of specimens contained a GCT, including teratoma differentiated (17 of 23 specimens). All three patients with residual NSGCT within the testis had histologically proven NSGCT at other sites of residual disease resected following chemotherapy. These patients have subsequently relapsed and died of progressive disease despite salvage therapy. All three patients with persistent SEM in the testis are currently alive and disease free although one has relapsed requiring salvage chemotherapy.

Forty-one patients (68 per cent) remain relapse free following initial chemotherapy and surgery although one patient has died from a primary brain tumour. Nineteen patients (32 per cent) relapsed following initial treatment; thirteen of these have been salvaged with further therapy giving an overall cure rate of 90 per cent.

Persistence of NSGCT at the site of the primary tumour post chemotherapy is associated with persistence of viable disease at other metastatic sites and poor prognosis. Post chemotherapy orchidectomy is recommended in all patients undergoing primary chemotherapy as a significant proportion (40 per cent) are left with viable disease that predisposes to subsequent relapse.

38. Organ Sparing Tumour Resection in Testicular Germ Cell Tumours (TGCT) – Long-term Follow-up

A. Heidenreich, for the German Testicular Study Group (GTCSG)

Department of Urology, Philipps-Universitat, Baldingerstrasse, 35043 Marburg, Germany

Purpose

Synchronous and metachronous bilateral TGCT occur in 2 to 5 per cent of patients. Bilateral radical orchiectomy has been the standard treatment resulting not only in infertility, but also in life-long dependency on exogenous testosterone substitution and major psychological disturbances due to bilateral castration at young age. Therefore, organ-sparing surgery has been proposed in small series of patients with either bilateral testis cancer or TGCT developing in a solitary testicle [1–3]. The aim of the current study was to evaluate the indications, surgical technique and outcome of organ preserving tumour enucleation rather than standard orchiectomy in patients with bilateral TGCTs or TGCT in a solitary testicle. We present the long term data of 73 patients included in our protocol.

Patients and Methods

Tumour excision resection was performed in 73 patients, 52 with metachronous and 17 with synchronous bilateral TGCT and four with GCT in a solitary testicle. Histology of the enucleated GCT revealed seminoma in 42 cases (57.5 per cent), embryonal carcinoma in 14 cases (19.2 per cent), mature teratoma in 11 cases (15.1 per cent), mixed and combined GCT in 6 cases (8.2 per cent). Mean tumour diameter was 15mm (5–30mm). Associated intratubular germ cell neoplasia (ITGCN) was diagnosed in 82 per cent of the cases, 82 per cent of the patients underwent local radiation with 18 Gy.

Results

After a median follow-up of 91 (3–191) months, 72 of the 73 patients (98.5 per cent) have no evidence of disease and one patient has died of systemic tumour progression. Forty-six of 56 patients diagnosed with ITGCN were treated by local radiation; none of them developed local relapse, whereas four of 10 patients who were not irradiated developed local recurrences after 3, 6, 12, and 165 months respectively and all were salvaged by inguinal orchiectomy. Testosterone levels are normal in 62 (84.9 per cent) patients, seven patients (9.6 per cent) developed hypogonadism and four patients (6.3 per cent) retained their preoperatively low testosterone levels. Five of 10 patients who postponed local radiation for paternity reasons successfully fathered a child after organ sparing surgery.

Conclusions

After long-term follow-up of more than 7 years, organ sparing surgery appears as a viable therapeutic approach in bilateral TGCT with excellent postoperative outcome. Tumour enucleation might be considered as standard approach if the guidelines are respected: cold ischaemia, organ confined tumour less than 20mm, multiple biopsies of the tumour bed, adjuvant local irradiation postoperatively to avoid local recurrences, close follow-up and high compliance. The risk of local recurrence indicates that organ preserving surgery should only be performed in centres experienced in the management of TGCTs.

References

1. Heidenreich A, Bonfig R, Derschum W, von Vietsch H, Wilbert D. A conservative approach to bilateral testicular germ cell tumors. *J Urol* 1995;153:10-3
2. Weissbach L. Organ preserving surgery for malignant germ cell tumors. *J Urol* 1995;153:90-3
3. Heidenreich A, Höltl W, Albrecht W. Testis preserving surgery in bilateral testicular germ cell tumors. *Brit J Urol* 1997;79:253-7

39. Chemotherapy for Testis Conservation in Patients with Germ Cell Cancer (GCC): Is it Safe and Could Combination with Tumour Enucleation Increase the Frequency of Success?

V. Nargund[1], T. Lane[2], R.T.D. Oliver[2], J. Ong[2], M. Cullen, S.A. Sohaib[3], R.H. Reznek[3], D. Badenoch[1]

Departments of 1. Urology, 2. Medical Oncology and 3. Radiology, School of Medicine and Dentistry, St Bartholomew's and Royal London Hospitals, West Smithfield, London EC1A 7BE

Introduction

There is increasing evidence that the link between declining sperm count and rising incidence of testicular germ cell cancer (GCC) is due to testicular atrophy induced gonadotrophin drive [1]. The observation that two thirds of GCC patients have reduced sperm count and that patients are now presenting earlier with smaller tumours than previously [2] justify attempts to conserve germinal epithelium in GCC patients. This paper updates our experience.

Methods

Seventy-eight testicular GCC patients receiving chemotherapy with primary tumour in situ during 1978–2000 have been reviewed. Sixty-one had advanced metastatic disease and 17 had stage I. Details of treatment schedules and protocols of care have been published elsewhere [2, 3].

Table 39.1: Impact of stage and histology on outcome after attempted testes conservation with chemotherapy.

	Preserved testes	Potentialy preservable
Stage 1 Seminoma (n = 11)*	64%	91%
Stage 1 Non-Seminoma (n = 6)	17%	83%
Stage 2/3/4 Seminoma (n = 18)	50%	73%
Stage 2/3/4 Non-Seminoma (n = 43)	24%	55%

*7 based on histology from contralateral testes

Results

In 25 of 78 (32 per cent) patients, the testis returned to normal and was retained. These cases have been followed for a median of 144 months. A second GCC developed subsequently in five of these patients. Actuarial relapse free survival was 90 per cent at 5 years and 88 per cent at 10 years. There were no relapses in patients receiving BEP. All the relapses appeared to be new tumours based on size and location, and as they were all stage 1 disease and patients are now disease free after orchidectomy alone (14, 24, 36 and 121 months). Twenty-two additional patients (28 per cent) who underwent orchidectomy for apparent treatment failure had necrotic tissue or differentiated teratoma involving less than 50 per cent of the testis and could have been candidates for tumour enucleation (potentially preservable). Shrinkage on ultrasound of more than 20 per cent after chemotherapy predicted for tumour necrosis. There was a trend for higher frequency of being potentially preservable in patients with stage I disease. There has been one successful pregnancy to date in seven patients with stage I on follow-up and five of six have recovered sperm, albeit all below 20×10^6 per ejaculate.

Conclusion

This study suggests that up to 50 per cent of all cases and 70 per cent of cases with tumours less than 2cms could have testis conservation using chemotherapy alone for complete responders and tumour enucleation for incomplete responders with less than 50 per cent of testis affected by tumour. Clearly the number preserved so far (n = 25) is insufficient to have strong confidence that the long term actuarial prediction is accurate, though it approximates to the results reported by Christensen et al [4]. However given that second tumours can occur up to 30 years after treatment, lifelong follow up will be required.

References

1. Oliver, R.T.D., Atrophy, hormones, genes and viruses in aetiology of germ cell tumours, in *Cancer Surveys*. 1990. p. 263–268.
2. Oliver, RT, Ong J, Blandy JP, Altman DG. Testis conservation studies in germ cell cancer justified by improved primary chemotherapy response and reduced delay 1978–1994. *Br J Urol* 1996;78:119–124.
3. Ravi, R, Oliver RT, Ong J et al., A single-centre observational study of surgery and late malignant events after chemotherapy for germ cell cancer. *B J Urol* 1997;80:647–652.
4. Christensen TB, Daugaard G, Geertsen PF, von der Maase H. Effect of chemotherapy on carcinoma in situ of the testis. *Ann Oncol* 1998;9:1–4.

40. How Valid Is a Prediction Rule for Residual Retroperitoneal Mass Histology in NSGCT?

Y. Vergouwe, E.W. Steyerberg, J.D.F. Habbema

Department of Public Health, Erasmus Medical Center Rotterdam, P.O. Box 1738, 3000 DR Rotterdam, The Netherlands

A prediction rule is available to predict the histology of residual retroperitoneal masses in patients treated with chemotherapy for metastatic nonseminomatous germ cell tumours [1]. The rule provides the probability that retroperitoneal lymph nodes are totally benign and is intended as an aid in choosing the optimal postchemotherapy treatment. We assessed the external validity of the rule, i.e. its applicability to a separate patient group than the one in which it was developed.

Probabilities of benign tissue were calculated for three patient populations: i) the more recently treated patients who were similar to the patients used to develop the rule (treated 1980–1996, n = 172), ii) patients from Indiana University (treated 1985–1999, n = 276), iii) patients from an EORTC/MRC trial (treated 1995–1998, n = 105).

The predicted probabilities were in agreement with observed frequencies for the more recently treated patients [2]. They were systematically too high for patients from Indiana University [3]. Recalibration of the rule by adjusting the intercept might be considered for those patients [4]. For patients from the EORTC/MRC trial, predicted probabilities above 10 per cent were reliable.

The ability of the model to distinguish patients with different outcomes (discrimination) was assessed using the area under the receiver operating characteristic curve (AUC). AUC was around 0.8 for all three populations. This indicates that the rule is better able to distinguish benign tissue from other tissues than common resection policies based predominantly on the size of the residual mass (AUC around 0.7).

In conclusion, the prediction rule showed good discriminative ability in all three populations. The rule had sometimes to be recalibrated in order to obtain reliable center-specific predictions.

References

1. Steyerberg E, Keizer H, Fosså S. Prediction of residual retroperitoneal mass histology following chemotherapy for metastatic nonseminomatous germ cell tumor: multivariate analysis of individual patient data from six study groups. *J Clin Oncol* 1995;13:1177–1187
2. Steyerberg E, Gerl A, Fosså Sl. Validity of predictions of residual retroperitoneal mass histology in nonseminomatous testicular cancer. *J Clin Oncol* 1998;16:269–274
3. Vergouwe Y, Steyerberg E, Foster R, Habbema J, Donohue J. Validation of a prediction model and its predictors for the histology of residual masses in nonseminomatous testicular cancer. *J Urol* 2001;165:84–88
4. van Houwelingen HC, Thorogood J. Construction, validation and updating of a prognostic model for kidney graft survival. *Stat Med* 1995;14:1999–2008

41. Minimizing Morbidity from Surgery for Non-seminoma Testicular Cancer

M.A.S. Jewett, B. Shekarriz, A.Grabowski

Division of Urology, Department of Surgery, Princess Margaret, Toronto General Hospital and the University of Toronto, Canada

Introduction

Most patients with testis cancer are now cured. Efforts to improve treatment are therefore primarily directed to reducing morbidity while maintaining the excellent survival rate. The urological surgical aspects of treatment include the management of the primary tumour as well as retroperitoneal metastases. The concept of scrotal violation, the role for partial orchiectomy and even for percutaneous needle biopsy will be reviewed. The indications for and the necessary extent of retroperitoneal lymphadenectomy (RPL) with nerve sparing as definitive treatment for metastatic disease to the regional nodes have been defined and in general reduced. There is an emerging role for laparoscopic lymphadenectomy for staging and probably therapy. The post chemotherapy residual mass remains a surgical problem. Most patients with detectable disease should undergo surgery. These issues will be addressed.

Issues in the Management of the Primary Tumour

Most patients with testis cancer present with a testis mass but many scrotal masses are not tumours. Physical examination, scrotal ultrasound and inguinal orchiectomy establish the diagnosis. The inguinal approach is thought to be necessary to avoid tumour implantation in the scrotal incision or developing inguinal metastases. The term "scrotal violation" has been used for a transcrotal incision with biopsy or orchiectomy. Is this concern valid and if not, is there a role for transcrotal needle biopsy to establish the diagnosis and even plan treatment without orchiectomy? Is orchiectomy necessary for all patients or could some be managed by planned partial orchiectomy?

Scrotal Violation and the Role for Transcrotal Needle Biopsy

Review of the literature is difficult due to the changes in terminology. Prior to 1940, simple orchiectomy referred to an orchiectomy through an inguinal incision and the term radical orchiectomy was reserved for an orchiectomy with a concomitant unilateral lymph node dissection [1]. The concept of an inguinal approach is therefore long established. Scrotal incision for suspected testis tumour is generally discouraged. A re-examination of the scrotal violation literature suggests that this is less of a concern than once thought. In Capeoluto and colleagues 1995 meta-analysis of all scrotal violation series between 1953 and 1993, a local recurrence risk of 2.9 per cent was seen in 206 patients, as opposed to a 0.4 per cent local recurrence risk in 976 patients treated by an inguinal orchiectomy [2]. Of note, there was no difference in survival or distant recurrence. Kennedy reviewed 210 patients with Stage 1 testicular tumours, of whom 26 had scrotal violation, managed by surveillance and noted no local recurrences [3]. Similarly, Aki reviewed 75 patients with stage 1 non-seminomas treated with surveillance [4]. Thirteen of these patients had scrotal violation and none developed a local recurrence. These results contrast to the often quoted 25 per cent local recurrence rate reported by Markland which was based on 3 recurrences in 12 patients referred specifically for management of scrotal violation [5]. Markland's high local recurrence rate may be a result of referral bias. In another widely quoted study, Dean reported a 24 per cent recurrence rate in 63 patients undergoing a "simple orchiectomy" [1]. This is not a contemporary series and may reflect the advanced stage of some patients.

In addition, there is considerable experience with transcrotal fine needle aspiration (FNA) of suspected testis tumors for cytology with little evidence for tumour implantation [6]. Only one seminoma was implanted but histological interpretation of the biopsy material is difficult and sampling errors are possible. The greatest degree of accuracy is obtained with seminomas [7,8]. While there is little evidence for wound implantation with a #23 gauge needle aspiration or transcrotal incisional biopsy, there is insufficient reported experience with needle core biopsy of invasive tumours to assess accuracy and safety. Nevertheless, needle biopsy remains an attractive possibility for the diagnosis of testis masses and for the diagnosis of seminoma if primary radiation or chemotherapy are being considered. At the present time, preemptive treatment of the scrotum with radiation or partial scrotectomy is unnecessary after violation unless there is a clinical recurrence.

Partial Orchiectomy

The current standard of care for germ cell testicular cancer is radical inguinal orchiectomy. However, there are a number of recent reports of success with organ sparing surgery for patients with bilateral tumours or tumours in solitary testes [9–11]. Although the prevalence of synchronous bilateral disease is only 0.4–1.3 per cent with 2.6–5 per cent for metachronous contralateral tumours, these occurrences have provided the impetus to explore this procedure [12].

There are a number of potential benefits with organ sparing partial orchiectomy. Ultimately, the major benefit may be for patients with benign lesions who may avoid unnecessary orchiectomy when their urologists feel more comfortable with excisional biopsy. The potential to preserve androgen production and fertility in patients with solitary testes and diminishing the psychosocial impact of the surgery are the major reasons to explore the safety of partial orchiectomy.

Partial orchiectomy was first reported by Richie in a 27-year-old man with synchronous bilateral seminoma who received adjuvant radiotherapy, showed no recurrences at 30 months and had good testosterone levels without hormone replacement [13]. Weissbach reported the first series in 1993, which was updated in 1995 [10]. He described 10 out of 14 successful partial orchiectomies with no local recurrences and adequate hormonal status. He also established the prerequisites for organ preservation which included an inguinal approach with early cord clamping, a detailed knowledge of the vascular anatomy of the testis, organ confined tumours away from the rete testis, tumour diameter less than 20 mm, normal preoperative plasma testosterone level, multiple biopsies of the tumour bed and adjuvant local irradiation with 20 Gy for presence of carcinoma in situ (CIS). Heidenreich and colleagues published a series of reports on 13 patients who underwent partial orchiectomy for bilateral testicular germ cell tumours (TGCTs) with a follow up of 62 months [9]. One patient recurred locally and underwent curative orchiectomy. The other 12 patients were free of disease without hormonal replacement. Van der Schyff recently presented an update on this series showing a 6 per cent local recurrence rate in 63 patients with TGCT treated with partial orchiectomy after a mean follow up of 74 months [11]. Carcinoma in situ (CIS) of the testis, now more aptly termed, intratubular germ cell neoplasia (ITGCN) was found in 44/63 (70 per cent) of patients and 38 of these 44 received prophylactic radiation to that testicle. All of the patients that recurred had untreated ITGCN and were subsequently cured with a radical orchiectomy. Since ITGCN is associated with a 50 per cent progression to malignancy within 5 years, current practice has included irradiation of the testicle with 18–20 Gy, which has been shown to be effective treatment for this entity by destroying germ cell tissue.

We have reviewed our experience with organ sparing surgery for suspected testicular tumours at our institution and found that we could perform a partial orchiectomy in 15/18 patients based on Weisbach's criteria. Seven of 15 had malignant tumours but most importantly, eight had benign conditions and were spared orchiectomy by the initial conservative approach. We have had no local recurrences in the patients with malignancies after a median follow up of 3 years. In our series 5/7 patients with malignancies had concomitant ITGCN and all received prophylactic radiation.

A major concern with partial orchiectomy is that it violates the scrotum and increases the risk of local and regional recurrence. From the recent partial orchiectomy series, it appears that local recurrence is uncommon in well selected patients when appropriate intraoperative precautions are taken along with postoperative irradiation for ITGCN.

A major advantage of partial orchiectomy is that it avoids complete removal of the testicle for benign lesions. Published literature indicates that up to 31 per cent of scrotal explorations and subsequent orchiectomies are for benign disease. This is in keeping with our series in which 9/18 explorations were for benign lesions. Complete excision of the lesion with sparing of normal parenchyma can be used as a diagnostic and curative procedure in these cases, while avoiding unnecessary orchiectomy.

Another compelling argument for organ sparing orchiectomy is the preservation of hormonal function in men with solitary testes or bilateral testicular cancer. This approach may avoid the need for lifelong androgen replacement. This is especially important, as studies have shown that exogenous androgen replacement in these patients is often inadequate [14]. Unfortunately, after a unilateral orchiectomy 6–25 per cent of patients have elevated LH levels and 0–16 per cent have decreased testosterone levels, signifying some degree of Leydig cell dysfunction. In addition, since 75 per cent of patients harbour ITGCN in tissue surrounding testicular cancer, a large majority will have to undergo prophylactic radiation treatment if an organ sparing approach is employed. A total dose of 18–20 Gy has been shown to be effective treatment for ITGCN, but it also has an effect on Leydig cell function. Giwercman et al. studied hormonal function and the effects of radiation in men with solitary testes and ITGCN [15]. In this study, 8/20 men had impaired Leydig cell function even before radiation as demonstrated by either low serum testosterone and/or elevated LH values. Radiation with 20Gy eradicated ITGCN but produced a decrease in the basal testosterone levels from a mean of 13.3+/–6 to 10.8+/–6.4 nmol/L (p = 0.06) over 36 months. LH values also rose in the first 3 months of follow-up, from 10.4+/–5.4 to 15.6+/–7.3 IU/L (p < 0.0001). Interestingly, only two men received androgen supplementation for complaints of sexual dysfunction and low testosterone levels which started before their radiation treatment. Furthermore, results from partial orchiectomy series indicate that the majority of patients do not require hormonal replacement. Weissbach reported 11/14 (78 per cent) patients had normal testosterone levels after irradiation with 20Gy and van der Schyff reported that 56/63 (88 per cent) of patients had normal testosterone levels after partial orchiectomy [10, 11]. Patients who do require androgen supplementation avoid large swings in androgen levels because they still maintain some baseline androgen secretion.

Testicular cancer affects men between the ages of 15 and 35, when preservation of fertility is important. Unfortunately, infertility is also associated with testicular cancer, especially in men with bilateral tumours. Fordham et al. found that none of the 38 patients in their series who developed metachronous tumours 6 months to 14 years after the first tumour were able to produce a pregnancy [16]. This is most likely secondary to the presence of ITGCN in the contralateral testicle, which is associated with poor semen parameters. Seventy percent of men who undergo a partial orchiectomy are found to harbour ITGCN in the ipsilateral testicle and need postoperative irradiation as treatment for this. The radiation destroys all germinal epithelium rendering them infertile. However, testicular preservation in the 30 per cent who do not have concomitant ITGCN may be instrumental in achieving fertility. In addition, there are also reports of men with ITGCN fathering children. These reports provide a rationale for delayed scrotal irradiation along with close surveillance in men with ITGCN in the hope of achieving a pregnancy before progression to malignancy. This strategy can be coupled with new technologies, such as intracytoplasmic sperm injection (ICSI), to achieve a pregnancy.

Approximately 10 per cent of testicular cancer patients suffer from long term psychological problems and 15 per cent have some long term sexual dysfunction [17]. It seems intuitive that patients undergoing organ sparing surgery are likely to have improved body image and quality of life as a result of decreased need for androgen supplementation and increased fertility. Data on this however are lacking, although studies to answer this question are currently underway.

In summary, partial orchiectomy in carefully selected patients appears to be a viable and safe option that achieves good cancer control while avoiding unnecessary orchiectomy for benign lesions. Furthermore, it has the potential of preserving hormonal function and fertility in men who have bilateral tumours or solitary testes, thus improving their overall quality of life.

Issues in the Management of the Retroperitoneum

Indications and Extent of Retroperitoneal Lymphadenectomy(RPL) in Stage I and II Non-seminoma

Stage I Non-seminoma

The cure rates appear to be similar when patients with clinical stage I non-seminoma are initially managed by surveillance, RPL and chemotherapy. The issue is overall burden of therapy and long term safety. We have imperfect prognostic factors for progression resulting in overtreatment in many patients and undertreatment in some.

Surveillance studies have demonstrated that 30 per cent of patients are understaged and progress and usually require chemotherapy (Table 41.1). A study to compare the outcomes of surveillance and RPL would require too many patients to complete. If we were to look at the outcome of 100 hypothetical patients with clinical stage I disease who undergo RPL, 70 would have no evidence of metastases and about 30 would have positive nodes (Figure 41.1a). Approximately 10 per cent of patients with pathological stage I progress from occult, probable haematogenous metastases. Overall, 50 per cent of patients with pathological stage II will also progress if not given adjuvant chemotherapy due to incomplete surgery or occult systemic metastases so that only 15 patients of the total 100 operated upon will actually be cured with surgery alone (Figure 41.1b). However, accurate staging of the retroperitoneum will be achieved and many follow-up CT's will be unnecessary compared to patients on surveillance. It appears that the ultimate role of surgery is likely to be limited in this population. For the alternative management with surveillance, poor compliance to follow-up does not seem to seriously jeopardize outcome. The retroperitoneum requires close follow-up with imaging over at least 2 years, which is not necessary after surgery, and late relapse is possible. Refinements in risk assignment are possible and initial treatment can be reserved for those at higher risk of progression on the basis of primary tumour pathology. With this philosophy of risk stratification, initial treatment with chemotherapy or surgery has been proposed for those with pure embryonal carcinoma or vasculo-lymphatic invasion in the primary tumour. In the future, laparoscopic RPL may alter the way we stage and initially manage these stage I patients with surgical staging in the high risk patients who may also receive a therapeutic benefit from the lymphadenectomy.

Mortality due to retroperitoneal lymphadenectomy is rare and the procedure has an acceptable morbidity. In a review of primary RPL for clinical stage I disease from Indiana University, the survival rate was 99.2 per cent for pathological stage I, 98.4 per cent for pathological stage II without chemotherapy and 100 per cent for pathological stage II after adjuvant chemotherapy [18]. Although there is a significant treatment burden, the results are impressive.

Table 41.2 demonstrates the results of RPL in pathological stage I disease. The most common site of relapse after RPL is the lung and retroperitoneal recurrences are rare

Table 41.1: Results of recent surveilance protocols for Stage I non-seminoma. (FU = follow-up in months)

Reference	Number	FU	Relapses (%)	Mortality (%)
Roth et al [59]	77	64	30	0
Roth et al [60]	373	60	27	1
Swanson et al [61]	99	81	27	2
Ondrus et al [62]	90	83	36	5
Nicolai et al [63]	85	132	29	4
Gels et al [64]	154	84	27	1
Sogani et al [65]	105	134	26	3
Hao et al [66]	76	46	37	3
Colls et al [67]	248	53	28	2
Sharir et al [68]	170	76	28	1
Total	1477		28.3	2

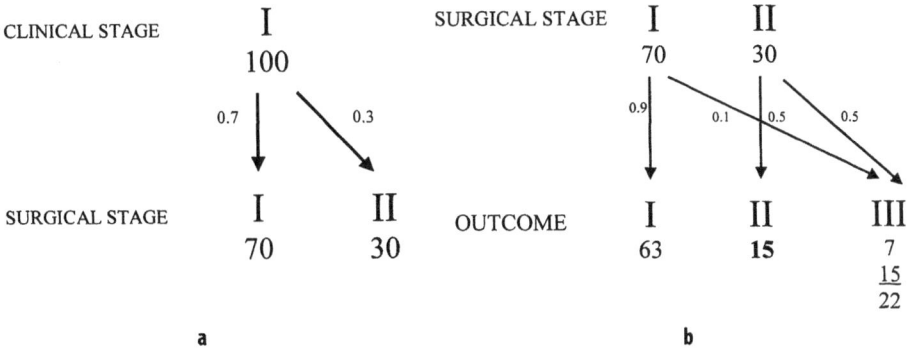

Figure 41.1: Expected outcomes for 100 men with clnical stage I non-seminoma undergoing RPL in terms of pathological stage (a) and ultimate outcome (b). Stage I is no evidence of metastases, Stage II with retropritoneal nodal metastases and Stage III refers to systemic metastases, usually to lung.

(0–3 per cent) [19–23]. In those patients who are pathological stage II and who are not treated with adjuvant chemotherapy, the relapse rate may be as low as 30 per cent. This indicates that approximately 70 per cent of patients with minimal nodal metastasis are cured with lymphadenectomy alone. This is unique in solid tumours and is a major impetus to address the utility of a minimally invasive approach with laparoscopy.

Stage II Non-seminoma

The role of primary RPL for management of clinical stage II disease is controversial. Data from Indiana University demonstrated that primary RPL alone was curative in 65 per cent of stage II patients [24]. Since this series includes patients from the 1960's and 1970's, bilateral complete RPL was performed in 83 per cent and modified unilateral dissection was performed in 17 per cent of these patients. A nerve-sparing technique was used in only 12 per cent. In a sub-group of 140 patients in the post-cisplatinum era, 23 per cent had pathological stage I disease. Of the remaining patients, 49 received primary RPL alone and 18 (37 per cent) relapsed. In contrast, none of the 59 patients who received adjuvant chemotherapy relapsed. The authors emphasized the importance of adjuvant chemotherapy in patients with retroperitoneal disease at RPL. The documented morbidities included pulmonary

Table 41.2: Results of retroperitoneal lymphadenectomy for pathological stage I non-seminoma.

References	Number	FU	Relapse RP (%)	Relapse Other (%)	Mortality (%)
Javadpour et al [69]	54	26	2	7	0
Aass et al [20]	107	70	0	7	0
Klepp et al [21]	204	50	3	12	1
Richie et al [70]	64	38	0	6	0
McLeod et al [71]	264	63	3	8	2
Donohue et al [72]	266	71	0	12	1
Total	959		1	10	1

U = follow-up in months, RP = retroperitoneum

complications, bleeding, small bowel obstruction and pancreatitis. Data on ejaculation and fertility status were not provided. However, the fact that most patients had bilateral dissection without nerve sparing indicate that ejaculation was not likely preserved in the majority of these patients.

With the advent of nerve-sparing techniques, it became apparent that antegrade ejaculation could be preserved in the majority of patients with low volume stage II disease undergoing primary RPL. At the University of Toronto, primary RPL has been performed in patients with low volume (less than 5 cm) lymphadenopathy on CT scanning who have marker levels of less than 100. In a review of 40 patients, 16(40 per cent) had negative nodes illustrating the potential for overstaging [25]. Adjuvant chemotherapy was not routinely given in the remaining 24 patients, of whom 7 relapsed. These patients received chemotherapy and remain disease free.

Primary chemotherapy has been associated with similar cure rates. In a series from the Royal Marsden Hospital, 122 patients with retroperitoneal lymphadenopathy less than 5 cm in diameter, underwent primary chemotherapy. Thirty-five (28.7 per cent) required secondary RPL for residual disease. The overall 5-year survival was 97 per cent [26]. The ideal initial management remains controversial but we prefer primary nerve-sparing RPL in patients with limited nodal disease (less than 5 cm) and low tumour marker levels. Otherwise, primary chemotherapy is chosen since the chance of systemic disease is high in the presence of significant marker elevation or high volume nodal disease. We believe that this selective approach will decrease the morbidity associated with treatment in stage II non-seminoma.

Reducing Morbidity of RPL: Nerve Sparing and Evolution of Templates

Traditionally RPL was performed to remove all nodal tissue from the suprahilar region to the common iliac bifurcation bilaterally [27]. This approach was associated with retrograde ejaculation in almost all cases and was the most significant long-term surgical morbidity. Subsequent mapping studies demonstrated that a full bilateral dissection in stage I and low volume stage II disease is not necessary [28–30]. To reduce the rate of retrograde ejaculation or anejaculation in these patients, two strategies were proposed.

Nerve identification and sparing with bilateral dissection demonstrated that nerve sparing was feasible [31]. The second strategy was to reduce the extent of lymphadenectomy to the areas (templates) most likely to contain metastases [32]. Although nerves are preserved in the templates, nerves in the non dissected areas will also be preserved. Adjuvant chemotherapy may be employed with both strategies, which prevents true assessment of the therapeutic role of surgery.

Nevertheless, similar outcomes can be achieved using a modified template RPL while fertility can be preserved in the majority of cases [22, 33–36]. In a review of the Indiana University data for stage A disease, 140 patients underwent bilateral suprahilar or infrahilar dissection compared to 183 who had modified unilateral RPL. The relapse rate was 11 per cent in both groups. Similarly the relapse rate for stage B disease without adjuvant treatment was 41 per cent and 46 per cent for bilateral suprahilar and infrahilar dissection respectively, compared to 27 per cent for modified template dissection.

The technique of bilateral nerve-sparing RPL has been described in detail previously [37, 38]. In the Indiana university study, the nerve-sparing technique was primarily used in patients with stage I disease [32]. Of 75 patients, 73 had clinical stage I disease and 14 had pathological stage II disease. Four patients relapsed with marker elevation and only one had a retroperitoneal recurrence. Initially, Jewett et al reported nerve-sparing RPL in 20 patients of various stages [31]. Ejaculation was preserved in 95 per cent of these patients. Although nerve-sparing is possible in patients with stage II disease, the University of Toronto experience has been that this approach may not be feasible in up to 30 per cent of patients with grossly positive nodal disease [25].

It is apparent that the introduction of nerve-sparing technique has further improved the results with respect to ejaculatory function and fertility while maintaining good outcomes. Initial fears that the procedure would be less therapeutic have been unfounded.

Indications and Extent of Retroperitoneal Surgery for Postchemotherapy Residual Mass

The current questions include whether all masses need resection, what is the required extent of lymphadenectomy and is there a role for minimally invasive laparoscopic lymphadenectomy. It is well documented that the histological finding at post-chemotherapy RPL includes fibrosis/necrosis in approximately 50 per cent, teratoma in 35–45 per cent, and carcinoma in only 10–15 per cent [39]. The percentage of cancer in the post-chemotherapy RPL has decreased with current chemotherapy regimens. The 50 per cent of patients with fibrosis or necrosis only do not need resection if the pathology could be determined preoperatively. Postoperatively, observation only is required. Teratoma requires resection, not only to determine the pathology but also to prevent the growing teratoma syndrome and compression of surrounding tissue. Approximately 3 per cent are associated with malignant transformation along somatic lines as well. Cancer resection is therapeutic and usually followed by further chemotherapy although this is not always necessary and remains somewhat controversial.

The current standard for management of post-chemotherapy residual disease with normalized serum markers is secondary RPL [39]. Among patients with carcinoma, the addition of post-resection adjuvant chemotherapy is an important prognostic factor. In an early report from Indiana group, in 22 patients only 2 long-term survivals were noted in those who had no adjuvant chemotherapy after complete resection of retroperitoneal mass [40]. In a more recent series, however, 19/32(59 per cent) of patients who received 2 cycles of adjuvant chemotherapy survived while

Table 41.3: Surgical outcome of laparoscopic retroperitoneal lymphadenectomy for Stage II non-seminoma.

Reference	No	OR time (minutes)	Conversion (%)	Complications (%) Minor	Major
Gerber et al [73]	20	480	20	20	0
Klotz et al [74]	4	285	0	0	0
Rasswheiler et al [75]	34	248	13	9	5.9
Giusti et al [76]	6	325	0	16.7	0
Zhuo et al]77]	13	292	7	7	0
Nelson et al [78]	29	258	6.9	6.9	0
Janetschek et al]79]	76	294	2.6	5.3	0
Total	182	311	7	9.2	0.8

U = follow-up in months, RP = retroperitoneum

none of the nine patients with primary surgery alone survived [41]. Therefore, the standard today is 2 cycles of adjuvant chemotherapy in the presence of residual disease in retroperitoneum. A recent update from the Indiana University summarized their results with post-chemotherapy RPL in 870 patients. The risk factors identified in this review included the presence of cancer in the specimen, and post-chemotherapy tumor marker elevation. In the absence of these risk factors, the overall survival rate was 95.5 per cent compared to 67.5 per cent in patients with associated risk factors [42]. There have been a number of reports of prediction of the histology of the residual mass. At the present time, it is not possible to individualize the prediction of RP pathology.

Early studies have reported that the pattern of nodal metastasis after chemotherapy requires a full bilateral dissection to achieve the highest cure rate [43]. Subsequently, most North American surgeons performed a full bilateral RPL after chemotherapy, specifically in cases of high volume (stages IIc and III) disease. In a retrospective review from Memorial Sloan-Kettering of distribution of retroperitoneal metastasis in 113 patients, they concluded that a modified dissection and resection of residual mass would have resulted in a low 8 per cent rate of residual tumor in retroperitoneum. They concluded that a modified dissection with resection of the residual mass may be indicated in a select group of patients [44]. More, recently several groups have described modifications of surgical technique including a nerve-sparing approach, modified template, resection of retroperitoneal mass alone or in combination with intra-operative frozen sections to decrease morbidity.

Nerve-sparing techniques have been used for postchemotherapy RPL in selected patients [45, 46]. However, this approach can only be only used in a limited number of patients. Coogan et al performed 93 nerve-sparing RPLs after primary chemotherapy. At a median follow-up of 35 months, the ejaculation was preserved in 76 per cent and no retroperitoneal recurrence was noted. However, a nerve-sparing technique was only feasible in 20 per cent of their post-chemotherapy patients. In University of Toronto experience, a nerve-sparing approach is not feasible in approximately 30 per cent of post-chemotherapy RPLs.

Alternatively, excision of the residual mass with intraoperative frozen section has been reported [47, 48]. Based on the results of frozen section, a bilateral or modified dissection was performed if teratoma or carcinoma was found. Using this approach in 62 patients, Herr et al reported that all residual cancer was located within the boundaries of the residual mass. Frozen section analysis was falsely negative in four patients, of whom three had residual cancer and one had teratoma on the final pathology of the resected mass. At a median follow-up of six years, only one patient relapsed in the retroperitoneum with teratoma A more recent study reported excision of residual mass alone in 68 patients after primary high-dose chemotherapy [49]. Rabbani has recommended resection of the mass in combination with a modified dissection. In this study, one out of two patients who had resection of the mass alone presented with local recurrence due to incomplete resection [50].

Role of Laparoscopic Retroperitoneal Lymphadenectomy

Generally, the morbidity of retroperitoneal lymphadenectomy can be attributed to the laparotomy itself as well as to the specific aspects of the procedure and extent of dissection. The majority of these complications are minor and related to the laparotomy. Previous studies have reported the complication rate in large number of patients (Table 41.3) [51–53]. The rate of complications is less for low stage disease, modified unilateral lymphadenectomy, and nerve-sparing techniques [53]. Overall rates for low stage disease is 8 per cent–35 per cent. The most common complication for primary RPL is wound infection (4 per cent–5 per cent) followed by pulmonary complications (2 per cent) and small bowel obstruction (1 per cent) while the rate of pulmonary complication in post-chemotherapy RPL is 8 per cent–10 per cent. Similarly, the rate of small bowel obstruction (5 per cent), chylus ascites(1 per cent), and neurological injuries(1 per cent) has been higher in postchemotherapy patients. The overall complication rate was 20.7 per cent in the Indiana experience and up to 35 per cent in other series with a mortality rate of 0.8–1 per cent. Clearly, tumour size, location, adherence to vital structures along with inferior preoperative performance status contribute to higher rate of post-chemotherapy complications.

Aside from the reported surgical complications, the morbidity resulting from a large abdominal incision and pain in the immediate postoperative course is significant from the patient's view. Post-operative ileus may be prolonged and most patients are hospitalized for one week or longer and do not return to normal activity for several weeks.

Laparoscopic RPL offers an opportunity to reduce the general morbidity of RPL if its efficacy can be demonstrated. It was first reported in 1992 in a patient with stage I non-seminoma [54]. This technique was later popularized by Janetschek and colleagues [55]. While initially described for patients with clinical stage I disease as a diagnostic/staging modality, its use has recently been extended to include post-chemotherapy RPL in patients with clinical stage II disease [56]. Table 41.4 summarizes the reported results of laparoscopic RPL. Most series are small and the follow-up is short. The surgical technique used has been described previously [57]. In summary, a template dissection is performed similar to the open approach including interaortocaval and paraaortic nodes for right-sided tumors and paraaortic nodes for left sided tumors. This template is identical for stage I and stage II disease. A technical limitation of laparoscopic approach is the fact that a bilateral dissection is technically challenging and has not been performed routinely [58]. Furthermore, dissection of lymph nodes behind the vessels was not performed in the reported series. However, a recent study has demonstrated that dissection behind the vessels is not necessary during RPL since all metastasis are located anterior to the great vessels [58].

Janetschek reported on 76 patients with clinical stage I disease with a conversion rate of 2.6 per cent. With increasing experience, their operative time decreased to 219 minutes. The estimated blood loss was 152 mL and 25 per cent had positive histology. At a mean follow-up of 45.3 months, retroperitoneal recurrence occurred in 2 per cent and antegrade ejaculation was preserved in 98.3 per cent. In patients with stage

Table 41.4: Follow-up after laparoscopic retroperitoneal lymphadenectomy for Stage I non-seminoma.

Reference	No	F/U range (mean)	Ejaculation (%)	Local recurrence (%)	Distant metastasis
Gerber et al [73]	20	2–25 (10)	100	0	10
Rasswheile et al [75]	34	4–43 (27)	94.1	0	11.8
Giusti et al [76]	6	12–42 (27)	100	0	0
Nelson et al [7]	29	1–65 (16)	96.6	0	6.9
Janetschek et al [79]	76	10–87 (45)	98.7	1.3	0
Total	165	25	97.8	0.2	5.7

II (49 stage IIb, 14 stage IIc) disease after chemotherapy, the overall operating time was 226 minutes with no conversion to open surgery. The histological finding included: fibrosis in 63 per cent, germ cell malignancy in 2 per cent, and teratoma in 36.7 per cent. Overall these reports demonstrate that laparoscopic RPL can be diagnostic and therapeutic. Large volume retroperitoneal disease after chemotherapy, however, cannot be managed safely laparoscopically.

Complications of laparoscopic RPL in reported series are summarized in Table 41.3. The overall rate of minor and major complications was 7.8 per cent and 0.7 per cent, respectively, with a conversion rate of 5.2 per cent.

A recent review of patient-reported morbidity and quality of life after RPL compared 53 open and 59 laparoscopic RPL using a questionnaire [58]. Patients were questioned with regard to satisfaction, return to normal activity and other aspects of social and sexual life. In summary, the quality of life was superior in the laparoscopic group. The complete satisfaction rate with surgery and side effects was 80 per cent in the laparoscopic group compared to 54 per cent in the open group. The average time required to return to normal activity was 7.2 weeks for the laparoscopic group compared to 14.9 weeks for the open group.

A limitation of the laparoscopic approach to RPL is the fact that advanced laparoscopic skills are required and the learning curve is significant. The current dilemma arises from the fact that many centers that do not have the laparoscopic expertise are treating the majority of patients with testicular cancer and vice versa. It is obvious that if this procedure is not performed routinely at an institution, the risks of the laparoscopic approach outweigh the benefits. Furthermore, due to an increase in operative times in the beginning, a loss of productivity should be expected. Therefore, this procedure should be reserved for centers with a sufficient patient referral base and laparoscopic experience in order to remain competitive to the open surgical approach.

If similar results can be achieved with a significant reduction in the surgical morbidity, the laparoscopic technique for RPL may change our current management of non-seminoma testis cancer. In clinical stage I disease, specifically in high risk patients, the application of laparoscopic RPL may become an alternative to surveillance and may replace open RPL in those centers which routinely perform modified RPL for clinical stage I disease. Furthermore, with current modifications of the surgical template for post-chemotherapy RPL, the laparoscopic approach can be offered as a therapeutic option to selected patients who have limited retroperitoneal nodal disease.

Conclusion

Patients presenting with suspected tumours need not undergo initial radical orchiectomy until the diagnosis is established. There appears to be a role for partial orchiectomy in selected cases and the role for percutaneous needle biopsy should be investigated. The necessary extent of retroperitoneal lymphadenectomy with nerve sparing as definitive treatment for metastatic disease to the regional nodes has been defined and in general reduced. There is an emerging role for laparoscopic lymphadenectomy for staging and probably therapy. The post chemotherapy residual mass remains a surgical problem. Although the rate of residual cancer has decreased with more effective chemotherapy, no reliable means for pathological confirmation exists for the individual patient. Most patients with detectable disease should undergo surgery. The extent of the surgery, i.e. removal of the mass versus extended lymphadenectomy remains controversial.

References

1. Dean AL. The treatment of teratoid tumours of the testes with radium and the x-ray. *J Urol* 1925;13:149.
2. Capelouto CC, Clark PE, Ransil BJ, Loughlin KR. A review of scrotal violation in testicular cancer: is adjuvant local therapy necessary? *J Urol* 1995;153:981–985.
3. Kennedy CL, Hendry WF, Peckham MJ. The significance of scrotal interference in stage 1 testicular cancer managed by orchiectomy and surveillance. *Brit J Urol* 1986;58:705.
4. Aki FT, Bilen CY, Tekin MI, Ozen H. Is scrotal violation per se a risk factor for local relapse and metastases in stage 1 nonseminomatous testicular cancer? *Urology* 2000;56:459–462.
5. Markland C, Kedia K, Fraley EE. Inadequate orchiectomy in patients with testicular tumours. *JAMA* 1984;224:1025.
6. Verma K, Ram T, Kapila K. Value of fine needle aspiration cytology in the diagnosis of testicular neoplasms. *Acta Cytologica* 1989;33(5):631–634.
7. Linsk JA, Franzen S. *Clinical Aspiration Cytology* 1983.
8. Zajicek J. *Monographs in Clinical Cytology* 1979.
9. Heidenreich A, Bonfig R, Derschum W, von Vietsch H, Wilbert DM. A conservative approach to bilateral testicular germ cell tumors. *J Urol* 1995;153:10–13.
10. Weissbach L. Organ preserving surgery of malignant germ cell tumors. *J Urol* 1995;153:90–93.
11. van der Schyff S, Heidenreich A, Weibbach L, Hohlt W. Organ preserving surgery in testicular cancer. *J Urol* 2000;163(supp):145.
12. Bokemeyer C, Schmoll H, Schoffski P, al e. Bilateral testicular tumours: Prevalence and clinical implications. *Eur J Cancer* 1993;6:874.
13. Richie JP. Simultaneous bilateral tumors with unorthodox management. *World J Urol* 1984;2:74.
14. Fossa SD, Opjordsmoen S, Huang E. Androgen replacement and quality of life in patients treated for bilateral testicular cancer. *Eur J Cancer* 1999;35:1220–1225.
15. Giwercman A, von der Maase H, Berthelsen JG, Rorth M, Bertelsen A, Skakkebaek NE. Localized irradiation of testes with carcinoma in situ: effects on Leidig cell function and eradication of malignant germ cells in 20 patients. *J Clin Endocrinol Metab* 1991;73:596.
16. Fordham MVP, Mason MD, Blackmore C, Hendry WF, Horwich A. Management of the contralateral testis in patients with testicular germ cell cancer. *J Urol* 1990;65:290–293.
17. Heidenreich A, Hofmann R. Quality-of-life issues in the treatment of testicular cancer. *World J Urol* 1999;17:230–238.
18. Donohue JP, Thornhill JA, Foster RS, Rowland RG, Bihrle R. Retroperitoneal lymphadenectomy for clinical stage A testis cancer (1965–1989): modifications of technique and impact on ejaculation. *J Urol* 1993;149:237–247.
19. Pizzocaro G. Retroperitoneal lymphadenectomy in clinical stage I nonseminomatous germinal testis cancer. *Eur J Surg Oncology* 1986;12:25–28.
20. Aass N, Fossa SD, Ous S, et al. Is routine primary retroperitoneal lymph node dissection still justified in patients with low stage non-seminomatous testicular cancer? *Brit J Urol* 1990;65:385–90.
21. Klepp O, Olsson AM, Henrikson H, et al. Prognostic factors in clinical stage I nonseminomatous germ cell tumors of the testis: multivariate analysis of a prospective multicenter study. *J Clin Oncol* 1990;8:509–518.
22. Richie JP. Clinical stage I testicular cancer: the role of modified retroperitoneal lymphadenectomy. *J Urol* 1990;144:1160.
23. McLeod DG, Weiss RB, Stablein DM, et al. Staging relationships and outcome in early stage testicular cancer: a report from the Testicular Cancer Intergroup study. *J Urol* 1991;145:1178–1183.
24. Donohue JP, Thornhill JA, Foster RS, Bihrle R, Rowland RG, Einhorn LH. The role of retroperitoneal lymphadenectomy in clinical stage B testis cancer: the Indiana University experience (1965 to 1989). *J Urol* 1995;153:85–9.
25. Jewett MA, Incze P. Retroperitoneal lymphadenectomy: the traditional treatment option. *Semin Urol Oncol* 1996;14:24–9.
26. Horwich A. Primary chemotherapy: how does it compare with surgery? *Semin Urol Oncol* 1996;14:34–5.
27. Foster RS, Donohue JP. Retroperitoneal lymph node dissection for the management of clinical stage I nonseminoma. *J Urol* 2000;163(6):1788–92.

28. Ray B, Hajdu SI, Whitmore WFJ. Distribution of lymph node metastases in testicular germinal tumors. *Cancer* 1974;33:340–348.
29. Donohue JP, Maynard B, Zachary M. The distribution of nodal metastases in the retroperitoneum from nonseminomatous testis cancer. *J Urol* 1982;128:315–320.
30. Weissbach L, Boedefeld EA.. Localization of solitary and multiple metastases in stage II nonseminomatous testis tumor as basis for a modified staging lymph node dissection in stage I. *J Urol* 1987;138:77–82.
31. Jewett MA, Kong YS, Goldberg SD, et al. Retroperitoneal lymphadenectomy for testis tumor with nerve sparing for ejaculation. *J Urol* 1988;139:1220–4.
32. Donohue JP, Foster RS, Rowland RG, Bihrle R, Jones J, Geier G. Nerve-sparing retroperitoneal lymphadenectomy with preservation of ejaculation. *J Urol* 1990;144:287–91; discussion 291–2.
33. Fossa SD, Klepp O, Ous S, et al. Unilateral retroperitoneal lymph node dissection in patients with non-seminomatous testicular tumor in clinical stage I. *Eur Urol* 1984;10:17–23.
34. Pizzocaro G, Salvioni R, Zanoni F. Unilateral lymphadenectomy in intraoperative stage I nonseminomatous germinal testis cancer. *J Urol* 1985;134:485–9.
35. Doerr A, Skinner EC, Skinner DG. Preservation of ejaculation through a modified retroperitoneal lymph node dissection in low stage testis cancer. *J Urol* 1993;149:1472–1474.
36. Donohue JP. Nerve-sparing retroperitoneal lymphadenectomy for testis cancer. Evolution of surgical templates for low-stage disease. *Eur Urol* 1993;23:44–6.
37. Jewett MA, Kong YS, Goldberg SD, et al. Retroperitoneal lymphadenectomy for testis tumor with nerve sparing for ejaculation. *J Urol* 1988;139:1220–4.
38. Jewett MA. Nerve-sparing technique for retroperitoneal lymphadenectomy in testis cancer. *Urol Clin North Am* 1990;17:449–56.
39. Sheinfeld J, Bajorin D. Management of the postchemotherapy residual mass. *Urol Clin North Am* 1993;20:133–43.
40. Einhorn LH, Williams SD, Mandelbaum I, Donohue JP. Surgical resection in disseminated testicular cancer following chemotherapeutic cytoreduction. *Cancer* 1981;48:904–8.
41. Fox EP, Weathers TD, Williams SD, et al. Outcome analysis for patients with persistent nonteratomatous germ cell tumor in postchemotherapy retroperitoneal lymph node dissections. *J Clin Oncol* 1993;11:1294–9.
42. Donohue JP, Foster RS. Retroperitoneal lymphadenectomy in staging and treatment. The development of nerve-sparing techniques. *Urol Clin North Am* 1998;25:461–8.
43. Donohue JP, Rowland RG. The role of surgery in advanced testicular cancer. *Cancer* 1984;54:2716–21.
44. Wood DP, Jr., Herr HW, Heller G, et al. Distribution of retroperitoneal metastases after chemotherapy in patients with nonseminomatous germ cell tumors. *J Urol* 1992;148:1812–5; discussion 1815–6.
45. Wahle GR, Foster RS, Bihrle R, Rowland RG, Bennett RM. Nerve sparing retroperitoneal lymphadenectomy after primary chemotherapy for metastatic testicular carcinoma. *J Urol* 1994;152:428–430.
46. Coogan CL, Hejase MJ, Wahle GR, et al. Nerve sparing post-chemotherapy retroperitoneal lymph node dissection for advanced testicular cancer. *J Urol* 1996;156:1656–8.
47. Aprikian AG, Herr HW, Bajorin DF, Bosl GJ. Resection of postchemotherapy residual masses and limited retroperitoneal lymphadenectomy in patients with metastatic testicular nonseminomatous germ cell tumors. *Cancer* 1994;74:1329–34.
48. Herr HW. Does necrosis on frozen-section analysis of a mass after chemotherapy justify a limited retroperitoneal resection in patients with advanced testis cancer? *Br J Urol* 1997;80(4):653–7.
49. Ozen H, Ekici S, Sozen S, Ergen A, Tekgul S, Kendi S. Resection of residual masses alone: an alternative in surgical therapy of metastatic testicular germ cell tumors after chemotherapy. *Urology* 2001;57:323–7.
50. Rabbani F, Gleave ME, Coppin CM, Murray N, Sullivan LD. Teratoma in primary testis tumor reduces complete response rates in the retroperitoneum after primary chemotherapy. The case for primary retroperitoneal lymph node dissection of stage IIb germ cell tumors with teratomatous elements. *Cancer* 1996;78:480–6.
51. Jewett MAS, Wesley-James T. Early and late complications of retroperitoneal lymphadenectomy. *Can J Surg* 1991;34:368–373.
52. Baniel J, Foster RS, Rowland RG, Bihrle R, Donohue JP. Complications of post-chemotherapy retroperitoneal lymph node dissection. *J Urol* 1995;153:976–80.
53. Baniel J, Sella A. Complications of retroperitoneal lymph node dissection in testicular cancer: primary and post-chemotherapy. *Semin Surg Oncol* 1999;17:263–7.
54. Rukstalis DB, Chodak GW. Laparoscopic retroperitoneal lymph node dissection in a patient with stage 1 testicular carcinoma. *J Urol* 1992;148(6):1907–9.

55. Janetschek G, Hobisch A, Holtl L, Bartsch G. Retroperitoneal lymphadenectomy for clinical stage I nonseminomatous testicular tumor: laparoscopy versus open surgery and impact of learning curve. *J Urol* 1996;156:89–93.
56. Janetschek G, Hobisch A, Hittmair A, Holtl L, Peschel R, Bartsch G. Laparoscopic retroperitoneal lymphadenectomy after chemotherapy for stage IIB nonseminomatous testicular carcinoma. *J Urol* 1999;161:477–81.
57. Janetschek G, Hobisch A, Peschel R, Bartsch G. Laparoscopic retroperitoneal lymph node dissection. *Urology* 2000;55:136–40.
58. Janetschek G. Laparoscopic retroperitoneal lymph node dissection. *Urol Clin North Am* 2001;28:107–14.
59. Rorth M, Jacobsen GK, von der Maase H, et al. Surveillance alone versus radiotherapy after orchiectomy for clinical stage I nonseminomatous testicular cancer. Danish Testicular Cancer Study Group. *J Clin Oncol* 1991;9:1543–8.
60. Read G, Stenning SP, Cullen MH, et al. Medical Research Council prospective study of surveillance for stage I testicular teratoma. *J Clin Oncol* 1992;10:1762–68.
61. Swanson D. The case for observation of patients with clinical stage I noseminomatous germ cell testicular tumors. *Semin Urol* 1993;11:92–98.
62. Ondrus D, Hornak M. Orchiectomy alone for clinical stage I nonseminomatous germ cell tumors of the testis (NSGCTT): a minimum follow-up period of 5 years. *Tumori* 1994;80:362–4.
63. Nicolai N, Pizzocaro G. A surveillance study of clinical stage I nonseminomatous germ cell tumors of the testis: 10-year followup. *J Urol* 1995;154:1045–9.
64. Gels ME, Hoekstra HJ, Sleijfer DT, et al. Detection of recurrence in patients with clinical stage I nonseminomatous testicular germ cell tumors and consequences for further follow-up: a single-center 10-year experience. *J Clin Oncol* 1995;13:1188–94.
65. Sogani PC, Perrotti M, Herr HW, Fair WR, Thaler HT, Bosl G. Clinical stage I testis cancer: long-term outcome of patients on surveillance. *J Urol* 1998;159:855–8.
66. Hao D, Seidel J, Brant R, et al. Compliance of clinical stage I nonseminomatous germ cell tumor patients with surveillance. *J Urol* 1998;160:768–71.
67. Colls BM, Harvey VJ, Skelton L, et al. Late results of surveillance of clinical stage I nonseminoma germ cell testicular tumours: 17 years' experience in a national study in New Zealand. *BJU Int* 1999;83:76–82.
68. Sharir S, Jewett MAS, Sturgeon J, et al. Progression detection of stage I nonseminomatous testis cancer on surveillance: Implications for the follow up protocol. *J Urol* 1999;161:472–476.
69. Javadpour N, Canning DA, O'Connell KJ, Young JD. Predictors of recurrent clinical stage I nonseminomatous testicular cancer. A prospective clinicopathologic study. *Urology* 1986;27:508–11.
70. Richie JP. Clinical stage 1 testicular cancer: the role of modified retroperitoneal lymphadenectomy. *J Urol* 1990;144:1160–3.
71. McLeod DG, Weiss RB, Stablein DM, et al. Staging relationships and outcome in early stage testicular cancer: a report from the Testicular Cancer Intergroup Study. *J Urol* 1991;145:1178–83.
72. Donohue JP, Thornhill JA, Foster RS, Rowland RG, Bihrle R. Primary retroperitoneal lymph node dissection in clinical stage A non-seminomatous germ cell testis cancer. Review of the Indiana University experience 1965–1989. *Br J Urol* 1993;71:326–35.
73. Gerber GS, Bissada NK, Hulbert JC, et al. Laparoscopic retroperitoneal lymphadenectomy: multi-institutional analysis. *J Urol* 1994;152:1188–91.
74. Klotz L. Laparoscopic retroperitoneal lymphadenectomy for high-risk stage 1 nonseminomatous germ cell tumor: report of four cases. *Urology* 1994;43:752–6.
75. Rassweiler JJ, Frede T, Lenz E, Seemann O, Alken P. Long-term experience with laparoscopic retroperitoneal lymph node dissection in the management of low-stage testis cancer. *Eur Urol* 2000;37:251–60.
76. Giusti G, Beltrami P, Tallarigo C, Bianchi G, Mobilio G. Unilateral laparoscopic retroperitoneal lymphadenectomy for clinical stage I nonseminomatous testicular cancer. *J Endourol* 1998;12:561–6.
77. Zhuo Y, Klaen R, Sauter TW, Miller K. Laparoscopic retroperitoneal lymph node dissection in clinical stage I nonseminomatous germ cell tumor: a minimal invasive alternative. *Chin Med J (Engl)* 1998;111:537–41.
78. Nelson JB, Chen RN, Bishoff JT, et al. Laparoscopic retroperitoneal lymph node dissection for clinical stage I nonseminomatous germ cell testicular tumors. *Urology* 1999;54:1064–7.
79. Janetschek G, Hobisch A, Peschel R, Hittmair A, Bartsch G. Laparoscopic retroperitoneal lymph node dissection for clinical stage I nonseminomatous testicular carcinoma: long-term outcome. *J Urol* 2000;163:1793–6.

Section 6

Quality of Life

42. Quality of Life in Patients with Good Prognosis Metastatic Germ Cell Tumours: Comparison of Four Chemotherapy Schedules (EORTC 30941/MRC TE20)

S.D. Fosså[1], L. Collette[2], N. Aaronson[3], R. deWit[4], J.T. Roberts[5], on behalf of the EORTC GU Group and the MRC Testicular Cancer Working Party

1. The Norwegian Radium Hospital, Oslo, Norway, 2. The European Organisation for Research and Treatment of Cancer Data Center, Brussels, Belgium, 3. The Netherlands Cancer Institute, Amsterdam, The Netherlands, 4. The Rotterdam Cancer Institute and University Hospital, Rotterdam, The Netherlands, 5. Northern Centre for Cancer Treatment, Newcastle upon Tyne, United Kingdom

Abstract

Aim: To compare Quality of Life (QL) in patients with metastatic testicular cancer (TC) receiving 3 or 4 cycles of cisplatin-based chemotherapy (BEP), given over 3 or 5 days.

Methods: QL was prospectively evaluated before chemotherapy and at 3 and 12 months in 666 patients receiving one of 4 different equally dosed BEP schedules (4 cycles/5 days [standard]; 4 cycles/3 days; 3 cycles/5 days; 3 cycles/3 days). The EORTC QLQ-C30 was used together with a specific TC module.

Results: The 3 day schedule lead to increased toxicity at three months, which was "clinically" significant (see below) for nausea/vomiting and tinnitus if each of 4 cycles was given over 3 days. At one year, no schedule-related difference was detectable except for tinnitus, which was worst after 4 cycles/3 days. Ototoxicity, peripheral neuropathy and Raynaud`s phenomena remained a clinical problem. Compared to baseline QL had slightly improved.

Conclusion: The 5 days BEP schedule is preferable if 4 cycles are planned to avoid excessive short-term and 1 year subjective toxicity.

Introduction

The scientific evaluation of health-related Quality of Life (QoL) has become a challenging research issue in clinical oncology, at a similar level to the consideration of survival and response rates. The multi-dimensional concept of QoL describes a cancer patient's psychosocial and physical well-being. In clinical practice, QoL is most often assessed by patient-completed questionnaires, which fulfil clearly defined psychometric criteria as to reliability, validity and responsiveness. Although QoL research still presents multiple methodological problems, consideration of QoL assists clinicians in therapeutic decisions regarding palliative and curative treatment modalities, and may be of importance when health economic aspects are discussed.

Cancer treatment affects both short-term and long-term QoL. For several years attention has focussed on the avoidance of long-term impairment of QoL. On the other hand, oncologists have more easily accepted reduction of short-term QoL, and severe, but transient toxicity is often viewed as an inevitable complication of intensive treatment of cancer. However, severe acute toxicity may lead to reduced patient compliance with therapy, and may also have negative long-term consequences after treatment discontinuation. If possible, even short-term toxicity should be avoided as much as possible.

Many cross-sectional studies have reported aspects of long-term QoL and long-term toxicity in patients with malignant germ cell tumours (GCT) [1–4]. Oncologists have become aware of the fact that the > 90 per cent cure rate obtained in recent years has probably been obtained by "over-treatment" of a substantial number of these patients. Some of today's aims of clinical research are therefore to define treatment modalities and treatment combinations, which maintain high cure rates, but leave the patient with optimal short and long-term QoL.

So far there is limited experience from prospective studies of short-term QoL after different treatment options for testicular cancer (TC), which is the most frequent presentation of GCT. In this situation, surgeons tend to argue for extended use of surgery, whereas oncologists have tried to apply less surgery and, during the last decade even less chemotherapy and radiotherapy. During recent years health economic considerations have also been put forward when the optimal treatment of TC has been discussed, such as the cost of necessary follow-up examinations and the number of days of hospitalisation required. Most of these discussions have been based on doctors' observations of objective side effects, whereas the patients' own perception of his QoL during the different treatment modalities has been less thoroughly investigated in prospective studies, except for one recent report by Weissbach et al. [5].

With this background the EORTC GU group decided in 1994 to investigate QoL in patients with good prognosis metastatic GCT, who were entered into trial 30941. The results of this trial have been published elsewhere [6] showing that the 2 year progression-free survival after 3 cycles of BEP chemotherapy (Bleomycin, Etoposide, Cisplatin) is equivalent to that after 4 cycles, and that the survival rates are not related to the schedule of Platinum chemotherapy (3 versus 5 days). In the present report, some observations concerning QoL are discussed.

Patients and Methods

Patients with good prognosis metastatic GCT [7] were randomised to receive 4 or 3 cycles of BEP with a further randomisation between equivalent drug doses administered over 5 or 3 days (2 x 2 factorial design) (Table 42.1). If 4 cycles were given, Bleomycin was omitted during the last course of chemotherapy. The hydration schedule during each cycle was standardised in the protocol and was similar in all patients. Post-chemotherapy residual tumour masses were to be resected surgically. Patients were followed-up at 3–6 months intervals after the end of all treatment.

Table 42.1: EORTC Trial 30941/MRC TE20

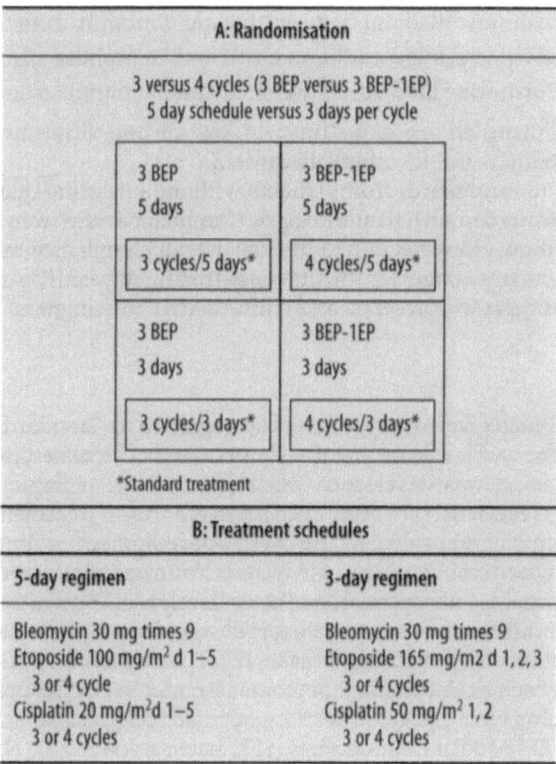

A: Randomisation

3 versus 4 cycles (3 BEP versus 3 BEP-1EP)
5 day schedule versus 3 days per cycle

3 BEP	3 BEP-1EP
5 days	5 days
3 cycles/5 days*	4 cycles/5 days*

3 BEP	3 BEP-1EP
3 days	3 days
3 cycles/3 days*	4 cycles/3 days*

*Standard treatment

B: Treatment schedules	
5-day regimen	**3-day regimen**
Bleomycin 30 mg times 9	Bleomycin 30 mg times 9
Etoposide 100 mg/m^2 d 1–5	Etoposide 165 mg/m2 d 1, 2, 3
3 or 4 cycle	3 or 4 cycles
Cisplatin 20 mg/m^{2}d 1–5	Cisplatin 50 mg/m^2 1, 2
3 or 4 cycles	3 or 4 cycles

QoL Assessment

Questionnaires: QoL was evaluated by the EORTC QLQ C-30 version 2 [8], supplemented by a published TC module [9]. The latter asked for TC specific side effects and expected treatment induced toxicity such as disturbance of sexual life, fertility, development of hearing loss, tinnitus, peripheral neuropathy and /or Raynaud's phenomena.

The scales of the EORTC QLQ C-30 were transformed according to the published scoring guidelines [8]. Functional scales ranged from 0 (worst) to 100 (best), and symptom scales from 0 (best) to 100 (worst). The transformation of the responses to the items from the TC module was similar to that of the symptom scales, except for the two items: "Have you been happy with the medical management?" and "Has the sexual relationship with your partner been satisfactory?" The scores of these 2 questions were transformed as done for functional scales.

Timing: Patients were asked to complete the questionnaire before randomisation and then 3, 6, 12 and 24 months after the start of treatment. The available questionnaires were grouped within the following time windows:

• Baseline if the assessment was done before the start of the treatment and within 15 days of entry on study.

- Month 3 if the form was filled out between 2 and 4,5 months from entry.
- Month 6 if the form was filled out between 4,5 and 9 months from entry.
- Month 12 if the form was filled out between 10 and 16 months from entry.
- Month 24 if the form was filled out between 20 and 30 months from entry.

Whenever several forms fell in a same time window, the one closest to the pre-defined time point was retained and the others discarded.

Post-treatment questionnaires from patients without a baseline questionnaire were excluded as were forms completed after relapse. Compliance rates were similar between the 4 treatment groups. However, due to the low overall compliance rate at 2 years (47 per cent), QoL was analysed only for the first post-treatment year. The dropout patterns did not, however, suggest the presence of an informative "missingness" pattern.

Statistics

Four cycles of BEP, each given during 5 days was regarded as "standard treatment" and the average score for each scale of the questionnaire was calculated for this schedule. A mixed effects model was developed which assessed the changes of scale scores within the same treatment schedule and between the 4 treatment schedules, at baseline, and 3 months and evaluated the overall development of dimensions during the first year (Longitudinal analysis). Any effects of interaction were also analysed. (This statistical model is sub-optimal for the evaluation of 6 months changes). Only clinically relevant differences were considered significant. These were defined as changes of ≥ 10 points of the individual scale [10]. The dimension of Global quality of life (QL) was regarded as the principal outcome parameter. For the present report the following dimensions were selected for more detailed longitudinal analysis: Physical (PF), emotional (EF), social functioning (SF), nausea/vomiting (N/V), peripheral sensory neuropathy in hands and/or feet (PHF), Raynaud`s phenomena (CHF: Cold hands and/or feet), hearing loss (HL: Hearing loss) and tinnitus (TN: Tinnitus). In addition the 1-year change of scores from baseline were compared. Due to multiple comparisons a p-value < 0.01 was regarded as statistically significant.

Results

For the final analysis a total of 2180 forms from 666 of the 812 randomised patients were used (Table 42.2). A total of 23 per cent of the patients had a pure seminoma, the remainder a non-seminoma, evenly distributed among the 4 treatment groups.

Table 42.2: Demographics

	3 cycles		4 cycles		Total
	3 days	5 days	3 days	5 days	
Entered	233	173	237	169	812
Evaluable					
Number of patients	183	142	200	141	666
Number of forms	593	478	635	474	2180
Median age (or years)	32	32	31	30	31
(Range)	(16–69)	(16–62)	(16–60)	(16–63)	(16–63)

At <u>baseline</u> patients described emotional problems, fatigue, pain and sleeplessness as their main problems (Figure 42.1a). They were highly worried about the outcome of their malignancy, about future fertility and their future sexual life (Figure 42.1b).

At <u>3 months</u> standard BEP chemotherapy (4 cycles/5 days) led to a decrease of the QL score by 9.6 points and of social (10.8 points) and physical (13.5 points) functioning (Figure 42.2a). For these functional scales no *clinically significant* differences between the 4 treatment schedules were detected, though the 4 cycles/3 days regimen resulted in *statistically* worse scores at 3 months. The EF scale had improved at 3 months.

Increased nausea/vomiting was reported at 3 months, but neither after 4 nor after 3 cycles did the changes from baseline reach the level of clinical relevance, as long as chemotherapy was given over 5 days during 4 or 3 cycles. If each of 4 cycles were given during 3 days, the increase of gastro-intestinal toxicity was on average 19.3 points. The analogue figure after 3 cycles was 8.7 points.

After 4 cycles symptoms of peripheral neuropathy reached their maximum at 6 months, and this was also observed regarding Raynaud`s phenomena (Figure 42.2).

Clinically relevant differences became evident for these two dimensions comparing 3 versus 4 cycles, 4 cycles appearing to be worse, but not between 3 versus 5 days. Three months after start of BEP chemotherapy tinnitus had become a clinically relevant problem, independent of the treatment schedule, but was worst if 4 cycles/3 days were applied. Hearing loss was perceived by the patients at a much lesser degree than tinnitus, but was most pronounced after 4 cycles/3 days.

The mixed effect model revealed a clinically relevant improvement of the emotional function at <u>1 year</u>, but deterioration of peripheral neuropathy and Raynaud phenomena. Overall QL had improved by 7.2 points on average. One year improvement/deterioration of the scales of the QLQ-C-30 and of the TC model was independent of the treatment schedule, except for tinnitus. For the latter, the 4 cycles/3 days schedule resulted in clinically relevant deterioration after 1 year (12 points), whereas the development of tinnitus was comparable to only 6 points after each of the 3 other treatment schedules.

Comparison Between Scores at Baseline and 1 Year

Comparison of the baseline scores with those obtained at 1 year confirms the improvement of emotional distress and a moderate increase of global QL (Figure 42.1). Symptom scales such as fatigue, pain and sleeplessness had improved, together with reduction of concerns about fertility. The symptoms of both peripheral neuropathy and Raynaud`s phenomena were maximal at six months following 4 cycles of chemotherapy. The increased 1-year scores of peripheral neuropathy, Raynaud`s phenomena and tinnitus support the results of the longitudinal analysis as to induction of these side effects.

Discussion

This prospective randomised study shows that 3 or 4 cycles of BEP chemotherapy lead to a significant reduction of QoL with gradual improvement thereafter. As expected 4 cycles result in more 3-month toxicity than 3 cycles. (In the latter case the patients have been off treatment for 3–4 weeks when completing the questionnaire whereas only for a few days have elapsed since last chemotherapy for patients

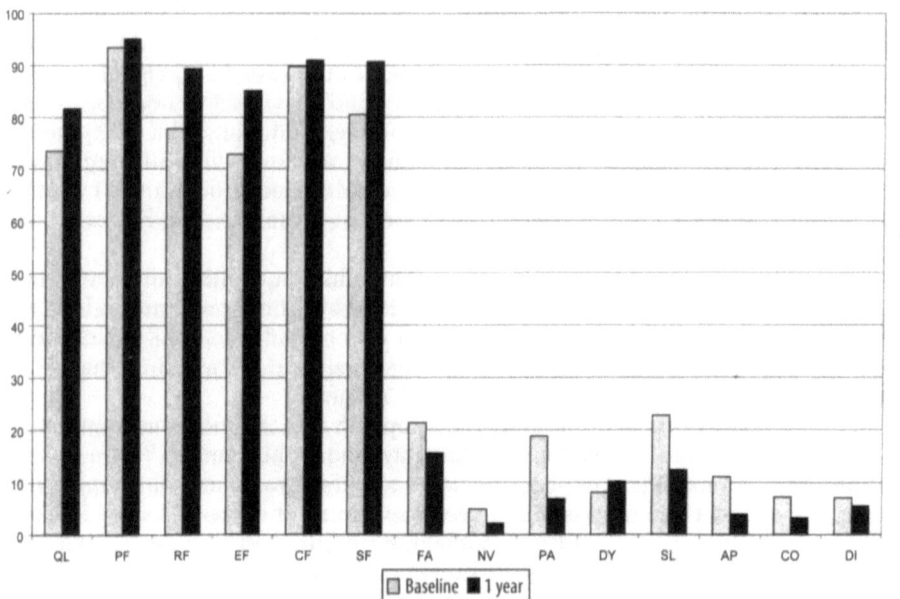

QL: Quality of Life; PF: Physical function; RF: Role function; EF: Emotional function; CF: Cognitive function; SF: Social function; FA: Fatigue; NV: Nausea/Vomiting; PA: Pain; DY: Dyspnoea; SL: Sleeplessness; AP: Appetite loss; CO: Constipation; DI: Diarrhoea.

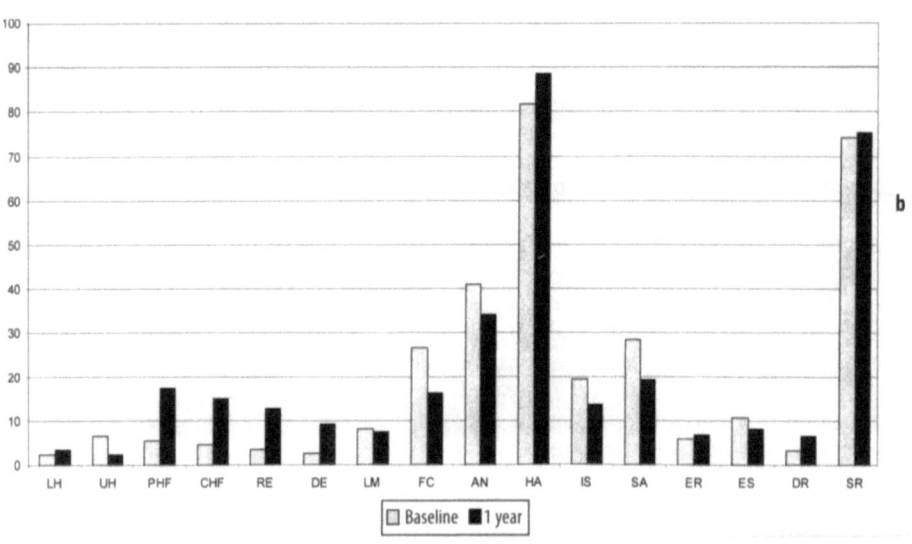

LH: Loss of Hair; UH: Upset by hair loss; PHF: Peripheral neuropathy in hands/feet; CHF: Pale/cold hands/feet; TN: Tinnitus; HL: Hearing loss; LM: Less masculine; FC: Fertility concerns; AN: Anxiety as to recurrence; HA: Happy with medical management; SI: Reduced sexual interest; SA: Reduced sexual activity; ER: Difficult erectile function; ES: Reduced sexual pleasure; DR: Dry ejaculation; SR: Satisfying sexual relationship with partner.

Figure 42.1: Mean quality of life scale scores at baseline ☐ and 1 year after ■ BEP chemotherapy. **a** EORTC QLQ C-30 **b** Testicular Cancer module

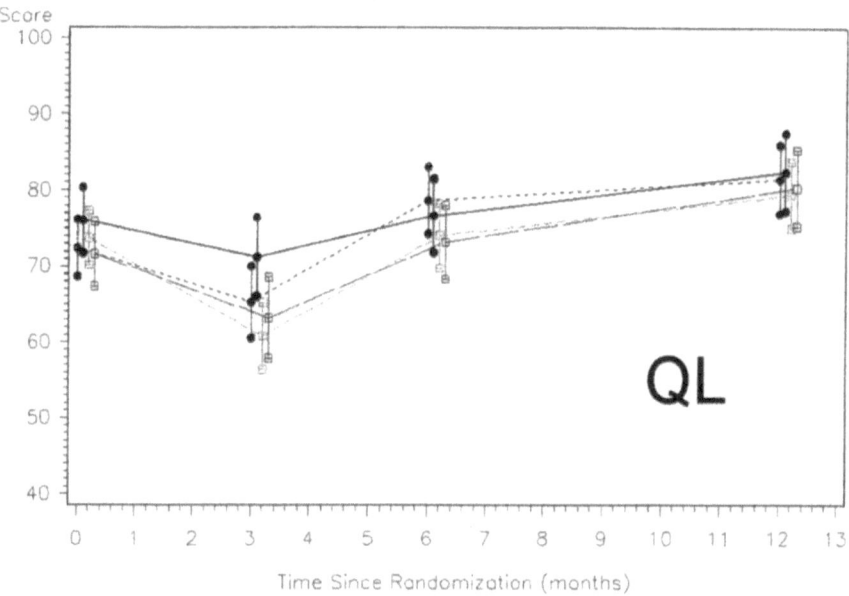

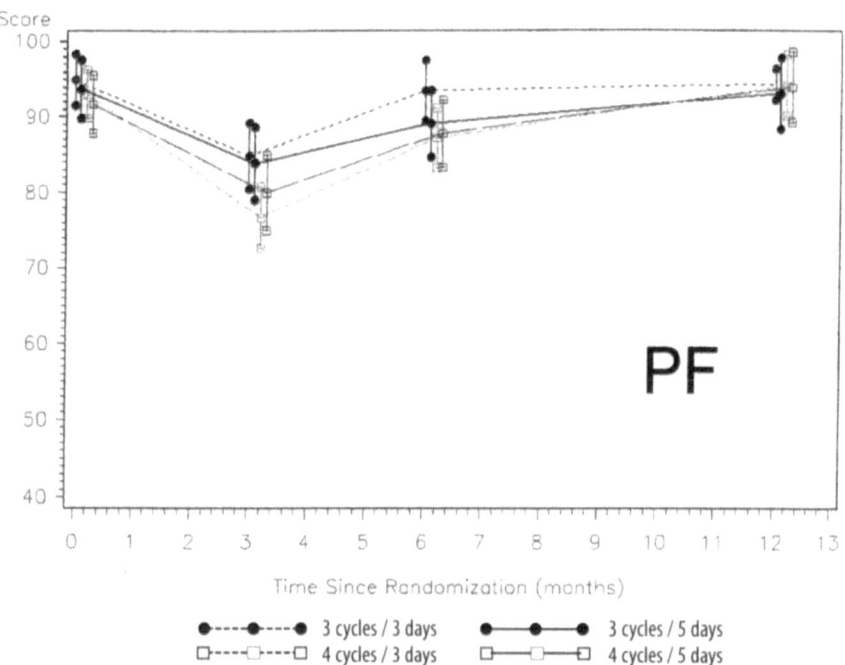

Figure 42.2a: 1-year profile of selected qualify of life scales. **a** EORTC QLQ C-30 **b** Testicular Cancer module.

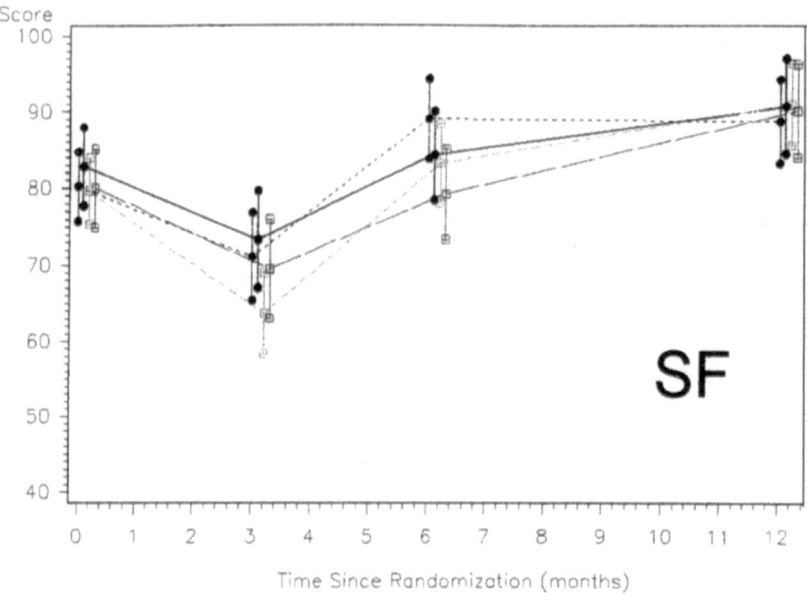

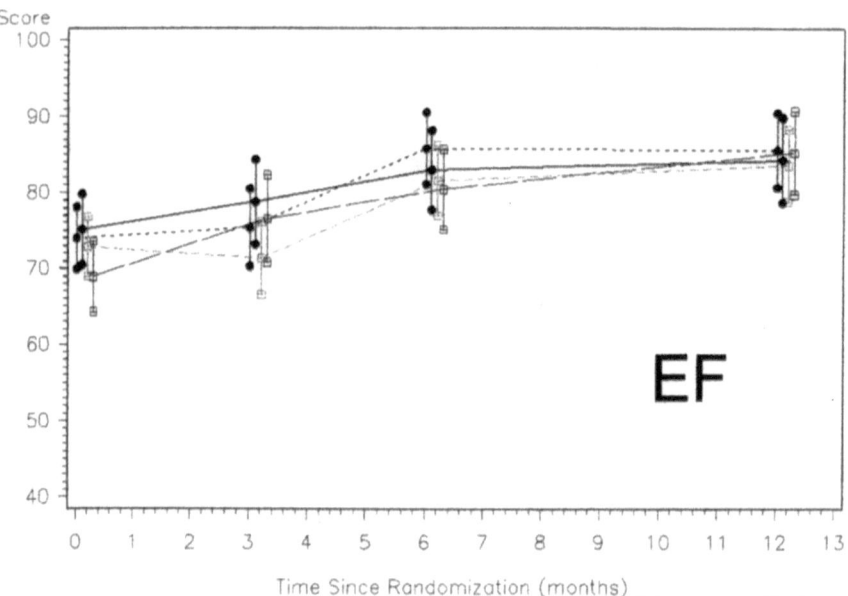

Figure 42.2a *(continued)*

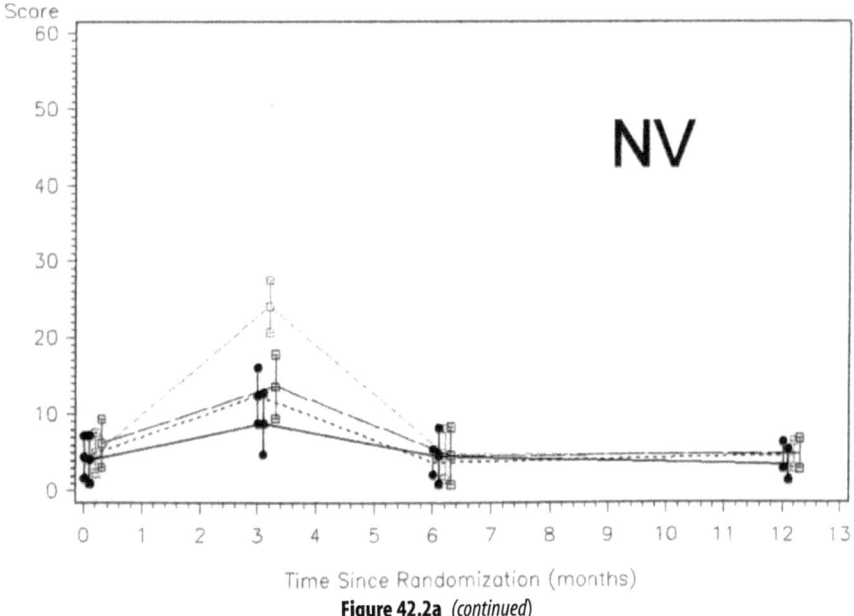

Figure 42.2a *(continued)*

QL: Quality of Life; PF: Physical function; EF: Emotional function; SF: Social function; NV: Nausea/Vomiting.

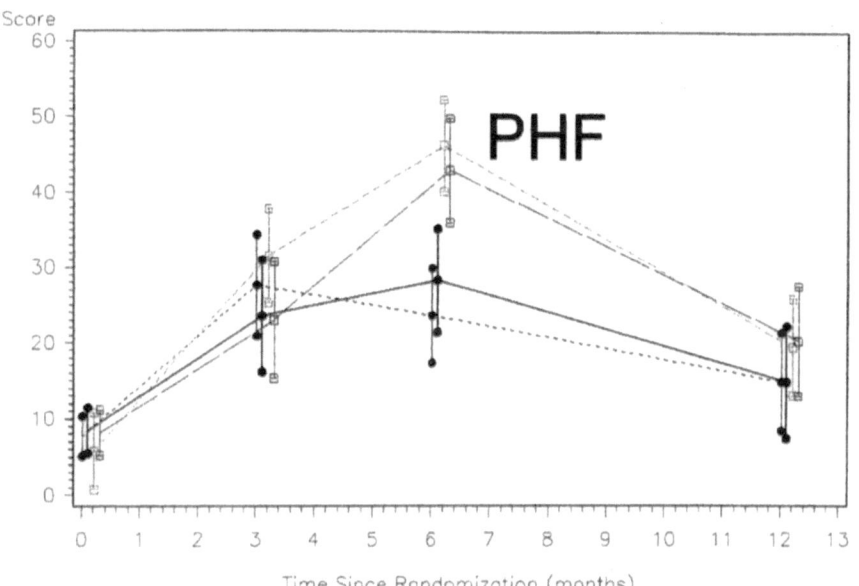

Figure 42.2b: PHF: Periphral neuropathy in hands/feet; CHF: Pale/cold hands/feet; TN Tinnitus; HL: Hearing loss.

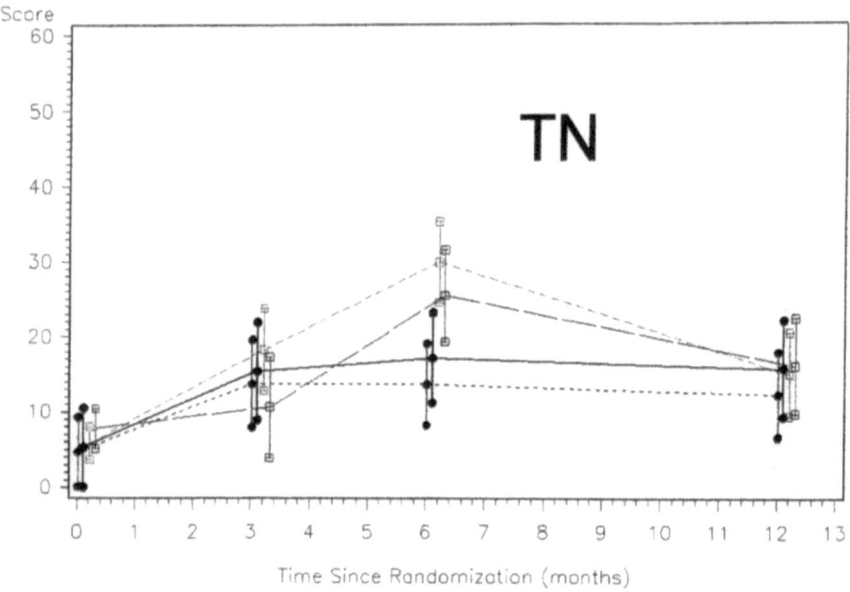

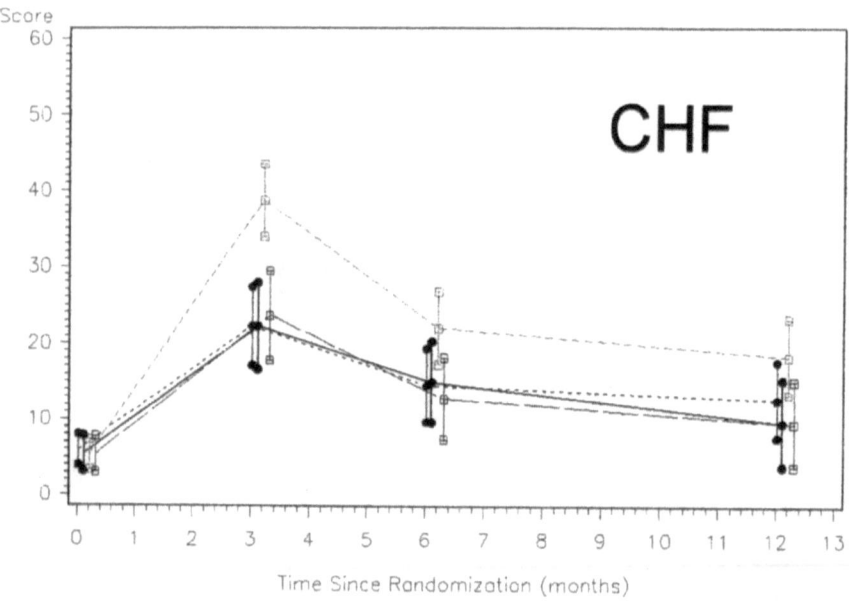

Figure 42.2b *(continued)*

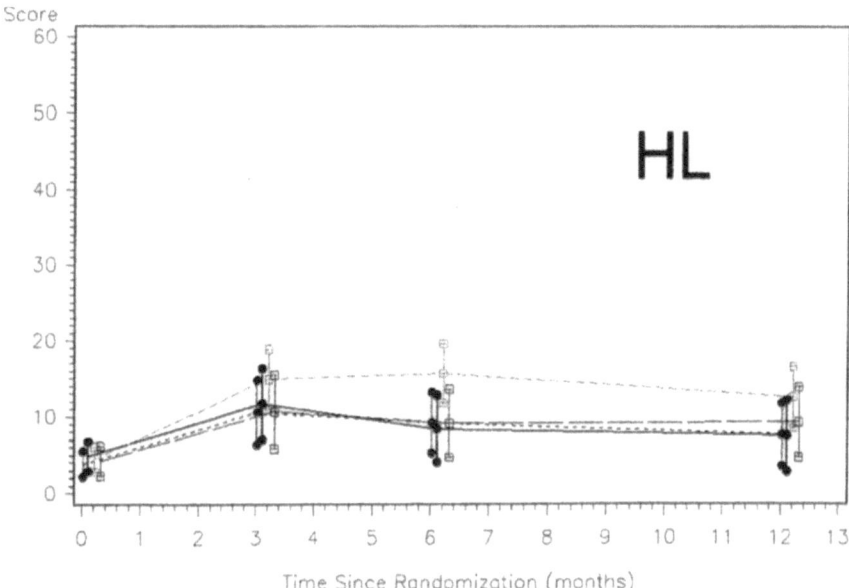

Figure 42.2b *(continued)*

receiving 4 cycles). Furthermore, the 4 cycles/3 days schedule of BEP is followed by more clinically relevant short-term and long-term toxicity (tinnitus) than the 3 other treatment schedules. There is a tendency towards more short-term gastro-intestinal side effects if each of 3 cycles was given over 3 days.

Our results confirm the clinical experience of the development of acute and sub-acute peripheral neurotoxicity and Raynaud phenomena. At 3–6 months the severity of these side effects is primarily dependent on the cumulative dose of cisplatin with some, but incomplete recovery thereafter. Different serum concentrations of cisplatin, reflected by the 3 versus 5 days application, are also of some relevance for the short-term toxicity, in particular if 4 cycles are given. If differences of 10 points or more were chosen as the cut-off point for clinical relevance, the 3 days regime does not result in additional toxicity at 1 year, except for tinnitus.

The 3 days regimes has undoubted administrative and health economic advantages, particularly since the 3-day chemotherapy schedule theoretically can be given as outpatient treatment. However, our results show that these cost-effective schedules may impose greater treatment burden for the patients with more, though often reversible, toxicity.

Even though some recovery is observed at 1 year for most of the chemotherapy induced side effects, 20–30 per cent of the patients have residual complaints of ototoxicity, neuropathy and Raynaud's phenomena. These observations are also in agreement with clinical experience and previous reports [2,4]. In spite of these side effects QL improves or remains reasonably good in the majority of patients, confirming the results of cross-sectional studies performed in treated TC patients.

Weissbach et al. [5] applied an ad hoc designed questionnaire in their study in which some of the dimensions were based on the QLQ C-30: Though this theoretically facilitates some inter-study comparison, we are reluctant to do this at the present time. Their prospective study was not completely randomised and different types of chemotherapy were applied. Furthermore, the authors' report does not allow an estimate of the compliance rates at the different times of assessments nor the evaluation of the pattern of absence of forms. We have not conducted any comparison with published European normative data either [11–14]. Fayers [15] has recently emphasised significant cross-national differences for some of the dimensions of the QLQ-C-30 instrument, which have so far not been explained and which prompt reluctance to perform cross-cultural, cross-lingual comparisons in our study.

Some methodological limitations of our study should be considered: There is no module for QoL assessment that has been developed according to the EORTC guidelines [16]. No TC module has been developed in accordance with these guidelines. When the trial was started one had to select "the next best" instrument [9]. Furthermore, as in many QoL studies, compliance was a problem in the present study report. Our baseline versus 1-year comparison is limited by a compliance rate of only 62 per cent at 12 months. Although absence of forms was most probably a random event in the present study, our baseline versus 1-year comparison may be flawed because of missing forms.

Our data allow us to conclude that the 5 day BEP regime is preferable if 4 cycles are to be given to patients with GCT. If only 3 cycles are planned the 3 day schedule may be appropriate although it produces increased acute but reversible gastro-intestinal toxicity.

Future analysis of our data should identify those baseline QL and clinical parameters, which influence the 1-year QoL. A long-term follow-up study of our patients would be of interest to investigate the changes in QoL and in side effects over several years.

References

1. Bloom JR, Fobair P, Gritz E et al. Psychosocial outcomes of cancer: a comparative analysis of Hodgkin's disease and testicular cancer. *J Clin Oncol* 1993;11:979.
2. Aass N, Kaasa S, Lund E, Kaalhus O, Heier MS, Fossa SD. Long-term somatic side effects and morbidity in testicular cancer patients. *Br J Cancer* 1990;61:151.
3. Kaasa S, Aass N, Mastekaasa A, Lund E, Fossa SD. Psychosocial well-being in testicular cancer patients. *Eur J Cancer* 1991;27:1091.
4. Bokemeyer C, Berger CC, Kuczyk MA, Schmoll HJ: Evaluation of long-term toxity after chemotherapy for testicular cancer. *J Clin Oncol* 1996;14:2923.
5. Weissbach L, Bussar-Maatz R, Flechtner H, Pichlmeier U, Hartmann M, Keller L: RPLND or primary chemotherapy in clinical stage IIA/B nonseminomatous germ cell tumors? Results of a prospective multicenter trial including quality of life assessment. *Eur Urol* 2000;37:582.
6. De Wit R, Roberts T, Wilkinson P et al. Equivalence of three or four cycles of Bleomycin, Etoposide and Cisplatin chemotherapy and of a 3- or 5-day schedule in good-prognosis germ cell cancer: A randomised study of the European Organisation for Research and Treatment of Cancer Genitourinary Tract Cancer Cooperative Group and the Medical Research Council. *J Clin Oncol* 2001;19:1629.
7. International Germ Cell Consensus Classification: a prognostic factor-based staging system for metastatic germ cell cancers. International Germ Cell Cancer Collaborative Group. *J Clin Oncol* 1997;15:594.
8. Aaronson NK, Ahmedzai S, Bergman B et al. The European Organization for Research and Treatment of Cancer QLQ-C30: a quality-of-life instrument for use in international clinical trials in oncology. *J Natl Cancer Inst* 1993;85:365.
9. Fossa SD, Moynihan C, Serbouti S. Patients' and doctors' perception of long-term morbidity in patients with testicular cancer clinical stage I. A descriptive pilot study. *Support Care Cancer* 1996;4:118.

10. Osoba D, Rodrigues G, Myles J, Zee B, Pater J. Interpreting the significance of changes in health-related quality-of-life scores. *J Clin Oncol* 1998;16:139.
11. Hjermstad MJ, Fayers PM, Bjordal K, Kaasa S. Health-related quality of life in the general Norwegian population assessed by the European Organization for Research and Treatment of Cancer Core Quality-of-Life Questionnaire: the QLQ = C30 (+ 3). *J Clin Oncol* 1998;16:1188.
12. Schwarz R, Hinz A: Reference data for the quality of life questionnaire EORTC QLQ-C30 in the general German population. Eur J Cancer 37:1345, 2001
13. Klee M, Groenvold M, Machin D. Quality of life of Danish women: population-based norms of the EORTC QLQ-C30. *Qual Life Res* 1997;6:27.
14. Michelson H, Bolund C, Nilsson B, Brandberg Y. Health related quality of life measured by the EORTC QLQ-C30 – reference values from a large sample of the Swedish population. *Acta Oncol* 2000;39:477.
15. Fayers PM. Interpreting quality of life data: Population-based reference data for the EORTC QLQ-C30. *Eur J Cancer* 37:1331, 2001
16. Sprangers MA, Cull A, Groenvold M, Bjordal K, Blazeby J, Aaronson NK. The European Organization for Research and Treatment of Cancer approach to developing questionnaire modules: an update and overview. EORTC Quality of Life Study Group. *Qual Life Res* 1998;7:291.

43. Introducing the Measurement of Quality of Life into Clinical Practice: Technology and Mechanisms

R. Sanders, G. Velikova, A. Smith, D. Stark, E.P. Wright, J. Randerson Moor, D.T. Bishop, P. Selby

Imperial Cancer Research Fund Clinical Centre in Leeds, Cancer Research Building St James's University Hospital, Beckett Street, Leeds, LS9 7TF, UK

Introduction

Health-related quality of life (QL) is a recognised and important patient-related outcome of anti-cancer treatment, which can be measured by carefully developed, psychometrically robust, questionnaires. Although the validity and sensitivity of the cancer QL questionnaires is now widely accepted and they are frequently used in therapeutic clinical trials, they have yet to impact fully on patients' care and are little used by practising oncologists. Several barriers have hampered the practical use of QL measures for individual patients, including the logistic barrier of collection and analysis of large amounts of data, the conceptual barrier of determining the clinical meaning of QL scores, the theoretical concerns over whether instruments developed for group comparisons can be used for individual patients, and the lack of research data on the possible benefits for individual patients. Thus, whilst oncology professionals are broadly convinced of the value of the concept and measurement of QL and its utilisation in clinical trials is increasing, its impact on routine clinical practice remains small.

However, many cancer patients face significant psychosocial difficulties. Patients with testicular cancer, for example, face several especially severe psychosocial challenges. The disease is life threatening, treatments are toxic, and the occurrence is at a time of life when emotional and social pressures may be especially great. In the face of high cure rates, which mean many patients have long survival with associated long-term morbidity and uncertainty, quality of life and its application to clinical practice is increasingly important.

Formal assessment of QL of individual cancer patients in everyday clinical practice can provide clinicians with additional information, which may aid earlier detection of morbidity and result in earlier intervention. Several studies were conducted towards the end of the last century, which addressed the impact of patient-based health status reports on patient's care and QL [1, 2]. They all assessed patients with chronic diseases causing functional impairments, such as rheumatoid arthritis, general medical illness and epilepsy. Those studies suggested that the health status reports provided accurate and useful information, and facilitated communication, but in general did not improve patient's functional status or QL; suggesting that merely collecting accurate and useful information is not by itself sufficient to facilitate clinically effective change.

The evaluation of routine QL measurement by carefully designed, randomised trials aimed at assessing impact on care and outcomes, is essential to the integration of QL and psychosocial instruments into routine clinical practice. This must take place with a full consideration of the mechanisms, both environmental and genetic, which influence quality of life, and an acknowledgement of the practical constraints of time and cost facing modern oncology clinics.

This chapter describes the work of our group in this field. The main focus of our work is to introduce QL instruments and psychosocial screening into routine oncology practice through utilising, and adapting, existing instruments, or, where essential, developing new ones. This leads naturally to a consideration of the mechanisms, both environmental and genetic, which influence quality of life and we will introduce some new approaches to understanding these mechanisms. Our group recognises these practical and theoretical goals by emphasising both automation and evaluation. Indeed, the use of automated means to measure QL allows for repeated measurements and for the delivery of results to healthcare professionals to inform their interactions with patients without excessive paperwork and cost.

Developing an Automated System

In developing such a system our group initially reviewed several available automated methods, and carried out a pilot study with 213 patients and several technologies. This resulted in the touch screen (TS) monitor and optical reading of paper forms being selected for more detailed evaluation. A computer programme for recording QL data from the TS monitor with immediate analysis and display of the data was designed, and a randomised crossover trial was conducted in which 149 patients completed the EORTC QLQ-C30 [3] and the Hospital Anxiety and Depression Scale (HADS) [4] on paper and touch screen in order to compare the two presentations (Figure 43.1). A different group of 81 cancer inpatients completed the electronic (TS) version of the questionnaires twice with a time interval of three hours to assess reliability.

Computer-touch screen QL questionnaires demonstrated good reliability and were generally equivalent to the paper forms with a possible minor tendency of more positive responses on the touch screen. Similar to recent data from a study in Canada we found that the computerised measurement of QL using the touch screen system was well accepted by the patients [5].

A field test of the feasibility and compliance that can be achieved using the computer touch screen system and the factors that will influence these was conducted in 1,563 patients who made 1,950 touch screen QL assessments. In a prospective cohort who gave informed consent, overall compliance was poor (median 40 per cent, mean 43 per cent) and it deteriorated steadily with longer follow up. We then tried an alternative approach, in which all of the patients attending clinics were offered QL assessment on a touch screen as part of clinic routine, (an "all-patients" approach). The overall compliance was greatly increased (median 100 per cent, mean 72 per cent) and compliance was retained over multiple visits [6].

The screening properties of several instruments (HADS, MHI-5) [7], Maguire's concerns checklist [8] and the Emotional Functioning Questions from the EORTC QLQ-C30, administered electronically by TS for detection of psychological morbidity were also assessed. The primary aim of the study was to evaluate the validity of using touch screen computers for screening clinically significant levels of

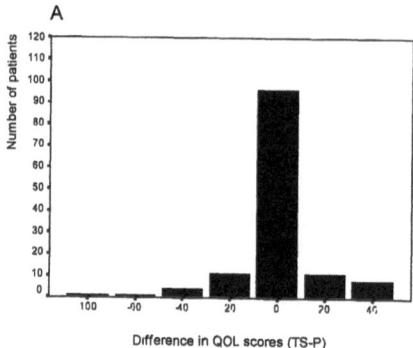

Difference in QOL scores (TS-P)

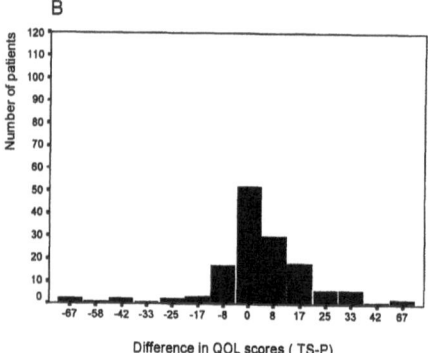

Difference in QOL scores (TS-P)

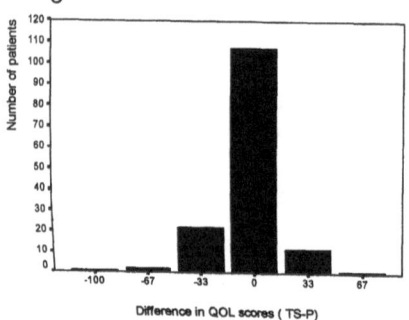

Difference in QOL scores (TS-P)

Figure 43.1: Comparison of Touchscreens with paper QL questionnaires

Examples of the range of variation of the differences in EORTC QQ-C30 scores on the physical function scale (A), emotional function scale (B) and appetite item (C). QOL, qualify of life; TS, touchscreen version; P, paper version.

distress among cancer patients in routine oncology practice. Its secondary aim was to begin to develop expertise in the use of the TS system for psychological screening – but not to provide a test of a definitive system for this purpose. A standard psychiatric interview (Present State Examination-PSE) [9] was conducted within a week of the second assessment to identify psychiatric "caseness" i.e. disorders sufficiently severe to justify intervention. On interview, 23 per cent of patients were identified as 'cases'. Using the available data (questionnaires, socio-demographic details, self-reported past psychiatric history), the best clinical screening strategy was to use combined

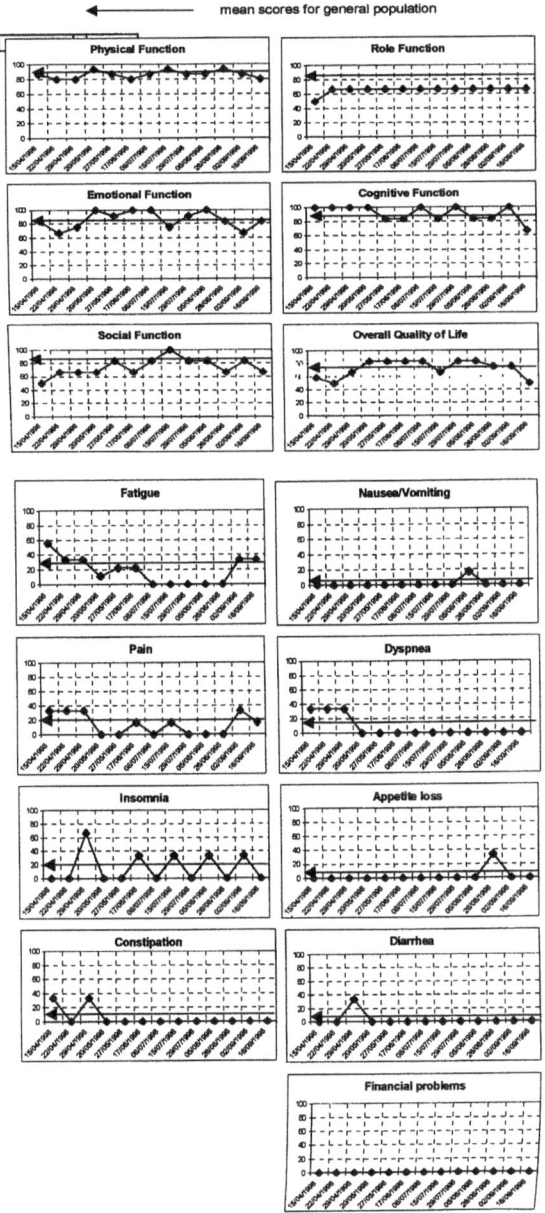

Figure 43.2: An individual patient profile: an example from the group with overall good QL with improvement over time. The QL profile reflects well this patient's disease history – minimal initial symptoms, rapid clinical response to chemotherapy, some treatment toxicity and problems aftr a liver biopsy at the end of treatment

Function scales (top 6): higher scores mean better function' symptom scales (lower 9): higher scores mean worse symptoms.

scores from MHI-5 and HADS, though further work is needed to develop optimal choice of screening questions for this purpose [10].

These studies suggested that the system was feasible, reliable and valid. To evaluate its impact and relationship to the medical interviewing processes, the concordance of results obtained using the automated QL measurement system with disease course and with medical records was assessed. One hundred and fourteen consecutive patients in our clinics completed the EORTC QLQ-C30 on a touch screen computer over six months and the results were compared with corresponding medical records at individual and group level. For individual patients the serial measurement of QL allowed recognition of patterns over time corresponding to disease course (Figure 43.2). At group level, a higher proportion of patients reported problems on EORTC QLQ-C30, than were mentioned in the medical records. The QL profiles had more information on symptoms and particularly on functional issues, such as emotional distress and physical performance [11].

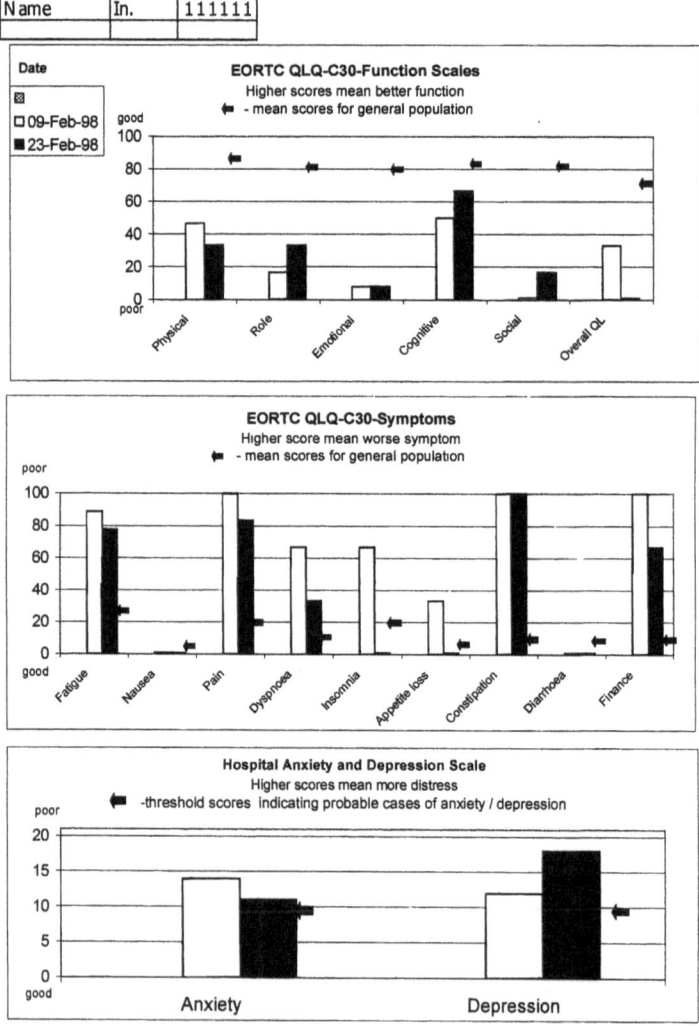

Figure 43.3: Quality of Life Study Form
Example of the graphic print-out of the quality of life results. Normal values are for the Norwegian population

Next, the feasibility of using the computer administered systems to assess individual quality of life and the impact of this information on consultations was evaluated in a prospective non-randomised intervention study in which the intervention consisted of the completion of QL questionnaires before the consultations and then informing clinicians of the results. The effects were measured by pre-test – post-test within subject comparisons and also the collection of views from the clinicians involved. Figure 43.3 shows the data as presented to clinicians.

The clinicians perceived that the QL data broadened the range of the clinical enquiry and helped them identify issues for discussion, resulting in more issues being discussed in the clinic. Having symptoms and functional problems expressed quantitatively on a scale was found to be useful for detection of change over time. We concluded computer based individual QL assessments in oncology clinics with feedback of results to clinicians was feasible. The availability of QL data during consultations led to an increase in the total number of issues discussed, and, specifically, increased enquiring about daily activities, emotional problems, and work related issues. Thus QL data may have a positive effect on doctor-patient interactions [11].

These encouraging results showed the considerable clinical potential of this approach but required confirmation in a randomised prospective trial. Therefore, we are currently assessing the impact of both QL measurement and information transfer to clinicians on the process of medical care, and investigating the potential benefits for the patients. The objective of the trial is to test the hypothesis that regular automated collection and transfer of QL questionnaire data to oncologists treating patients with palliative chemotherapy would have a positive impact on the process and outcome of care. The efficacy of the intervention is evaluated in terms of two primary outcomes: 1) increased number and range of issues discussed during the consultations and 2) patients' QL over time. The efficacy is also evaluated in terms of potential impact on the process of medical care (requested tests, prescribed drugs, referrals) and patients' perceptions of continuity of care and satisfaction. There has been an accrual of 287 patients completed to the end of June 2001, with a follow up to December 2001 in progress.

Applications of an Automated System

Integrating the automated system into routine practice will require further evaluation and development. Its effectiveness will be impacted by the manner in which it is implemented in routine practice, and in particular it has to fit comfortably and pragmatically into existing routines and be widely accepted by clinicians. It is our belief that for such a system to be accepted it must be perceived to confer benefits to the process of medical care without adding to clinicians' workload. One method of easing this transition is to present clinicians with a package of data containing both QL information and clinical information. For this, the combining of QL data and other clinical elements, such as the scoring of toxicity in chemotherapy patients, should increase its accessibility and its perceived utility, and provide a context for the QL data. Its continued use in general oncology practice to identify patients at risk of psychological and social problems, to monitor both quality of life and symptoms, and to hopefully improve the outcome of care will need further evaluation on a longitudinal basis.

As an example, high dose chemotherapy (HDC) with peripheral blood stem cell transplant (PBSCT) is increasingly used to treat patients with lymphoma with poor prognosis indicators, and its efficacy has been studied in other solid tumours. Despite significant improvement in the supportive treatment during the transplant period and reduction in transplant related mortality, HDC remains an aggressive procedure associated with significant acute, intermediate and long-term toxicity. An extensive body of work on quality of life in this context has been carried out to assess the impact of this intensive approach to treatment. However, in their excellent review of this subject, McQuellon and Andrykowski [12] concluded, "very little empirical research has addressed the psychosocial complications associated with the acute phase of the bone marrow transplant and its immediate aftermath".

A longitudinal prospective study addressing this issue and using touch screen technology found that the majority of patients reported a statistically significant deterioration in symptoms (fatigue and gastrointestinal toxicity) during weeks 1 and 2 after the HDC. Physical, social, cognitive and role function, HADS depression and overall quality of life scores were all reported to be at their lowest during this same period. Emotional distress and anxiety did not change significantly during the in-patient treatment. All symptoms and functional impairments resolved rapidly one to two months after discharge including improvement in emotional function and HADS anxiety. Further gradual improvement was noted over the following months.

The severe toxicity during high dose chemotherapy with PBSCT has significant effects on patients functioning and quality of life, and is associated with depression during the acute phase of treatment. The recovery period after discharge is 1–2 months. Such data could be used to give patients accurate information pre-transplant and help them plan accordingly.

Biochemical and Molecular Genetic Determinants of Psychosocial Morbidity

The behavioural response to any stress is the result of a complex mix of both environmental and genetic factors. The cancer patients' response to their situation will be influenced, either directly or indirectly, by many factors, including their psychological and social environment, in addition to the disease. Many of these factors will be influenced, at least in part, by the genetic makeup of the patient and it is important to recognise the importance of genetic influences in the behavioural response of the patient, as well as the environmental ones.

Despite a substantial body of research, there remains only a limited understanding of the factors that may determine the development of psychological distress in cancer patients. Hospitalisation status (in-patient versus out-patient) explains little of the large variance in depression prevalence [13]. Greater physical disability has been associated with increased prevalence of depression [14], as has advanced disease stage with prevalences in patients with advanced cancer ranging from 23 per cent to 53 per cent [15, 16]. By contrast, there appears to be no relationship either between anxiety prevalence and cancer site, or between anxiety prevalence and disease stage [17], though, of course, different cancer sites, and their concomitant treatments, each bring their own unique psychological stressors to bear upon the individual patient. Interestingly, the slightly higher prevalence of anxiety and depression in females in the general population is not observed in cancer populations [18] suggesting that psychological morbidity in cancer patients may be subject to additional influences over and above psychological morbidity in the general population. Previous psychiatric history, however, remains a highly significant predictive factor in anxiety and depression in cancer patients [10].

Evidence for genetic involvement in psychological disorders comes from family, twin and adoption studies. Family studies of major depression, as defined using formal diagnostic criteria, demonstrate increased morbid risks for relatives of clinically depressed probands when compared with relatives of control probands. That is, major depression demonstrates familial aggregation, which of course, may be due to genetic or environmental factors, or a combination of both. In order to delineate genetic and environmental factors one must look to twin and adoption studies.

Twin studies all demonstrate higher concordance rates for depression among monozygotic rather than dizygotic twins [19, 20], which is suggestive of genetic influences. Indeed, estimates of heritability of major depression using these data range from 17 per cent to 78 per cent. A meta-analysis of these data results in an estimated heritability of major depression of 37 per cent (95 per cent CI = 31 per cent–42 per cent) with individual-specific environmental effects accounting for 63 per cent (95 per cent CI = 58 per cent–67 per cent) of the total variance, and shared environmental effects being negligible 0 per cent (95 per cent CI = 0 per cent–5 per cent) [21]. Sullivan and colleagues however, suggest that this may be an underestimate of heritability given the possibility of error in detecting cases of major depression.

There are an increasing number of behavioural-genetic studies and some have identified several genes or loci putatively involved in the heritability of major depression, including 5HT-5a, D10S1423, tryptophan hydroxylase, the G-protein beta-3 sub unit, Gamma-aminobutyric receptor, alpha-5 sub unit [22], and two polymorphisms of the serotonin transporter (5HTT) gene involving a variable number tandem repeat (VNTR) [23] and a 44 base pair insertion/deletion in the 5HTT linked polymorphic region (5HTTLPR) [24].

Genetic research on anxiety disorders has tended to polarise around either panic disorder or phobic disorders. Family studies of panic disorder utilising a direct interview approach have all demonstrated that panic disorder is familial [25, 26]. Similarly, the fewer number of family studies of phobic disorders have demonstrated familial patterns for simple phobia and social phobia [27, 28]. This polarisation of the literature reflects the observation that both panic and phobic disorders tend to 'breed true', that is, relatives are at highest risk of the proband's disorder; though, interestingly, generalised anxiety disorder does not appear to share familial determinants with either panic or phobic disorders [29].

Agoraphobia, however, shares symptoms with both panic disorder and phobic disorder. One family study [30], which included agoraphobia, showed that relatives of probands with agoraphobia were at increased risk of both agoraphobia and panic disorder, whilst relatives of probands with panic disorder were at increased risk for panic disorder but not agoraphobia. This led the authors to conclude that agoraphobia represents a more severe form of panic disorder but others have reported conflicting results [31]. Thus the genetic nosology of anxiety disorders is far from simplistic. Indeed, Maier and colleagues [32] showed that relatives of probands with panic disorder were at an increased risk of major depression, whilst others have demonstrated that depression shares familiality with generalised anxiety. However, one should bear in mind that familiality may also reflect shared environmental factors in addition to, or instead of, genetic factors.

Results from large twin studies demonstrate heritability estimates of 44 per cent for panic disorder, 39 per cent for agoraphobia, 32 per cent for generalised anxiety disorder, 32 per cent for animal phobias, and 30 per cent for social phobia [33–35]. An increasing number of genetic studies have implicated several genes or loci involved in panic disorder with or without agoraphobia, specifically: the adenosine A_1 receptor, and the adenosine A_{2A} receptor [36], MAOA [37], D10S220, D12S368 and GATA136b01 [38] and D13S779 [39]. Fewer studies have been done to implicate genetic loci in generalised anxiety disorder or phobic disorder, though there are some, notably, the oestrogen receptor ESR1 [40] and 5HTTLPR [41].

An opportunity is therefore presented by the sequencing of the human genome, and its variations, to explain, at least in part, why some cancer patients develop psychological disorders but many do not. Workers in the fields of general psychiatry and behavioural genetics have already made some progress, through studies of associations between genetic polymorphisms and disorders, toward answering such questions. However, we have, to date, been unable to identify any information that specifically relates to the psychological functioning of cancer patients.

Studies in psychiatric genetics are so far not conclusively able to associate specific genetic polymorphisms with specific disorders. They are beset by problems of study design, statistical power, differing populations and varying definitions of caseness or phenotype. This is compounded by the probable multi-factorial polygenic nature of such disorders. Indeed, the gene-environment interactions that influence psychological morbidity will be complex with multiple genes and multiple environmental influences. Ultimately large numbers of patients combined with good DNA storage and carefully defined phenotypes will be required to investigate the functional role of genetic polymorphisms.

This is illustrated by the associations reported for two polymorphisms in the human serotonin transporter gene, which we are using to begin our programme (Figures 43.4 and 43.5). The serotonin transporter is an excellent candidate gene because it is both biologically and medically plausible, and the site of action of selective serotonin re-uptake inhibitors, a successful class of major antidepressants. While some associations for the serotonin transporter gene look consistent, for example the SS genotype of 5HTTLPR with bipolar disorder, and the STin2.12 allele of the VNTR with bipolar disorder [24], others show apparent conflict, for example both the SS and the LL genotypes of 5HTTLPR have been associated with alcoholic disorders [42, 43].

The interest and potential of these analyses are illustrated in a paper by Coyle and colleagues [44], who studied polymorphisms in the serotonin transporter gene using the VNTR polymorphism in intron-2. They reported a marked over-representation of genotypes bearing the ST2.12 allele in a group of 97 patients with puerperal psychosis. The presence of at least one ST2.12 allele was associated with a relative risk

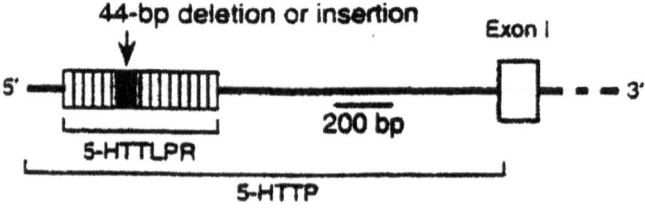

Figure 43.4: Schematic representation of the human serotonin transporter gene-linked polymorphic region (5HTTLPR). (From [48])

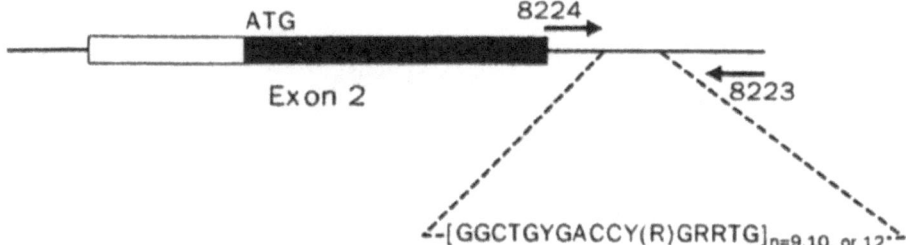

Figure 43.5: Schematic representation of the region of the human serotonin transporter gene containing a variable number tandem repeat (5HTT VNTR). (Form [23])

of 3.9 of developing puerperal psychosis. Interestingly in an exploratory analysis when the definition of the relevant phenotype was narrowed to include those who had experienced multiple episodes, the effect size increased with an odds ratio of 9.2. These are very large risk factors that clearly require confirmation in larger studies. However, they do illustrate not only the potential of genotypic analysis to indicate risks of the development of psychological disorders but also the importance of a precisely defined, and sometimes rather narrow, definition of the phenotype.

Using an automated touch screen system we can define and evaluate the phenotype of cancer patients, and thus make comparisons with patient's genotypes quantified in the laboratory. Figure 43.6 gives an example of such genotyping of the 5-HTT VNTR polymorphism. This consists of a variable number of 17bp tandem repeats in the second intron of the transporter gene. Three alleles are observed representing 9 (Stin2.9), 10 (Stin2.10) or 12 (Stin2.12) repeats. So far there is no human evidence to suggest a functional implication for the polymorphism and evidence for association to mood disorders is inconsistent [45]. The observed Stin2.12 allele frequency (57.9 per cent) (Table 43.1) is consistent with those reported in other Caucasian populations (54–62.5 per cent) [23, 24]. However, the frequency of the Stin2.9 allele (3.4 per cent) is higher than that reported in the literature (1–2.9 per cent) [46, 47]. This discrepancy is probably due to the small sample size used in the pilot study. A full analysis of the entire control population should result in more accurate estimates of allele frequency.

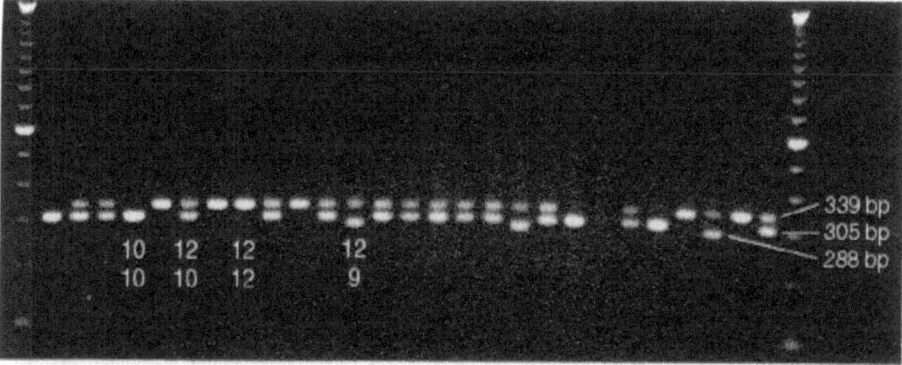

Figure 43.6: Example of 5HTT VNTR assay. PCR products are separated on a 2% agarose gel against a 100bp maker ladder to resolve the 17bp difference between the alleles. Four of the possible genotypes identified by this assay are indicated.

Table 43.1: Genotype and allele distributions (n, % in parentheses) fr the 5-HTT VNTR polymorphism in a pilot control population (n = 44).

	Genotype Distribution			
	STin2.9/ others	STin2,10/ STin2.10	STin2.10/ STin2.12	STin2.12/ STin2.12
Controls	3 (6.8)	6 (13.6)	22 (50.0)	13 (29.5)

	Allele Distribution		
	STin2.9	STin2.10	STin2.12
Controls	3 (3.4)	34 (38.6)	51 (57.9)

We are currently engaged in a prospective longitudinal study, which will allow us to define the psychological phenotype of cancer patients using an automated system and to collect DNA samples. This will allow us to compare patients' psychological phenotypes with selected candidate genes and begin to answer the question of why some cancer patients develop psychological disorders but many do not.

Conclusions

Measuring QL in practice using new technologies has the potential to help improve the interaction between healthcare professionals and patients with all kinds of cancer – perhaps especially men with testicular cancer, many of whom face long survival with associated long term morbidity and uncertainty. An automated system of QL assessment can provide more information on symptoms and functional issues, can broaden the range of clinicians' enquiries and aid in the identification of issues for discussion, and can thus have a positive effect on doctor-patient interactions. Of course, the introduction of such a system into routine clinical practice must be done pragmatically and with due consideration of the practicalities and demands of the modern oncology clinic. Indeed, new technologies such as those created by the human genome project can offer novel approaches to our understanding, and new avenues of investigation, which will ultimately benefit the cancer patient.

References

1. Lohr KN. Applications of health status assessment measures in clinical practice: Overview of the third conference on advances in health status measurement. *Med. Care* 1992;30:MS1–MS14 (suppl. 5).
2. Lohr KN. Advances in health status assessment: Overview of the conference. *Med.Care* 1989;27:S1–S11 (suppl. 3).
3. Aaronson NK, Ahmedzai S, Bergman B et al. The European Organisation for Research and Treatment of Cancer QLQC30: A quality of life instrument for use in international clinical trials in oncology. *J. Natl. Cancer Inst.* 1993;85:365–376.
4. Zigmond A, Snaith R. The hospital anxiety and depression scale. *Acta Psychiatr Scand* 1983;67:361–7.
5. Velikova G, Wright EP, Smith AB et al. Automated collection of quality of life data: A comparison of paper and computer touch-screen questionnaires. *J. Clin. Oncol.* 1999;17:998–1007.
6. Wright EP, Selby PJ, Gillibrand A et al. Feasibility and compliance of automated measurement of quality of life in oncology practice. *Submitted to J. Clin. Oncol.*
7. Berwick DM, Murphy JM, Goldman PA, Ware JE, Barsky AJ, Weinstein MC. Performance of a five item mental health screening test. *Med. Care* 1991;29:169–176.

8. Harrison J, Maguire P, Ibbotson T, Macleod R, Hopwood P. Concerns, confiding and psychiatric disorder in newly diagnosed cancer patients: A descriptive study. *Psycho-Oncology* 1994;3:173–9.
9. Wing JK, Cooper J, Sartorius N. *Measurement and classification of psychiatric symptoms.* Cambridge University Press, Cambridge, 1974.
10. Cull A, Gould A, House A et al. Validating automated screening for psychological distress by means of computer touchscreens for use in routine oncology practice. *Submitted to Br. J. Cancer.*
11. Velikova G, Wright EP, Smith AB et al. Self-reported quality of life of individual cancer patients: Concordance of results with disease course and medical records. *J. Clin. Oncol.* 2001;19:2064–2073
12. McQuellon RP, Andrykowski M. *Psychological complications of hematopoietic stem cell transplantation. In: Clinical bone marrow and blood stem cell transplantation.* K Atkinson (Ed) Cambridge University Press, Cambridge, 2000.
13. Massie MJ, Popkin MK. Depressive disorders In: *Psycho-oncology*, JC Holland (Ed), Oxford University Press, 1998.
14. Bukberg J, Penman D, Holland JC. Depression in hospitalised cancer patients. *Psychosom. Med.* 1984;46:199–212.
15. Plumb M, Holland JC. Comparative studies of psychological function in patients with advanced cancer I: Self-reported depressive symptoms. *Psychosom. Med.* 1977;39:264–276.
16. Craig TJ, Abeloff MD. Psychiatric symptomatology among hospitalised cancer patients. *Am. J. Psychiatry* 1974;131:1323–1327.
17. Noyes RN, Holt CS, Massie MJ. Anxiety disorders In: *Psycho-oncology*, JC Holland (Ed), Oxford University Press, 1998.
18. Stark DPH, House A. Anxiety in cancer patients. *Br. J. Cancer* 2000; 83:1261–1267.
19. McGuffin P, Katz R, Watkins S, Rutherford J. A hospital based twin register of the heritability of DSM-IV unipolar depression. *Arch. Gen. Psychiatry* 1996;53:129–136.
20. Kendler KS, Prescott CA. A population based twin study of lifetime major depression in men and women. *Arch. Gen. Psychiatry* 1999;56:39–44;correction 57:94–95.
21. Sullivan PF, Neale MC, Kendler KS. Genetic epidemiology of major depression: Review and meta-analysis. *Am. J. Psychiatry* 2000;157:1552–1562.
22. Oruc L, Verheyen GR, Furac I et al. Positive association between the GABRA5 gene and unipolar recurrent major depression. *Neuropsychobiology* 1997;36:62–64.
23. Ogilvie A, Battersby S, Bubb VJ et al. Polymorphism in serotonin transporter gene associated with susceptibility to major depression. *Lancet* 1996;347:731–733.
24. Collier DA, Stober G, Heils A et al. A novel functional polymorphism within the promoter of the serotonin transporter gene: Possible role in susceptibility to affective disorders. *Mol. Psychiatry* 1996;1:453–460.
25. Crowe RR, Noyes R, Pauls DL, Slymen D. A family study of panic disorder. *Arch. Gen. Psychiatry* 1983;40:1065–1069.
26. Fyer AJ, Mannuzza S, Chapman T, Lipsitz J, Martin L, Klein D. Panic disorder and social phobia: Effects of comorbidity on familial transmission. *Anxiety* 1996;2:173–178.
27. Fyer AJ, Mannuzza S, Gallops S et al. Familial transmission of simple phobias and fears. *Arch. Gen. Psychiatry* 1990;47:252–256.
28. Stein MB, Chartier MJ, Hazen AL et al. A direct interview family study of generalised social phobia. *Am. J. Psychiatry* 1998;155:90–97.
29. Smoller JW, Tsuang MT. Panic and phobic anxiety: Defining phenotypes for genetic studies. *Am. J. Psychiatry* 1998;155 :1152–1162.
30. Noyes R, Crowe RR, Harris EL, Hampa BJ, McChesney CM, Chaudry DR. Relationship between panic disorder and agoraphobia: A family study. *Arch. Gen. Psychiatry* 1986;43:227–232
31. Mendlewicz J, Papadimitriou G, Wilmotte J. Family study of panic disorder: A comparison with generalised anxiety disorder, major depression and normal subjects. *Psychiatr. Genet.* 1993;3:73–78
32. Maier W, Minges J & Lichtermann D. The familial relationship between panic disorder and unipolar depression. *J. Psychiatr. Res.* 1995;29:375–388.
33. Kendler KS, Neale MC, Kessler RC, Heath A, Eaves L. The genetic epidemiology of phobias in women. *Arch. Gen. Psychiatry* 1992;49:273–281.
34. Kendler KS, Neale MC, Kessler RC, Heath A, Eaves LJ. Panic disorder in women: A population based twin study. *Psychol. Med.* 1993;23:397–406.
35. Kendler KS, Pedersen NL, Neale MC, Mathe A. A pilot Swedish twin study of affective illness including hospital- and population-ascertained subsamples: Results of model fitting. *Behav. Genet.* 1995;25:217–232.
36. Deckert J, Nothen MM, Franke P et al. Systematic mutation screening and association study of the A_1 and A_{2A} adenosine receptor genes in panic disorder suggest a contribution of the A_{2A} gene to the development of disease. *Mol. Psychiatry* 1998;3:81–85.

37. Deckert J, Catalano M, Syagailo YV et al. Excess of high activity monoamine oxidase A gene promoter alleles in female patients with panic disorder. Hum. Mol. Genet. 1999;8:621–624.
38. Smoller J, Acierno JS, Rosenbaum JF et al. Targeted genome screen of panic disorder and anxiety disorder proneness using homology to murine QTL regions. Am. J. Med. Genet. (Neuropsychiatric Genetics) 2001;105:195–206.
39. Weissman M, Fyer A, Haghighi F et al. Potential panic disorder syndrome: Clinical and genetic linkage evidence. Am. J. Med. Genet. (Neuropsychiatric Genetics) 2000;96:24–35.
40. Comings DE, Muhleman D, Johnson P, MacMurray JP. Potential role of the estrogen receptor gene (ESR1) in anxiety. Mol. Psychiatry 1999;4:372–377.
41. Jorm AF, Prior M, Sanson A, Smart D, Zhang Yorkgate, Eateal S. Association of a functional polymorphism of the serotonin transporter gene with anxiety-related temperament and behaviour problems in children: A longitudinal study from infancy to the mid-teens. Mol. Psychiatry 2000;5:542–547.
42. Sander T, Harms H, Dufeu P et al. Serotonin transporter gene variants in alcohol-dependent subjects with dissocial personality disorder. Biol. Psychiatry 1998;43:908–12
43. Schuckit MA, Mazzanti C, Smith TL et al. Selective genotyping for the role of 5-HT2A, 5-HT2C, and GABA alpha 6 receptors and the serotonin transporter in the level of response to alcohol: a pilot study. Biol. Psychiatry 1999;45:647–651.
44. Coyle N, Jones I, Robertson E, Lendon C, Craddock N. Variation at the serotonin transporter gene influences susceptibility to bipolar affective puerperal psychosis. Lancet 2000;356:1490–1. 1998;81:58–63.
45. Spencer SM, |Carver CS Price AA Psychological and social factors in adaptation. In: Psycho-oncology, JC Holland (Ed), Oxford University Press, 1998
46. Bellivier, F, Henry C,k Szoke A t al. Serotonin transporter gene polymorphisms in patients with unipolr or bipolar depression. Neurosci Lett 1998;255:143–6
47. Furlong RA Ho L, Walsh C et al. Analysis and meta-analysis of two serotonin transporter gene polymorphisms in bipolar and unipolar affective disorders. Am J Med Genet 1998;81:58–63
48. Lesch K-P, Bengel D, Heils A et al. Association of anxiety-related traits with a polymorphism in the serotonin transporter gene regulatory region. Science 1996;274:1527–1531.

44. Mortality Rates in Patients with Malignant Germ Cell Tumours (MGCT) with Emphasis on Second Cancer and Cardiovascular Mortality

N. Aass[1], S.D. Fosså[1], S. Harvei[2], S. Tretli[2]

1. The Norwegian Radium Hospital, 2 The Cancer Registry of Norway (CRN)

Aim

To assess mortality rates in patients with MGCT, and compare them with figures from the general population. Emphasis is put on second cancer and cardiovascular disorders.

Methods

Patients up to the age of 55 diagnosed with MGCT between 1962–1993 were included in the study. All patients were followed until death or to 1997. The patients were grouped according to the year of diagnosis, which mirrored the main treatment modalities:

Group 1: 1962–1969: Radiotherapy
Group 2: 1970–1979: Radiotherapy +/– available chemotherapy
Group 3: 1980–1993: Surgery only. Radiotherapy only. Cisplatin-based chemotherapy
          +/– surgery/radiotherapy

The total number of patients was 487, 823 and 1990 for groups 1, 2 and 3, respectively.
   Mortality rates up to 1997 were obtained from the CRN and compared to figures for the age-matched general population. Patients dying from MGCT were excluded from the analysis.

Results

There was a significant increase in mortality for patients cured of MGCT compared to age-matched men in the general population (Table 44.1). This was primarily related to non-germ cell second tumours, especially gastric, pancreatic and lung cancer. The MGCT patients had a significantly increased mortality due to gastrointestinal disorders and cardiovascular disorders in general, but not to myocardial infarction. Other non-cancer causes of death were similarly distributed in the general population and the MGCT patients.

Table 44.1

		Mortality			
		Group 1	Group 2	Group 3	Total
All causes except germ cell tumours	O	103	123	72	298
	E	93.3	75.5	51.1	219.9
	SMR	1.1	1.6*	1.4*	1.4*
Second cancer	O	32	56	28	116
	E 24.9	20.2	11.8	56.9	
	SMR	1.3	2.8*	2.4*	2.0*
All causes except cancer	O	71	67	43	181
	E	68.4	55.3	39.3	163
	SMR	1.0	1.2	1.1	1.1
Cardiovascular disorders	O	50	40	17	17
	E	42.5	31	14.9	88.4
	SMR	1.2	1.3	1.1	1.2*
Gastrointestinal disorders	O	3	7	3	14
	E	2.6	2.4	1.8	6.7
	SMR	1.2	3*	2.2	2.1*

O: Observed; E: Expected; SMR: Standardised mortality ratio; * < p0.05

Conclusion

Patients cured of MGCT have a significantly higher mortality than age-matched men in the general population. The increased mortality is primarily due to non-germ cell second cancers, but also to non-malignant gastrointestinal and cardiovascular disorders.

45. Cardiovascular Disease as a Long Term Complication of Treatment for Testicular Cancer

R.A. Huddart[1,2], A. Norman[1], M. Shahidi[2], A. Horwich[1,2], D. Coward[2], J. Nicholls[2], D. Dearnaley[1,2]

1. The Royal Marsden Hospital and 2. The Institute of Cancer Research, Sutton, Surrey, SM2 5PT, UK

Purpose

Effective multi-agent chemotherapy means that most patients with testicular cancer are now cured and have a long potential life expectancy. Long term toxicity is therefore an important consideration. Some groups have reported an increased risk of cardiovascular disease in testicular cancer survivors. We have investigated whether such a risk exists by undertaking a cross sectional study of cardiovascular morbidity and risk factors in patients treated at our institution between 1982 and 1992.

Patients and Methods

All UK resident male patients registered between 1982–1992 were eligible for this study. Eligible patients attending for follow up were contacted by post 2 weeks before their visit and asked to complete written consent, a current health questionnaire and quality of life questionnaire (EORTC QLY C-30). On attendance, clinical review was undertaken along with haematological, biochemical and hormonal profiles. For patients not under routine review, follow up information was sought from their general practitioner and mortality data from the Office of National Statistics. Descriptive analysis was performed on all variables and comparisons made between patients treated by orchidectomy and follow up only (S), chemotherapy alone(C), radiotherapy alone (RT) and radiotherapy and chemotherapy (C/RT). Categorical data was compared using Chi squared test and continuous variables by the Mann Whitney non parametric test. Univariate and multivariate analysis was performed using logistic regression analysis.

Results

Data on cardiovascular events were available on 992 patients. After a median follow up of 10.2 years; 68 events had been reported including 18 sudden/cardiac deaths, 41 patients with angina and 9 myocardial infarctions. After adjusting for age and by comparison with surveillance alone (S), increased risk for cardiac events was seen after C (RR 2.89, 95 per cent confidence intervals (C.I.) 1.34–6.25, p = 0.007), RT (RR 2.32, C.I. 1.06–5.05, p = 0.035) and C/RT (RR 2.08, C.I. 0.85–5.12, p = 0.11). There was a trend towards higher cholesterol levels in the RT group (mean 5.51, standard deviation 0.99 versus 5.38, standard deviation 0.95 for surveillance, p = 0.09) but there were no other significant differences in risk factors such as smoking history, hypertension, body mass index and cholesterol. Treatment was associated with significant differences in urea (C, RT, C/RT), creatinine (C, C/RT), calculated creatinine clearance (C/RT), sodium (RT), potassium (C, RT), magnesium (C/RT), albumin (C) and total protein (C). On univariate analysis, age, radiotherapy treatment and LH, free thyroxine, sodium, urea, protein, albumin and cholesterol levels were significantly associated with developing cardiovascular disease. On multivariate analysis of the full data set, age and treatment group were associated with cardiovascular disease. In a multivariate analysis of the subgroup that had full information, age, free thyroxine, protein and magnesium levels were associated with cardiovascular disease.

Conclusion

We observed a two fold or greater risk of developing cardiovascular disease in long term survivors of testicular cancer. This was not due to increases in cardiac risk factors, suggesting that a direct or indirect treatment effect may be responsible. This data supports the continued research into the minimisation of treatment in good prognosis testicular cancer.

46. Fertility and Quality of Life after Treatment for Testicular Cancer

R.A. Huddart[1,2], A. Norman[1], C. Moynihan[2], D. Coward[2], J. Nicholls[2], G. Jay[2], M. Shahidi[2], A. Horwich[1,2], D. Dearnaley[1,2]

1. The Royal Marsden Hospital and 2. The Institute of Cancer Research, Sutton, Surrey, SM2 5PT, UK

Aims and Methods

Modern treatments cure most testicular cancer patients so an important goal is to minimise toxicity. We have undertaken a cross-sectional study to evaluate the quality of life (Qol) of long-term survivors of testicular cancer. Six hundred and fify four patients treated between 1982 and 1992 completed the EORTC Qly-C-30 (QC30) questionnaire, the associated testicular cancer specific module and a general health and fertility questionnaire. Patients have been subdivided according to treatment received: orchidectomy either alone (surveillance, S), with chemotherapy only (C), radiotherapy only (R), or both chemotherapy and radiotherapy (C/RT).

Results

Only 221 (30 per cent) patients reported attempting conception after treatment. When attempted, the success rate was high with 178 (81 per cent) reporting success, only 12 of which required infertility treatment. Forty-three (19 per cent) were unsuccessful, with or without fertility treatment. There was a trend to lower success rate after C (75 per cent) ($p = 0.133$) compared to S (85 per cent). Impaired spermatogenesis as indicated by raised FSH levels was common (S 43 per cent) and marginally worse after chemotherapy (C 50 per cent, C/RT 71 per cent, $p < 0.005$). Overall Qol was good with mean scores in the all domains of the QC30 in the range of 80–95, equivalent to or better than both pre-treatment testicular patients and normal population reference scores. Treated patients had a higher chance of impaired social functioning (S 95, RT 92 ($p = 0.24$), C/RT 89 ($p = 0.003$), C 92 ($p = 0.056$)) and marginally lower scores for physical functioning after C (S 96.1, C 94.6 ($p = 0.039$), C/RT 92.9 ($p = 0.12$)). Compared to S, patients after C were more likely to report tingling ($p = 0.001$), pale cold hands ($p = 0.001$), ringing in the ears ($p = 0.05$); dyspnoea ($p = 0.05$) and worries about fathering ($p = 0.009$) and in the C/RT concerns about hair loss ($p = 0.017$) and less interest in sex ($p = 0.01$). RT alone was associated with reduced sexual activity/enjoyment ($p = 0.05$)). Fifty-three per cent of patients reported anxiety regarding recurrence, which was moderate to severe in 11 per cent, especially in patients receiving treatment (C 13 per cent, C/RT 10 per cent, RT 13 per cent, S 5 per cent) and 16 per cent felt their disease had affected their relationship (especially after C 17 per cent (p = 0.175), C/RT 23 per cent (p = 0.022) v S 13 per cent). Forty-two percent of patients reported difficulties with work or obtaining insurance/mortgages especially after C (S 37 per cent C 46 per cent). After treatment more patients were unable to work (C 9 per cent, C/RT 11 per cent, RT 9 per cent v S 5 per cent).

Conclusion

The majority of long term survivors have a good quality of life. Most patients retain their fertility but the risk of infertility is increased by chemotherapy. However, patients can suffer from long term effects of treatment and psychosocial sequelae, including difficulties in obtaining insurance.

47. The Prevalence of Avascular Necrosis in Patients Treated with Chemotherapy for Testicular Tumours

A.M. Cook[1], A.S.K. Dzik-Jurasz[2], A.R. Padhani[2], A. Norman[3], R.A. Huddart[1]

1. Academic Department of Radiotherapy & Oncology, 2. Department of X-Ray, 3. Department of Computing and Information, The Royal Marsden NHS Trust, and Institute of Cancer Research, Downs Road, Sutton, Surrey SM2 5PT, UK

Purpose

Avascular necrosis (AVN) has been described as a complication of combination chemotherapy, especially where it includes intermittent high dose corticosteroids. We have recently reported five patients treated with chemotherapy for testicular tumours who developed symptomatic avascular necrosis following chemotherapy with steriods used as an antiemetic [1]. In this study we aim to assess the prevalence of avascular necrosis in patients who have received first line chemotherapy for testicular tumours.

Methods

Patients who had completed at least 2 cycles of first line chemotherapy in the five years prior to the start of the study who have remained relapse free and had at least six months follow up (March 1993–September 1997) were asked to participate in this study. Patients completed a questionnaire regarding hip pain and risk factors for AVN and invited to have a T1 coronal magnetic resonance imaging (MRI) scan. Time to AVN was calculated using the methods of Kaplan and Meier using the time from chemotherapy to diagnosis of AVN as the endpoint. Patients with no AVN were censored on the date of enrolment to the study.

Results

Of the 103 eligible patients who were contacted, 63 returned questionnaires. The median follow up of patients invited for screening was 32 months (range 7.1–65 months). Sixteen patients did not have MRI scans because of failure to attend or being unsuitable due to metallic implants. The frequency of AVN in the patients undergoing MR examination was 4/47 (9 per cent, confidence interval (CI) 2–20) including two from our previous case series who were in the defined cohort. All four patients with AVN had had bilateral hip pain. Two additional patients described bilateral hip pain but did not attend for MRI scanning. AVN was diagnosed at a median of 21 months (range 14–32 months) after commencement of chemotherapy. If it is assumed that all affected patients were symptomatic and that all symptomatic patients attended for MR examination the overall prevalence was 4/103 (3.8 per cent, CI 1–10 per cent). As not all patients had completed the at risk period this equates to a 3 year actuarial risk of 6.3 per cent (95 per cent CI 2.4–16.1).The affected patients received BEP chemotherapy either 4 cycles or 3 cycles and received total steroid doses equivalent to 2.97g, 2.49g, 3.3g and 1.45g of prednisolone respectively (mean 2.55g) compared to a mean of 2.25g for all patients. The patient who received the equivalent of 1.45g of prednisolone had a high alcohol intake, a known predisposing factor to AVN.

Conclusions

Avascular necrosis is uncommon but significant complication of chemotherapy for testicular cancer when dexamethasone is used as an antiemetic. Efforts should be made to minimise the dose of steroids administered and patients warned of this potential complication. Patients developing hip pain especially when bilateral should have radiological investigations to exclude AVN as the cause.

Reference

1. Cook AM, Patterson H, Nicholls J, Huddart RA. Avascular necrosis in patients treated with BEP chemotherapy for testicular tumours. *Clin Oncol* 1999;11:126–7.

48. Factors Associated with Bleomycin Lung Toxicity in Germ Cell Tumour Patients Treated at the Royal Marsden Hospital Between 1982 and 1999

J.M. O'Sullivan, A.R. Norman, J. Nicholls, R.A. Huddart, D.P. Dearnaley, A. Horwich

1. Department of Clinical Oncology, 2. Department of Computing and Information, 3. Bob Champion Research Unit, Institute of Cancer Research/ Royal Marsden N.H.S. Trust, Sutton, Surrey, SM2 5PT, UK

Background

Bleomycin is a polypeptide antibiotic, anti-neoplastic agent, which has been used in the treatment of germ cell tumours for over 20 years. Pulmonary toxicity has been known since the early clinical trials in the 1960's. There are a surprisingly few large studies examining risk factors for bleomycin lung toxicity in germ cell cancers. Suggested risk factors include cumulative dose, reduced renal (EDTA) clearance, raised creatinine, age of patient, and major surgery.

Materials and Methods

We examined the prospectively collected Bob Champion Unit testicular cancer research database, and identified 1047 patients (mean age 29.5 (95 per cent CI 12.6–46.4), range: 10–62) treated with bleomycin containing regimens for germ cell tumours between January 1982 and December 1999.

Results

Sixty-eight (6.5 per cent) patients had bleomycin lung toxicity (BPT) ranging from X-ray/CT changes to dyspnoea. There were 13 deaths (1.2 per cent of patients treated) directly attributed to BPT. The mean time from bleomycin administration to documented lung toxicity was 4.2 months (range 1.4–82). In uni-variate analysis, more than four courses of bleomycin containing regimens, stage IV disease, and age 40 or more, had a statistically significant association with an increased risk of both fatal and non-fatal BPT, while lowest recorded GFRs of 80ml/min or more were protective. On multivariate analysis, only lowest recorded GFR of 80ml/min had a statistically significant association with altered risk of toxicity.

217

Conclusion

This study illustrates the need for careful assessment of renal function, dose limitation, and caution in patients aged over 40 with germ cell tumours being considered for bleomycin.

49. The Provision of an Adolescent Service to Patients Aged up to 25 Years Attending the Germ Cell Tumour Service, Leeds

S. Morgan

Teenage Cancer Trust Unit, St James's University Hospital, Leeds, UK

It has been well recognised that adolescents with cancer have specific needs, which must be met within the Cancer Centre [1]. These include the provision of psychosocial support, access to peer support networks and attention to their educational needs [2]. Indeed, the entire family requires support when a young person is diagnosed with a malignancy.

The Germ Cell Tumour Service (GCTS) at the Leeds Cancer Centre is a well-established tertiary centre, which receives many referrals, including young men under the age of 25 years diagnosed with testicular cancer. Patients referred to the GCTS receive all of their care and chemotherapy within an adult ward, by an adult team. The Adolescent Service consists of a small group of professionals whose main base of work in within a Teenage Cancer Trust Unit (TCTU), St James's University Hospital, and who have now joined forces with the GCTS. This Unit is an integral part of the Paediatric Oncology Unit. Two of these professionals, a Macmillan Clinical Nurse Specialist and a Sargent Cancer Care Social Worker, now provide a peripatetic service, which reaches out to the young people who are not treated on the TCTU. This goes some way to ensuring equality of supportive care offered to young patients throughout the region.

These professionals attend the GCT clinic on a weekly basis, where they are referred all patients under the age of 25 years. The service offered provides psychosocial support for the family/carers as a whole, provides them with access to a young persons support group and a developing peer network, financial/benefit advice, educational advice and support, and bereavement work. The team also has established links to access other professionals who are experienced in caring for young adults i.e. psychologists, dietitians etc. These professionals are not experts in Germ cell Tumours, although they have a working knowledge of the subject. However, they do have expertise in adolescent cancers, and an understanding of adolescents and the issues, which may affect them during their illness. The team works within a family – centred model of care on a Teenage Cancer Trust Unit with its own uniquely adolescent environment. The skills obtained within this field are transferable to young adults with all forms of cancer.

The provision of this service to the young adults commenced in March 2000. Since then the service has received 20 referrals, all of who have been offered financial, practical and psychosocial support and access to a young adult cancer support group, along with information about the disease, its treatment and side effects. Other interventions have included liaison with the probation service, benefits arranged with Macmillan and Sargent, discussions with employers and colleges and home visits. Three referrals have also resulted in the patients, due to their young age and disease status, being cared for on the Teenage Cancer Trust Unit. Some of these young men have required little input from this service, but, at the very least, have had the option of help if needed. Others have benefited from this service, along with their families and/or partners, and have made good use of the facilities and support services offered to them.

References

1. Department of Health (1995) A policy framework for commissioning cancer services. A report by the Expert Advisory Group on Cancer to the Chief Medical Officers of England and Wales. (Calman Hine) London DoH
2. Lewis, I.J. Cancer in Adolescence. *Brit Med Bull 1996;* 52 :887–897

Section 7

Current Status Non Surgical

50. Chemotherapy for Germ Cell Tumours in the United States

Craig R. Nichols

Oregon Health & Science University, 3181 SW Sam Jackson Park Road, OP28 Portland, OR 97201, USA

Introduction

The therapeutic success of chemotherapy for advanced germ cell tumours over the last several decades has resulted in extension of the use of chemotherapy, from a modality used strictly as primary therapy of surgically unresectable disease or disease outside the confines of radiation therapy port, to the modern use which includes consideration of the use of chemotherapy as an adjuvant for fully resected pathological stage II non-seminomatous germ cell tumour, certain rare situations with clinical stage I non-seminoma and of course extension of chemotherapy into a role for secondary therapies after failure of primary chemotherapy. Herein we will review the current standard usage of chemotherapy in the United States as primary therapy for disseminated disease, its use as a post-surgical adjuvant in resected stage II non-seminoma, its rare usage in seropositive clinical stage I non-seminoma and the myriad of salvage chemotherapy approaches for patients with recurrent disease.

Primary Therapy for Disseminated Disease

Good Risk Disease

For patients with disseminated good risk disease by the International Germ Cell Cancer Consensus prognostic system, standard therapy in the United States of America is three cycles of bleomycin, etoposide and cisplatin (BEP) (Table 50.1) [1]. An alternative is four cycles of etoposide and cisplatin in standard doses as with BEP. Equivalence is suggested by the studies by Memorial Sloan Kettering Cancer Center and the randomized trial from the French testis study group[2, 3]. Again as listed in Table 50.1, BEP or EP are given in "American" doses with etoposide at $100mg/m^2$ daily for five days along with cisplatin $20mg/m^2$ daily for five days. It has become more common practice for patients with disseminated seminoma to opt for four cycles of etoposide and cisplatin, omitting bleomycin. While this has not been subjected to scrutiny in a randomized trial, the equivalence suggested above is reassuring. In practice patients with disseminated seminoma are frequently older, often have had radiation therapy, and tolerate bleomycin less well. A secondary concern is that frequently in patients with disseminated or bulky seminoma, the radiological response is in evolution at the time of the third cycle and practitioners are

Table 50.1: Standard cisplatin-based chemotherapy

BEP
Bleomycin 30 units weekly day 1, 8 & 15
Etoposide 100mg/m^2 daily 1–5
Cisplatin 20mg/m^2 day 1–5
Cycles repeated every 21 days for three to four cycles
VIP
Etoposide 75mg/m^5 daily day 1–5
Ifosfamide 1.2gm/m^2 daily day 1–5
Cisplatin 20mg/m^2 day 1–5
Salvage Chemotherapy
VeIP
Vinblastine 0.11mg/kg day 1, 2
Ifosfamide 1.2gm/m^2 day 1–5
Cisplatin 200mg/m^2 day 1–5
Repeat every 21 days times 4 cycles

uncomfortable discontinuing chemotherapy when there is significant bulk remaining. Accordingly, Indiana University, Memorial Sloan Kettering Cancer Center and Oregon Health & Sciences University have adopted four cycles of etoposide and cisplatin as standard therapy for disseminated seminoma.

Intermediate Risk Disease

Patients with intermediate risk disseminated germ cell tumour by the IGCCC prognostic system are generally entered into the randomized trial of standard BEP times 4 versus 2 cycles of BEP followed by 2 high-dose cycles of carboplatin, etoposide, and cyclophosphamide. Off protocol, these patients should receive 4 cycles of BEP.

Poor Risk Disease

Patients who have poor risk disease by IGCCC prognostic system again are preferentially entered into the Intergroup randomized trial of standard chemotherapy versus brief standard chemotherapy followed by high dose chemotherapy. Off protocol, those patients should receive 4 cycles of BEP. Alternatives to BEP are the regimen of VIP with etoposide, ifosfamide and cisplatin. (Table 50.1). The equivalence of BEP and VIP were demonstrated in the Intergroup randomized trial [4]. While the regimens were therapeutically equivalent at the time of the study, VIP was slightly more toxic, particularly in terms of haematological toxicity. It must be noted that however, that this trial was done before the era of haematopoietic growth factors.

Chemotherapy After Resection of Residual Disease

It cannot be emphasized enough in that patients with residual radiological abnormalities after initial chemotherapy should undergo consideration of resection to render them surgically free of disease. This is a particularly a vexing clinical setting and requires a great deal of experience to gauge the appropriateness of surgery, extent of surgery, and post surgery management. It is appropriate to emphasize at this juncture that this situation is not appropriate for attempts at minimizing surgical morbidity, such as laparoscopy, biopsy only, or significant attempts at nerve sparing procedures. These surgeries should be performed by experienced urological and thoracic surgeons with extensive experience in these techniques. Also, the availability of a multidisciplinary team to carefully evaluate the timing, extent and order of surgeries adds immeasurably to the care of these complex patients.

For the 10–15 per cent of patients with resected residual viable malignancy after primary chemotherapy, the tradition has been to apply post-operative chemotherapy. The recurrence rate after resection of residual viable disease after primary chemotherapy is 30–50 per cent [5]. Accordingly, two cycles of etoposide and platinum have been routinely applied in this setting. There are very few data to measure the exact contribution of the role of the additional chemotherapy, but this had long been the practice in the USA.

Several reviews and recent investigations have suggested that the impact of subsequent chemotherapy after resection of residual disease in the salvage setting is not warranted [5, 6]. The majority of these patients relapse and it is not standard practice to administer chemotherapy in this setting.

Stage II Non-seminoma

In patients with clinical stage II non-seminoma, the majority of oncologists in the United States would recommend chemotherapy for patients with greater than 2cm disease. Such an approach enhances the chances of curing the patient with a single modality of treatment. Approximately 80 per cent of the patients with small volume stage II disease treated with chemotherapy will not require post chemotherapy surgery. Such patients are given three cycles of chemotherapy in most instances (depending on the IGCCC stage). Cure rates in this setting exceed 90 per cent.

In those patients who undergo primary retroperitoneal lymphadenectomy and are found to have pathological stage II disease, adjuvant chemotherapy is frequently applied. Approximately 60–70 per cent of patients with resected stage II disease are cured with surgery alone. The application of two cycles of adjuvant cisplatin-based therapy in this setting assures that the patient will not experience recurrence. In most circumstances, two cycles of BEP at 3-week intervals are given and the cure rate is near 100 per cent [7]. There is a single reported experience with two cycles of etoposide and cisplatin that had similar good results, but this trial was underpowered to provide confidence of its equivalence to two cycles of BEP[8, 9].

Clinical Stage I Disease

In the US, the single circumstance that triggers primary chemotherapy is when the patient has persistently elevated blood markers after orchiectomy despite negative radiological evaluations. Particularly with persistent elevated alpha-fetoprotein, the chance of surgical cure is remote and patients should receive three cycles of BEP.

Salvage Therapy

The situation of recurrent germ cell tumour after primary chemotherapy requires significant thought and experience to sort through a number of subtle clinical scenarios that may mimic relapse. If the patient is proven to have recurrent disease by persistently rising markers or biopsy after BEP, most clinicians would consider VeIP times 4 cycles. Cure rates for patients who do not have manifest cisplatin refractory disease (progression on or within 4 weeks of last cisplatin dose) is approximately 25–30 per cent [8]. With such relatively low expectations of cure, many investigators have chosen to incorporate high dose chemotherapy in this setting. Two cycles of VeIP followed by two high dose cycles with carboplatin and etoposide has been reported to cure approximately 50 per cent of patients with recurrent non-cisplatin refractory disease [10]. There are no randomized studies comparing salvage therapy without transplant to therapy incorporating transplant to date.

Third-line therapy for non-cisplatin refractory patients consists of high dose chemotherapy with stem cell support in patients who have not had this as part of initial therapy, or Taxol-based or oral etoposide-based palliative chemotherapy [11, 12]. Such approaches can be useful in delivering disease control with low toxicity, but these are not felt to be curative approaches.

It is appropriate to remember that there are significant non-chemotherapy options that are associated with cure. For patients with localized chemotherapy-refractory disease, desperation surgery can in some circumstances cure the patient [13]. Again, centers with multidisciplinary teams and experienced urological surgeons are necessary to maximize surgical cures of refractory disease.

There is one exception to consideration of the early application of high dose chemotherapy and stem cell support in recurrent disease. For patients with seminoma, four cycles of standard dose VeIP have reported cure rates in excess of 50 per cent [14]. In such patients, it is appropriate to give four cycles of standard salvage therapy and reserve high dose chemotherapy and stem cell support for those recurring after conventional dose of salvage therapy.

Practical Tips on Giving BEP

Patients received BEP for three or four cycles should receive such therapy every 21 days. Therapy is not delayed for low white blood cell counts, vacations, or other reasons. Therapy should be started irrespective of the white blood cell count and dosage should not be reduced or delayed for asymptomatic granulocytopenia.

The use of growth factors is not warranted for patients with good risk disease receiving three cycles of therapy. For patients with intermediate or poor risk disease receiving 4 cycles of therapy, the addition of haematopoietic growth factors with GCSF is appropriate.

In patients receiving 4 cycles of chemotherapy and for whom surgery after chemotherapy is anticipated, it is frequently recommended that the last two doses of bleomycin (week 11 and 12) be deleted. Again, while there are no randomized trials supporting this minor deviation, it seems prudent in light of the extensive surgeries these patients face.

Conclusions

Chemotherapy is broadly applied for germ cell tumours in the United States. However, it is not felt to be appropriate for high risk stage I disease and certainly is optional in patients with small volume resected clinical stage II disease. BEP is standard therapy in most settings but VIP could be considered in special circumstances.

Salvage chemotherapy is most commonly VeIP for four cycles but many centres are incorporating early high dose therapy in this setting. Therapy after bone marrow transplant is largely palliative and, as such, the premium should be on well-tolerated chemotherapy.

References

1. International Germ Cell Consensus Classification: A Prognostic Factor-Based Staging System for Metastatic Germ Cell Cancers. *J Clin Oncol* 1997;15:594–603
2. Bajorin DF, Sarosdy MF, Pfister DG et al. Randomized Trial of Etoposide and Cisplatin versus Etoposide and Carboplatin in Patients With Good-Risk Germ Cell Tumors: A Multiinstitutional Study. *J Clin Oncol* 1993;11:598–606
3. Culine, S., et al., Are 3 Cycles of Cleomycin, Etoposide and Cisplatin (3BEP) or 4 Cycles of Etoposide and Cisplatin (4EP) Equivalent Regimens for Patients with Good-Risk Metastatic Non Seminomatous Germ Cell Tumors (NSGCT)? Preliminary Results of a Randomized Trial. America Society of Clinical Oncology, 1999
4. Nichols CR, Catalano PJ, Crawford ED, Vogelzang NJ, Einhorn LH, Loehrer PJ. Randomized comparison of cisplatin, etoposide and either bleomycin or ifosfamide in treatment of advanced disseminated germ cell tumors: An Eastern Cooperative Oncology Group, Southwest Oncology Group and Cancer and Leukemia Group B study. *J Clin Oncol* 1998;16:1287–1293
5. Fox EP, Weathers TD, Williams SD et al. Outcome Analysis for Patients with Persistent Germ Cell Carcinoma in Post Chemotherapy Retroperitoneal Lymph Node Dissections. *J Clin Oncol* 1993;11: 1294–1299
6. Foster R et al., Results of post chemotherapy retroperitoneal lymph node dissection for patients with persistently elevated tumor markers. *Proc Am Soc Clin Oncol* 2001;20:179a
7. Behnia M et al., Adjuvant bleomycin, etoposide, and cisplatin in fully resected stage B nonseminomatous testicular cancer. *Proc Am Soc Clin Oncol* 1996;14:249
8. Motzer R, Sheinfeld J, Mazumdar M et al. Etoposide and cisplatin adjuvant therapy for patients with pathologic stage II germ cell tumors. *J Clin Oncol* 1995;13:2700–4
9. Nichols C, Gonin R, Foster R. Defining new standards for adjuvant therapy of testis cancer. *J Clin Oncol* 1995;13:2681–2683
10. Bhatia S et al., High dose chemotherapy with peripheral stem cell or autologous bone marrow transplant as initial salvage chemotherapy for testicular cancer. *Proc Am Soc Clin Oncol* 1998;17: 321A, #1239
11. Nichols C, Andersen J, Lazarus HMl. High-Dose Carboplatin and Etoposide with Autologous Bone Marrow Transplantation in Refractory Germ Cell Cancer: An Eastern Cooperative Oncology Group Protocol. *J Clin Oncol* 1992;10:558–563
12. Bokemeyer C, Beyer J, Metzner B et al. Phase II study of paclitaxel in patients with relapsed or cisplatin-refractory testicular cancer. *Ann Oncol* 1996;7:31–4
13. Murphy BR, Breeden ES, Donohue JP et al., Surgical salvage of chemorefractory germ cell tumors. *J Clin Oncol* 1993;11:324–329
14. Miller KD, Loehrer PJ, Gonin R, Einhorn LH. Salvage Chemotherapy With Vinblastine, Ifosfamide, and Cisplatin in Recurrent Seminoma. *J Clin Oncol* 1997;15:1427–1431

51. The Current Status of Radiotherapy in the Management of Germ Cell Tumours

M. Mason

University of Wales College of Medicine, Velindre Hospital, Whitchurch, Cardiff CF14 2TL, UK

Introduction

The classical role of radiotherapy in the management of germ cell tumours is in the adjuvant therapy of stage I seminoma. It is interesting that here, as in other instances, the role of radiotherapy has been challenged in recent years. However, the potential uses of radiotherapy also cover the treatment of testicular intratubular germ cell neoplasia, the primary treatment of stage II seminoma, consolidation therapy for residual seminomatous masses following primary chemotherapy, for metastatic nonseminoma, and for primary CNS germ cell tumours. The latter group are the subject of articles elsewhere in this volume, and are not further discussed here.

Adjuvant Therapy for Stage I Seminoma

Adjuvant radiotherapy has long been the mainstay of therapy for stage I seminoma, with a long and honourable pedigree dating back to the 1920s. It is associated with a cure rate of around 98 per cent, which would seem an unassailable record. However,

Table 51.1: Specified institutional 'standard' doses for adjuvant ratiothrapy of stage I seminoma (data from MRC Clinical Trials Unit)

Country	Total dose (Gy)	Fractions
UK	30	15
Austria	25	14
Serbia	30	15
Denmark	24	12
France	20	8
Israel	25	15
Italy	30	20
Netherlands		
Centre 1	30	15
Centre 2	25	16
Centre 3	26	13
Poland	24	12
Russia	30	15

surveillance studies have clearly shown that the majority (around 80 per cent) of patients treated with adjuvant radiotherapy do not, in fact, need it [1], and this, together with data on long-term side effects such as second malignancies, has put adjuvant radiotherapy somewhat under the critical spotlight [2].

One approach to this challenge is to reduce the extent and dose of adjuvant radiotherapy. The Medical Research Council performed a randomised trial, which indicated that a policy of para-aortic field (rather than the traditional and more extensive 'dogleg' field) was acceptable [3]. More recently, the Medical Research Council has conducted a further randomised trial, comparing a dose of 30Gy with a dose of 20Gy. Preliminary analyses suggest that the lower dose is acceptable [4].

Have we, with a para-aortic field, and a dose of 20Gy, reached the limit beyond which treatment cannot be further reduced? Certainly, comparing para-aortic fields with surgical dissection templates it is clear that adjuvant radiotherapy in the context of stage I seminoma treats a much larger volume of tissue than does surgery in the same context. Furthermore, with the imminent use of techniques such as Intensity Modulated Radiotherapy, there must be scope for further reductions in the volume of irradiated tissue.

An alternative approach is to replace radiotherapy altogether with other strategies. A multi-institutional analysis of surveillance has highlighted categories of patients at higher risk of relapsing on surveillance [5]. This could be used to select such patients

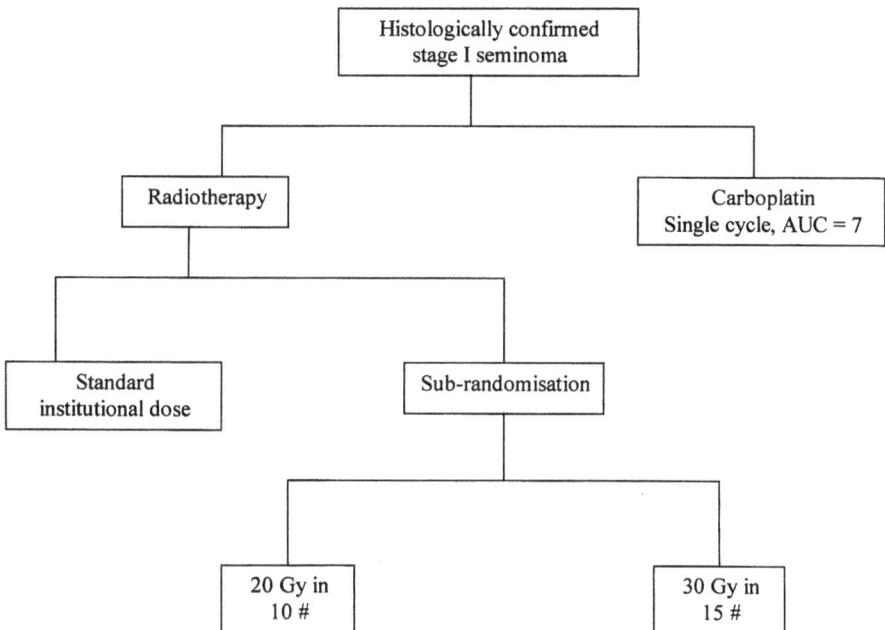

Figure 51.1: Schema of the MRC-EORTC randomised trial of adjuvant radiotherapy versus adjuvant carboplatin.

This study highlighted an enormous variation in the institutional definition of a standard dose for adjuvant radiotherapy in stage I seminoma. Centres had the option of entering patients into a sub-randomisation between 20Gy and 30Gy (to contribute to the MRC dose study) or to define their institutional dose if they chose not to do this. The range in specified doses is shown in Table 51.1. Admittedly, these data were collected long before the first analysis of the MRC dose study was presented, but they nonetheless highlight an uncomfortable truth about variations in medical practice.

for adjuvant therapy, leaving other patients to be managed by surveillance. The drawbacks of surveillance as a management strategy have been very extensively debated over the years, and a second alternative is to replace adjuvant radiotherapy with adjuvant carboplatin, as piloted by Oliver and colleagues [6]. This approach has been tested in a recently completed MRC-EORTC randomised trial, which compared adjuvant radiotherapy with a single cycle of adjuvant carboplatin (Figure 51.1). This study has accrued 1477 patients, and the first analysis will probably be in 2004.

Ablation of Intratubular Germ Cell Neoplasia

Around 5 per cent of patients with primary germ cell tumours of the testis have intratubular germ cell neoplasia (ITGCN) in the contralateral testis [7]. Unlike other epithelia, germinal epithelium, being highly sensitive, can be completely ablated by low-dose radiation. This underlies the evident success of low dose testicular irradiation in both eradicating ITGCN and in preventing its recurrence [7]. This is in contrast to chemotherapy, which manifestly does not always eradicate germinal epithelium, as evidenced by the recovery of fertility in some germ cell cancer patients, and which, similarly, does not always eradicate ITGCN, though it does so sometimes [8].

Is there a gradient in the radiosensitivity of seminoma compared with ITGCN? That a dose of 20 Gy (if substantiated) has been shown to eradicate the former and 18 Gy the latter does not, so far suggest any substantial difference in radiosensitivity between the two. Can doses of adjuvant radiotherapy, therefore be reduced still further from 20 Gy? Time will tell, but it is possible that doses much below 16Gy will lead to recurrence of ITGCN.

An unresolved issue is whether patients with primary testicular tumours should have routine contralateral biopsies, with radiotherapy offered to those found to have ITGCN (subsequent contralateral tumours being unlikely in the remainder).

Treatment of Stage IIA/IIB Seminoma

Stage II seminoma is relatively uncommon at presentation, and hence, although radiotherapy has been used for many years as definitive treatment, it is relatively hard to make definitive statements about its efficacy, and still harder to make comparisons with alternative options such as primary chemotherapy. A data review has been performed by von der Maase [9], from which a relapse rate of 7 per cent was estimated for combined stage I and II seminoma treated with radiotherapy, based on 22 recurrences in 313 patients reported in seven studies. It seems clear, however, that relapse rates for stage IIC seminoma are somewhat higher, justifying the approach commonly adopted of primary chemotherapy in this group of patients [9].

Do the small but not insignificant relapse rates for stage IIA or IIB seminoma justify attempts to reduce them? Biologically, relapses in most such patients result from occult micro-metastatic disease in mediastinal nodes, since this is the main site of relapse, relapse in an irradiated para-aortic field being uncommon. Using the same rationale as that applied to stage I seminoma, a pilot study has been performed in which definitive radiotherapy to a 'dogleg' field was preceded by a single cycle of carboplatin in 33 patients from 2 institutions [10]. Two patients relapsed, giving a 5 year relapse rate of around 3 per cent. This suggests that such an approach might be feasible, but its value would need to be tested in a large randomised study.

Consolidation Therapy for Residual Masses after Chemotherapy in Advanced Seminoma

Another controversy surrounding radiotherapy for seminoma is the question of its role in the management of residual masses following the completion of chemotherapy. Such masses can be large, and difficult to remove surgically, and a common, though unproven practice was to consolidate a chemotherapy response with radiotherapy. The efficacy of this approach has never been prospectively evaluated. However, Duchesne and colleagues performed a European retrospective study based on 174 patients with residual masses from 10 centres [11]. No significant benefit to consolidation radiotherapy was detected, absolute progression-free survival being 88 per cent, and the estimated, absolute benefit of radiotherapy being 2.3 per cent. This study represents the best available data addressing this question, and offers no support for a policy of routine post-chemotherapy irradiation of residual seminomatous masses.

Radiotherapy for Metastatic Nonseminoma

The optimum management of residual metastatic nonseminoma following chemotherapy is surgical excision. However, this is not possible in some patients, and unresectable masses are a potential source of residual active nonseminoma. Salvage chemotherapy remains the cornerstone of the management of patients with unresectable, active nonseminoma. Might there be a role for radiotherapy in selected patients? There is no direct evidence to inform this question. However, a randomised trial was reported comparing surveillance with adjuvant radiotherapy in patients with stage I nonseminoma, dating from a time when adjuvant radiotherapy was more commonly used in this setting [12]. It is interesting that, in this study, out of 150 patients, 14 retroperitoneal relapses were seen in the surveillance group, compared to none in the adjuvant radiotherapy group. While the study concluded, rightly, that surveillance was the preferred option for stage I nonseminoma, it did demonstrate that radiotherapy was capable of eradicating microscopic disease in the retroperitoneum, which must have been present in a proportion of irradiated patients. Furthermore, in a retrospective analysis of patients with isolated CNS relapse following first line chemotherapy for germ cell tumours [13], it appeared that radiotherapy was of significant benefit (in contrast to patients with CNS disease at presentation). Radiotherapy for metastatic nonseminoma will never have more than a limited role, but, though limited, it could be important in some patients, and that role deserves to be better defined.

Summary and Conclusions

The role of radiotherapy in germ cell tumours is changing. Over the next few years, its role in stage I seminoma could be challenged as the MRC/EORTC TE19 study is analysed. However, a cautionary note; encouraging early results of adjuvant carboplatin would not exclude the possibility of late relapses, if such relapses are merely delayed and not prevented by carboplatin. If radiotherapy has 'a diminishing role', to quote Duchesne, in some aspects, its roles in stage II seminoma and as a component of salvage therapy have the potential to expand. Defining these roles will inevitably require international collaboration, as no single country is likely to have adequate numbers of patients for a randomised trial.

References

1. Warde PR, Gospodarowicz MK et al. Results of a policy of surveillance in stage I testicular seminoma. *Int J Radiation Oncol, Biol, Phys* 1993;27:11–5
2. Grossfeld GD, Small EJ. Long-term side effects of treatment for testis cancer. *Urol Clin North America* 1998;25:503–15
3. Fossa SD, Horwich A, Russell JM et al. Optimal planning target volume for stage I testicular seminoma: A medical research council randomized trial. *J Clin Oncol* 1999;17:1146–1154
4. Jones WG, Fossa SD, Mead GM et al. Preliminary results of a international randomised trial of radiotherapy at two dose schedules of 20Gy versus 30Gy (at 2Gy/day) as adjuvant treatment of stage 1 seminoma testis, including morbidity and quality of life data (MRC study TE18). In this volume
5. Warde P, Maase Hvd, Horwich A, Gospodarowicz M, Panzarella T, Specht L. Prognostic factors for relapse in stage I seminoma managed by surveillance (meeting abstract). In: Proc Annu Meet Am Soc Clin Oncol; 1998: ASCO; 1998. p. A1188
6. Oliver RT, Boublikova L, Ong J. Fifteen year follow up of the Anglian Germ Cell Cancer Group adjuvant studies of carboplatin as an alternative to radiation or surveillance for stage 1 seminoma (meeting abstract). Proceedings of the American Society of Clinical Oncology 2001;20:196a
7. Dieckmann KP, Loy V. The value of the biopsy of the contralateral testis in patients with testicular germ cell cancer: the recent German experience. *Apmis* 1998;106:13–20;discussion 20–3
8. Dieckmann KP, Classen J, Souchon R, Loy V. Therapie der testikularen intraepitheilian Neoplasie (TIN) – eine Ubersicht auf Grunlage der evidenzbasierten Medizin (EBM) [Management of testicular intraepithelial neoplasia (TIN) – a review based on the principles of evidence-based medicine]. Wiener Klinische Wochenschrift 2001;113:7–14
9. von der Maase H. Editorial: Do we have a new standard of treatment for patients with seminoma stage IIA and stage IIB? *Radiotherapy and Oncology* 2001;59:1-3
10. Patterson H, Norman AR, Mitra SS et al. Combination carboplatin and radiotherapy in the management of stage II testicular seminoma: comparison with radiotherapy treatment alone. *Radiotherapy and Oncology* 2001;59:5-11
11. Duchesne GM, Stenning SP, Aass N et al. Radiotherapy after chemotherapy for metastatic seminoma – a diminishing role. MRC Testicular Tumour Working Party. *Eur J Cancer* 1997;33:829-35
12. Rorth M, Jacobsen GK, Von der Maase H et al. Surveillance alone versus radiotherapy after orchiectomy for clinical stage I nonseminomatous testicular cancer. *J Clin Oncol* 1991;9:1543–1548
13. Fossa SD, Bokemeyer C, Gerl A et al. Treatment outcome of patients with brain metastases from malignant germ cell tumors. Cancer 1999;85:988–97

52. Limited Volume Short Course Radiation for Stage I Seminoma of the Testis

J.P. Logue, J.E. Livsey

Department of Clinical Oncology, Christie Hospital, Manchester, M20 4BX

Methods

Between December 1988 and December 1998, 402 men with stage I seminoma of the testis received radiotherapy to the para-aortic area (20 Gy in 8 fractions over 10 days).

Table 52.1: Details of recurrent patients

Pattern	Time (months)	Site	Markers at presentation	Markers at relapse	Treatment at relapse
Markers only (n =1)	15	not applicable	AFP < 5 HCG 291	AFP < 10 HCG 191	BEP
Distant (n = 2)	9	1.5 cm lung Excision seminoma	AFP < 5 HCG < 5	AFP < 5 HCG < 10	BEP
	23	6 cm mass scapula Biopsy GCT Axillary nodes, lung	AFP < 5 HCG < 5	AFP 16 HCG 1546	PVE + XRT
Local (n = 1)	10	Scrotum Excision : seminoma	AFP < 5 HCG < 5	AFP < 5 HCG < 5	Surgry
Nodal (n = 9)	7	11 cm R iliac nodes 3.5 cm inguinofemoral nodes Biopsy : seminoma	AFP < 5 HCG < 5	AFP < 5 HCG < 5	XRT CE DIED
	9	8 x 9 cm pelvic nodes Biopsy : seminoma	AFP < 5 HCG 17	AFP 2 HCG 7	BEP
	9	5 x 9 pelvic nodes Biopsy : seminoma	AFP 5 HCG < 5	AFP < 5 HCG < 5	BEP
	12	5 cm inguinal mass Biopsy : seminoma	AFP < 5 HCG 6	AFP 35 HCG < 5	
	12	Pelvis	AFP < 5 HCG17	AFP8 HCG,5	BEP Surg
	26	2.5 cm left inguinal node Biopsy : seminoma	AFP < 5 HCG 49	AFP < 5 HCG 82	XRT
	31	3.4 x 4.6 cm iliac nodes	AFP < 5 HCG 31	AFP < 5 HCG 274	BEP
	36	5 cm left ext iliac biopsy Biopsy : seminoma	AFP < 5 HCG < 5	AFP < 5 HCG < 10	BEP NED 6 months
	63	1.8 cm para-aortic	AFP < 5 HCG < 5	AFP 9 HCG 45	BEP NED 5 months

Results

At a median follow up of 50 months thirteen patients (3.6 per cent) have developed recurrence of disease (Table 52.1). The median time to relapse is 12 months. On univariate analysis the presence of lympho-vascular invasion (p = 0.007), invasion of the tunica (p = 0.0001) and elevated HCG at presentation (p = 0.0001) were of prognostic significance. The disease free survival is 96.5 per cent. One patient died of disease.

Discussion

The ideal management in Stage I seminoma aims to achieve high cure rates while minimising morbidity. Surveillance, if successful, eliminates treatment but it is not a "no irradiation" option since it entails CT scanning for 10 years and a potential carcinogenic effect from the cumulative radiation exposure clearly remains.

The chemosensitivity of seminoma has led to the use of chemotherapy as adjuvant treatment in these patients. The initial results with one cycle of Carboplatin were promising. This led to the MRC TE19 study comparing chemotherapy and radiotherapy. The results of this study will not however be available for several years and in the interim the recent publication by Dieckmann [1] demonstrating a relapse rate of 8.6 per cent following a single course of Carboplatin suggests caution in utilising this treatment.

The relapse rate of 3.6 per cent in this study using a short course of limited volume radiotherapy compares favourably with both arms of the MRC adjuvant radiotherapy trial using longer radiation schedules with higher radiation doses. The data presented support this short duration limited field radiotherapy schedule as a valid and preferred protocol in the management of stage I seminoma patients.

Reference

1. Dieckmann KP, Bruggeboes B, Pichlmeier U et al. Adjuvant treatment of clinical stage I seminoma: Is a single course of Carboplatin sufficient? *Urology* 2000;55:102–6

53. A Randomised Trial of Two Radiotherapy Schedules in the Adjuvant Treatment of Stage I Seminoma (MRC TE18) – Preliminary Report

W.G. Jones, S.D. Fossa, G.M. Mead, J.T. Roberts, M. Sokal, S. Naylor, S.P. Stenning for the MRC Testicular Tumour Working Party

MRC Clinical Trials Unit, London

Background

Adjuvant post-orchidectomy radiotherapy cures the majority of patients with stage I seminoma, but as approximately 80 per cent would remain relapse-free on surveillance alone, minimising radiotherapy – and hence morbidity and second cancer risk – is a worthwhile aim. An earlier MRC trial (TE10) assessed the impact of reducing radiotherapy field size from the dog-leg field to the para-aortic strip only. This follow-on trial assessed the impact of reducing radiotherapy dose on relapse rates, acute morbidity and quality of life.

Methods

Patients were randomised within 8 weeks of orchidectomy to receive 20 Gy in 10 fractions over two weeks or 30 Gy in 15 fractions over three weeks. They were asked to complete a symptom diary card daily for four weeks after starting radiotherapy and weekly for a further eight weeks, and quality of life forms (EORTC QLQ-C30 and testis cancer module) at 0, 3, 6, 12 and 24 months. The primary endpoint was the relapse-free rate, and the trial was designed as an equivalence trial, powered to exclude differences in the relapse rate of 3–4 per cent at 2 years.

Results

Between Jan 1995 and Jan 1998, 625 patients were randomised from 45 centres worldwide. The groups were well balanced with respect to baseline characteristics. Compliance was high with over 98 per cent of patients in each treatment group receiving their allocated schedule. Based on assessments during radiotherapy, there were trends towards less nausea and vomiting (p = 0.06), and less severe leucopaenia (p = 0.02) in the 20 Gy group, although the incidence of CTC grades greater than 1 was rare in both groups.

Seventy-three percent of patients completed the daily diary cards. Based on this data, four weeks after the start of radiotherapy significantly more 30 Gy patients reported moderate or severe lethargy (20 per cent versus 5 per cent) and an inability to carry out normal work (46 per cent versus 28 per cent), but by 12 weeks, levels in the randomised groups were similar.

With a median follow-up time of 37 months, eight relapses have been reported in the 30 Gy group and 10 in the 20 Gy group (HR = 1.27, log rank p = 0.61, 90 per cent confidence interval (0.58, 2.8)). The difference in two year relapse rates is 0.3 per cent, (30 Gy: 97.3 per cent, 20 Gy: 97.0 per cent) with 90 per cent CI (–1.9 per cent, 2.5 per cent), hence the probability that the true difference exceeds 2.5 per cent is less than 5 per cent. Of the 18 relapsed patients, 16 are currently disease-free, one (20 Gy) has died from seminoma and another (30 Gy) has active disease.

A further 393 patients have so far been randomised with respect to the same radiotherapy doses within a subsequent trial (MRC TE19). Of these, six (five 30 Gy , one 20 Gy) have relapsed; analysing all 1018 patients, the difference in relapse rates at two years is 0.8 per cent in favour of the 20 Gy group, with the upper 90 per cent CI excluding differences of more than 1.3 per cent.

Conclusions

These preliminary results indicate that 20 Gy in 10 fractions is unlikely to produce relapse rates more than 2 per cent higher than for standard 30 Gy radiotherapy and reductions in morbidity enable patients to return to work more rapidly.

54. Metastatic Seminoma: Should Treatment Be Different from Non-seminoma?

J. Ong, R.T.D. Oliver, J. Shamash , M. Williams, B. Sizer, J. Ostrowski, J. Le Vay

St Bart's and London, Oldchurch, Addenbrookes Colchester, Norfolk & Norwich, and Ipswich Hospitals

Introduction

It is now more than 50 years since Friedman [1] first demonstrated that seminoma was more sensitive to radiation than non-seminoma and it has since been standard to give a different radiation dosage. In contrast, although our group first demonstrated 18 years ago that the chemosensitivity of metastatic seminoma to single agent cisplatin was so different to that of non-seminoma, that it might be safe to treat all metastatic seminoma with single agent and only use combination to salvage the minority who fail it [2, 3], BEP combination chemotherapy remains the standard of care. With new evidence from multivariate analysis demonstrating that pure seminoma histology predicts for a better relapse free survival after cisplatin based combination therapy than non-seminoma [4] and given the increased anxiety about late second malignant events after etoposide treatment [5], renewed interest in this issue is emerging. This paper updates the results from our studies and attempts to define a subgroup of seminoma patients in whom it may be safe to use single agent platinum therapy.

Patients and Methods

Patients treated from January 1980 to January 1999 have received either cisplatin (n = 19) or carboplatin (n = 34) as a single agent, or combination therapy with etoposide and cisplatin +/– bleomycin (n = 56). Details of patient selection and drug doses have been published elsewhere [2, 3].

Results

Relapse free and overall survival was 84 per cent and 84 per cent for cisplatin (n = 19), 82 per cent and 97 per cent for carboplatin alone (n = 34) and 95 per cent and 93 per cent for BEP/EP (n = 56). The poor survival in the cisplatin alone group was due to small sample size and accident of selection as one of the failures was aged 68 with a solitary lung lesion that could, in retrospect, have been a coincidental lung primary,

Table 54.1: Prognostic factors for relapse free survival

	Single Agent Cisplatin		Single Agent Carboplatin		BEP/EP		*statistics BEPEP v Carboplatin
	No. of cases	Continuous NEM	No. of cases	Continuous NEM	No. of cases	Continuous NEM	x^2
All cases	19	84%	34	82%	56	93%	3.82
Stage 2a/b	1	100%	12	100%	15	100%	
Stage 2c	5	100%	9	79%	19	95%	
Stage 2d	3	100%	6	67%	9	100%	1.28
All Stage 2	9	100%	27	85%	43	95%	2.49
Stage 3 + 4	10	7%	7	71%	13	92%	3.36
hCG negative	9	89%	30	83%	32	97%	0.95
hCG raised	10	80%	3	67%	18	89%	2.11
HD/LDH-ve	5	100%	9	89%	9	100%	2.11
HBD/LDH + ve	10	80%	12	67%	14	93%	2.57
≤ 40	10	100%	14	93%	24	96%	0
> 40	9	67%	20	75%	32	94%	5.12

the second failure was a schizophrenic who would not tolerate therapy and the third was a patient with advanced and atypical disease spread involving internal mammary lymph glands. The poorer overall survival after combination was due to treatment related deaths. For good risk patients with less than 10cm paraortic nodes or normal hCG or normal LDH and age 40 or less, relapse free survival after single agent carboplatin was in excess of 90 per cent (Table 54.1). There have been no relapses after 19 months (longest follow-up 20 years, median 68 months).

Conclusion

Although these data and the results from the recently completed randomized trials [5,6] suggest that the primary relapse free survival after single agent carboplatin is not as good as single agent cisplatin when matched stage for stage in poorer risk seminoma patients, in good risk patients the difference is so little that given the high salvage rate leading to equivalent overall survival to that achievable by BEP chemotherapy, it is clearly justified to continue exploration of this approach in research trials to reduce late treatment related toxicity. The availability of new, less toxic cisplatin analogues, some of which have demonstrated better activity than carboplatin in vitro [7] and new approaches to evaluating response such as d21 CT scan volume reduction measurements [8] and PET scanning [9] are providing additional justification and safeguards for such studies.

References

1. Friedman N. Supervoltage (1 million volts) roentgen therapy at Walter Reed General Hospital. *Surg. Clin. N. Am.* 1944;24:1424–32

2. Oliver RTD, Hope-Stone HF, Blandy JP. Justification of the use of surveillance in the management of stage 1 germ cell tumours of the testis. *Br J Urol* 1983;55:760–763
3. Oliver RTD, Love S, Ong J. Alternatives to radiotherapy in management of seminoma. *Br J Urol* 1990;65:61–67
4. Bajorin D, Mazumdar M, Meyers M et al. Metastatic germ cell tumours: modelling for response to chemotherapy. *J Clin Oncol* 1998;16(2):707–15
5. Horwich A, Oliver R, Wilkinson P et al. A Medical Research Council randomized trial of single agent carboplatin versus etoposide and cisplatin for advanced metastatic seminoma. *Br J Cancer* 2000;83: 1623–1629
6. Clemm T. Carboplatin versus Vinbloestin Ifosfamide and Cisplatin in Seminoma. *Proc Amer Soc Clin Onc* 2001
7. Dunn T, Schmoll H, Grunwald V, Bokemeyer C, Casper J. Comparative cytotoxicity of oxaliplatin and cisplatin in non-seminomatous germ cell cancer cell lines. *Invest New Drugs* 1997;15:109–14
8. Bozcuk H. Day 21 Post chemotherapy CT scan response: a predictor for need of post chemotherapy surgery in non-seminomatous germ cell cancer? In: BAUS 1998;1998;Harrogate;1998
9. Albers P, Bender H, Yilmaz H, Schoeneich G, Biersack HJ, Mueller SC. Positron emission tomography in the clinical staging of patients with Stage I and II testicular germ cell tumors. *Urology* 1999;53:808–11

55. GAMEC–a Novel Protocol for IGCCCG Poor Prognosis and Relapsing Germ Cell Tumours

J. Shamash, R.T.D. Oliver, J.P.C. Steele, W. Ansell, L. Millard

Department of Medical Oncology, St. Bartholomew's Hospital, London

The results of BEP chemotherapy for all cases of metastatic germ cell tumours (GCTs) remains to be bettered in any multicenter randomised controlled trial. However, less than half of patients with poor prognosis disease can expect to be cured with it. For salvage therapy a cisplatin and ifosfamide based treatment will cure 25–30 per cent of cases; alternatively a weekly-based therapy (m-BOP) [1] may achieve similar results. High dose therapy may be able to improve on this, although its exact role remains to be determined. The recognition that actinomycin and methotrexate have a role in salvage [2] has encouraged us to investigate these drugs with cisplatin and etoposide in a new schedule (GAMEC) – cisplatin 100mg/m^2 weeks 1, 3, 6, 8 and 10 with 50mg/m^2 on weeks 2 and 4. Etoposide 360mg/m^2 over 4 days on weeks 1, 3, 6, 8 and 10. Methotrexate with folinic acid rescue 10g/m^2 on weeks 1, 3, 6, 8 and 10 (with linear dose reduction for creatinine clearance of < 120ml/min). Actinomycin-D 1mg/m^2 on weeks 1, 3, 6, 8 and 10. Granulocyte colony-stimulating factor (GCSF) is given between courses. The proposed advantages of this therapy included the fact that it did not contain bleomycin and therefore would not be contra-indicated as a salvage regimen. It allowed the integration of high dose methotrexate and actinomycin, both active agents in GCTs, into a dose-dense high intensity cisplatin based regimen whilst maintaining the exposure to etoposide in a therapeutic dose without resorting to stem cell rescue.

Twelve untreated patients have received the treatment to date – 58 per cent are progression free by GAMEC and surgery, one relapsing patient received further therapy and is in remission making the current progression free survival for this poor prognosis group 67 per cent. Sixteen relapsing cases, 12 with a poor prognosis for salvage as identified by Fossa et al [3] (progression-free interval < 2 years and incomplete remission to initial therapy and raised markers at relapse –hCG >100 or AFP > 100). Eight patients (50 per cent) are currently progression free including six of the 12 with all three poor prognostic features.

Toxicity was considerable with the following grade 3/4 toxicities seen: anorexia 13 per cent; diarrhoea-10 per cent; constipation-1 per cent; infection-60 per cent; lethargy-32 per cent; mucositis-26 per cent; nausea and vomiting-7 per cent; neuropathy-1 per cent; renal dysfunction-2 per cent. There were a total of 3 treatment-related deaths. Extensive pharmacokinetic studies are on-going. To date a relationship between the 24 hour level of methotrexate and neutropenia has emerged.

Although toxic, the results in the salvage group of patients are encouraging. Patients with poor performance status and over 40 years of age seem to be most prone to life threatening side effects. Further refinement of the regimen is being undertaken to reduce the frequency of life threatening events.

References

1. Levi JA, Thomson D, Harvey V et al. Effective salvage chemotherapy with etoposide, dactinomycin and methotrexate in refractory germ cell cancer. *J Clin Oncol* 1990;8:27–32
2. Shamash J, Oliver RTD, Ong J et al. Sixty-percent salvage rate for germ cell tumours using sequential m-BOP, surgery and ifosfamide –based chemotherapy. *Ann Oncol* 1999;10:685–92
3. Fossa SD, Stenning SP, Gerl A et al. Prognostic factors in patients progressing after cisplatin-based chemotherapy for malignant non-seminomatous germ cell tumours *Brit J Cancer* 1999;80:1392–99

56. Adjuvant Chemotherapy in High-risk Stage I Non-seminomatous Germ Cell Tumours: the Spanish Germ Cell Cancer Group Experience

P. Maroto, X. García del Muro, M. Lomas, D. Almenar, J. Aparicio,
R. Bastús, M. López-Brea, R. Lasso de la Vega, J. Lizón, J. Terrasa, R. Pérez,
M. Tejedor, J.A. Arranz, E. Alba, P. Diz, L. Paz-Ares, J.F. Sancho,
J.R. Germa-Lluch, on behalf of Spanish Germ Cell Cancer Group

*Dr P Maroto, Medical Oncology Department, Hospital Sant Pau, Avda. Sant Antoni Ma Claret
167, Barcelona 08025, Spain*

Purpose

Patients with clinical stage I non-seminomatous germ cell tumour (NSGCT) with
pathological high-risk features have a risk of recurrence on observation of
approximately 40 per cent. This study evaluated the efficacy of adjuvant
chemotherapy in a large series of patients treated in a multi-institutional setting.

Material and Methods

From January 1994 to June 2001, 105 patients with clinical stage I NSGCT with
vascular invasion and/or tumour stage pT2 or greater (1992 TNM), were treated in 39
hospitals. Patients received 1-3 cycles of cisplatin 100 mg/m^2, etoposide 400-500
mg/m^2 and weekly bleomycin 30 mg (BEP).

Results

Median follow-up was 29 (1-76) months, 40 per cent of the patients being followed-up
for at least 2 years. All patients have remained alive and free of disease to date. The
actuarial event-free survival at 2 years was 100 per cent. Grade 3-4 toxicity was
observed infrequently, and consisted mainly of granulocytopenia. No significant long-
term sequelae were found. Sixteen patients fathered one child after treatment.

Conclusion

The administration of adjuvant chemotherapy is an alternative to surveillance or
retroperitoneal lymphadenectomy in clinical stage I patients with a high-risk of relapse.

57. Single Agent Carboplatin for Advanced Seminoma: Effective Initial Therapy

N.L. Fernie, V.J. Harvey

Department of Oncology, Auckland Hospital, Auckland, New Zealand

There remains controversy whether single agent carboplatin (SAC) can replace more toxic cisplatin based combination chemotherapy (CC) in the treatment of metastatic seminoma. In this retrospective review of our experience, 29 patients were treated with SAC and 26 with CC. There were 27 good prognosis and 2 intermediate prognosis patients in the SAC arm and 21 good prognosis and 5 intermediate prognosis patients in the CC arm (IGCCCG criteria). Median follow up was 48 months (range 4 to 178 months).

Results

In patients treated with SAC, 25 of 26 evaluable patients had a response (10 CR, 15 PR), one patient had progressive disease and three patients without measurable disease remain well. There were relapses in nine patients (36 per cent), 5 of whom are well following salvage therapy. There were five deaths, all from seminoma. Overall survival was 83 per cent (89 per cent for good prognosis patients).

In CC treated patients, 22 had a response (10 CR, 12 PR), three patients were un-evaluable and one had progressive disease. Eight patients died, five from seminoma and three from treatment related toxicity (one neutropenic sepsis, 2 bleomycin lung). Overall survival was 69 per cent (81 per cent for good prognosis patients).

Although the relapse rate of patients treated with SAC was high, salvage therapy was often effective and cure rates overall were good. Combination chemotherapy produced durable responses but deaths due to toxicity led to overall reduced survival in this series. SAC remains an effective initial therapy for selected patients with advanced seminoma.

58. Bleomycin in Combination Chemotherapy of Testicular or Extragonadal Germ Cell Tumours: a Review of Published Trials

L. Boublikova[1], R.T.D. Oliver[1], J. Shamash[1], R.G. Fish[2], M.D. Mason[2], S.P. Stenning[3,] L. Collette[4]

1 Department of Medical Oncology, St Bartholomew's Hospital, London EC1A 7BE, 2 Department of Clinical Oncology, Cardiff University, 3 MRC Clinical Trials Office, London, 4 EORTC Clinical Trials Centre, Brussels.

Introduction

Bleomycin, Etoposide and Cisplatin remain the standard chemotherapy for metastatic germ cell cancer, despite up to one third of patients having some evidence of lung toxicity [1]. Most large series report treatment related deaths due to Bleomycin lung but there are at least three clinical trials providing evidence that it is not safe to drop bleomycin [2–4]. Prompted by the need to find safe ways to reduce toxicity in good risk patients, this paper reviews the evidence for the benefit of Bleomycin in germ cell cancer and data from a series of sequential phase 2 studies undertaken by the Anglian Germ Cell Cancer Group developing new schedules aimed at reducing the risk of toxicity and maintaining or increasing its activity.

Materials and Methods

Data was extracted from the published articles from the 3 trials in which the same combination was studied with or without Bleomycin . Two compared BEP versus EP [2, 3] and one PVB versus PV [4]. Data from previously published Anglian Germ Cell Group sequential phase 2 studies comparing Bleomycin given as a 30mg bolus, 45mg infusion [5, 6] and 90 mg infusion [7] have been reviewed and updated. The scoring technique for CT scan assessment of bleomycin lung toxicity has been published elsewhere [6].

Results

In the 3 trials with and without Bleomycin, there were higher complete remissions (CR), less relapses and better disease free (DFS) and overall survival (OS) in the Bleomycin-containing arms. But the difference in CR was only statistically significant in one trial (92 vs. 85 per cent) [3]. The other two trials revealed statistically significant differences in DFS (86 versus 69 per cent and 84 versus 71 per cent) and OS

Table 58.1: Pooled results from comparing cisplatin based regimens with and without Bleomycin [2–4]

Outcomes	+ Bleomycin (n = 3961)	– Bleomycin (n = 3881)
Complete response	87%	81%
Relapse free survival at median follow up	89% in 3–7 years[a]	80"% in 3–7 years[b]
Overall survival at median follow up	94% in 3–7 years[c]	89% in 3–7 years[d]
Treatment related deaths	2%	0.26%

a versus b: p = 0.00098, c versus d: p = 00986

(95 versus 86 per cent and 90 versus 84 per cent) [2, 4]. Loehrer's study also showed significantly lower relapse rate (10 per cent versus 23 per cent) in patients treated with Bleomycin [2]. When the data was pooled statistically significant differences in CR, DFS and OS were confirmed (CR: p = 0.01036, DFS: p = 0.00098, OS: p = 0.00986– see Table 58.1). Bleomycin containing regimens produced significantly higher lung toxicity in all three trials and overall treatment related mortality was 2 per cent in the Bleomycin containing arm and 0.26 per cent in the arm without Bleomycin.

In the AGCCG studies the frequency of grade 1 change in patients receiving 30mg short infusion (30mins) was 69 per cent (n = 55 including 1 respiratory death). In patients receiving 15mg × 3 eight hourly the incidence was 44 per cent (n = 18) and in patients receiving 90mg infusions over 72 hours the frequency of grade 1 change was 18 per cent (n = 11). Comparison of results from a series of 77 patients receiving the 15 mg × 3 eight hour infusion schedule showed 81 per cent relapse free survival compared to 93 per cent in a series of 31 patients who had received the 90mg 72 hour infusion schedule.

Conclusion

This review of published trials data reinforces the generally held view on the beneficial role of Bleomycin despite the higher death rate from lung toxicity. Given the increasingly good results, there is a need for more effort to reduce these deaths, which could risk exceeding those from disease. The number of cases in the sequential phase 2 studies is too small to allow definitive conclusions but the data from five animal studies [8–11] and one previous clinical trial [12] provide additional encouragement that there could be therapeutic gain, with both reduced lung toxicity and increased therapeutic activity from use of prolonged infusion. A randomized trial to investigate this is now being launched.

References

1. Saxman SB, Nichols CR, Einhorn LH. Pulmonary toxicity in patients with advanced-stage germ cell tumors receiving bleomycin with and without granulocyte colony stimulating factor. *Chest* 1997;111(3):657–60
2. Loehrer P, Johnson D, Elson P, Einhorn L, Trump D. Importance of bleomycin in favorable prognosis disseminated germ cell tumours – an eastern-cooperative-oncology-group trial. *J Clin Oncol* 1995;13(2):470–476
3. de Wit R, Stoter G, Kaye SB et al. Importance of bleomycin in combination chemotherapy for good-prognosis testicular nonseminoma: a randomized study of the European Organization for Research

and Treatment of Cancer Genitourinary Tract Cancer Cooperative Group *J Clin Oncol* 1997;15(5):1837–43

4. Levi JA, Raghavan D, Harvey V et al. The importance of bleomycin in combination chemotherapy for good prognosis germ cell carcinoma. *J Clin Oncol* 1993;11:1300–1305

5. Oliver RTD, Dhaliwal HS, Hope-Stone HF, Blandy JP. Short course etoposide, bleomycin and cisplatin in the treatment of metastatic germ cell tumours. Appraisal of its potential as adjuvant chemotherapy for stage 1 testis tumours. *Br J Urol* 1988;61:53–58

6. Chisholm RA, Dixon AK, Williams MV, Oliver RTD. Bleomycin lung: the effect of different chemotherapeutic regimens. *Cancer Chemother Pharmacol* 1992;30:158–160

7. Shamash J, Oliver R, Reznek R, Chisolm R, Dixon A, Williams M. Bolus versus infusional bleomycin for Germ Cell Cancer. In: Proc ASCO; 1999: *J Clin Oncol*; 1999. p. Abst 1258

8. Sikic BI, Collins JM, Mimnaugh EG, Gram TE. Improved therapeutic index of bleomycin when administered by continuous infusion in mice. *Cancer Treat Rep* 1978;62(12):2011–7

9. Ekimoto H, Takahashi K, Matsuda A, Umezawa H. Changes of anticancer activity and pulmonary toxicity of bleomycins in differences of adminstration schedules and routes in mice. *Gan to Kagaku Ryoho* 1984;11:853–7

10. Peng YM, Alberts DS, Chen HS, Mason N, Moon TE. Antitumour activity and plasma kinetics of bleomycin by continuous and intermittent administration. Br J Cancer 1980;41(4):644–7

11. Osieka R. Comparison of a continuous infusion with a daily bolus injection of bleomycin in a heterotransplanted human testicular cancer. *Arzneimittel-Forschung.*4 1984: 34(4):460

12. Krakoff IH, Cvitkovic E, Currie V, Yeh S, LaMonte C. Clinical pharmacologic and therapeutic studies of bleomycin given by continuous infusion. *Cancer* 1977;40(5):2027–37

59. Long Term Follow Up of Anglian Germ Cell Cancer Group Studies of Chemotherapy for Stage 1 Non Seminoma

R.T.D. Oliver, J. Ong, R. Ravi, J. Shamash, J. Ostrowski, B. Sizer, T. Tahir, M. Williams, J. LeVay, P. Harper

St Bart's and London, Oldchurch, Norfolk & Norwich, Colchester, Addenbrookes, Ipswich and Guy's Hospitals

Introduction

Prior to the advent of cisplatin-based chemotherapy, there was prolonged debate over the relative merits of surgery versus radiotherapy for management of the retroperitoneum. Although the early results of surveillance [1] proved equivalent to previous surgical and radiotherapy results, late relapses and default from follow-up have led to increasing use of adjuvant chemotherapy for patients with a high risk of relapse. It is now 14 years since adjuvant chemotherapy with two courses of BEP was first used in stage I non-seminoma. Reports of leukaemia in patients receiving Etoposide [2] have led to the development of regimens substituting Vincristine for Etoposide. This paper reviews the long term impact of this policy in the global management of stage I non-seminoma.

Materials and Methods

Stage I non-seminoma patients treated by the AGCCG from 1978–2000 were reviewed. Details of the BEP regimen have been previously published [3]. The BOPq10 regimen consisted of Bleomycin 30mg days 1 and 10, Oncovin 2mg days 1 and 10 and Cisplatin 50mg/m2 days 1/2 and 10/11. CT scans were performed at 2–3, 10–12 and 18–24 months.

Results

From 1–78 to 12–83, 83 patients were entered into the surveillance study. Median follow-up was 125 months (range 4–196). Thirty patients (36 per cent) relapsed at a median of 7 months (2–87). One died of germ cell cancer at 18 months and one of heart failure at 57 months. Three patients developed a second germ cell primary at 21, 97 and 132 months, and one developed lymphoma at 36 months. From 1/86 to 6/2000, 148 patients received adjuvant chemotherapy (28 BEPx2 with one relapse, 46 BEPx1 with three relapses and 74 BOPq10 with two relapses, i.e. a total of 6 (4 per cent) relapsed, one (1 per cent) developed a second germ cell cancer and two patients died of germ cell cancer. During the adjuvant chemotherapy era, 151 patients were entered into surveillance based on patient preference or a less than 25 per cent risk of relapse. Median follow-up was 58 months (4–144). Forty patients (26.4 per cent) relapsed at a median of 5 months (2–19), and five died of germ cell cancer. One patient died of heart failure at 31 months, and two developed a second germ cell cancer. Overall, since the introduction of the policy of selective adjuvant chemotherapy, overall relapse rate was 46 of 299 (15 per cent). There have been no relapses after 24 months compared to 5 of 83 (6 per cent) in the unselected surveillance series.

Conclusion

In higher and intermediate relapse risk stage 1 non-seminoma patients, the use of adjuvant chemotherapy is safe and has a substantially lower risk of relapse than retroperitoneal lymphadenectomy. Given the high relapse risk and incidence of chemo-resistance after surveillance, there could be a case for more frequent usage of adjuvant treatment, particularly if the ability to improve prediction of relapse risk by PET scanning and laparoscopic sentinel node biopsy is confirmed.

References

1. Freedman LS, Parkinson MC, Jones WG et al. Histopathology in the prediction of relapse of patients with stage I testicular teratoma treated by orchidectomy alone. *Lancet* 1987;2:294–8
2. Boshoff C, Begent RH, Oliver RT et al. Secondary tumours following etoposide containing therapy for germ cell cancer. *Ann Oncol* 1995;6:35–40
3. Oliver RT, Dhaliwal HS, Hope-Stone HF, Blandy JP. Short-course etoposide, bleomycin and cisplatin in the treatment of metastatic germ cell tumours. Appraisal of its potential as adjuvant chemotherapy for stage I testis tumours. *Br J Urol* 1988;61: 53–8

Section 8

Practice Guidelines

60. Radiation Risk in the Follow-up of Early Stage Germ Cell Tumours and Newer Imaging Modalities

S. Swift

St James's and Cookridge Hospitals, Leeds, UK

Ionising radiation from diagnostic medical investigations is a major source of man-made radiation and adds approximately one sixth to the population dose from background radiation. The use of such examinations, however, is an accepted part of current medical practice and is justified in terms of the clear clinical benefits of the test outweighing the radiation risk. Justification is central to new legislation, the Ionising Radiation (Medical Exposures) Regulations that came into force in May 2001 in the UK, which define the responsibilities of anyone referring patients for investigation or treatment involving ionising radiation. Exposure of a patient to ionising radiation must be clinically justified, and such exposure in the absence of good clinical indication will be illegal and those responsible may be held criminally liable [1]. It will also be an offence for anyone who is not an authorised referrer to sign a request card. The task of justifying each exposure falls to the 'practitioner' i.e. the radiologist, however it is the responsibility of the referrer to provide the clinical information that the practitioner needs in order to justify the exposure. These regulations are in effect enshrining in law the previously existing requirements of good practice, the 'ALARA' principal (As Low As Reasonably Achievable).

One way of keeping radiation dose as low as possible is not to perform unnecessary examinations. Does the patient need imaging? When an investigation is required, the appropriate imaging modality should be selected. If there is a choice of examinations, select the modality most likely to solve the clinical problem and if it is one which involves ionising radiation, factors including collimation, technical parameters e.g. mAs and kV, and the use of modern equipment such as digital radiography where available, should be considered.

We strive to keep doses as low as reasonably achievable to minimise the effects of radiation. Stochastic effects are random and include cancer induction and genetic defects. The probability of a stochastic effect depends on the total radiation dose received but the severity is independent of dose and there is no threshold dose below which such effects do not occur. Deterministic effects are non-random, they are certain to occur if sufficient radiation dose is received, the severity depends on the dose, dose rate and fractionation and there is a threshold dose. Examples of deterministic effects are skin changes and cataracts.

To describe the risk of radiation in a quantitative manner weighting factors are involved to take account of different types of radiation, which have different biological effectiveness, and the different tissues, which have different susceptibility to radiation, involved an the exposure. For example the gonads are more susceptible than lung, which is more so than breast which is more so than skin etc. The effective dose for a radiological examination is the weighted sum of the doses to a number of body tissues and provides a single dose estimate related to total radiation risk. Effective doses are expressed in milli-sieverts (mSv). Examples of typical effective doses for chest X-ray (CXR) and Computed Tomography (CT) are as follow [2]:

CXR – 0.2 mSv
CT Chest – 8 mSv, i.e. 400 CXRs
CT Abdomen or Pelvis – 10 mSv, i.e. 500 CXRs

To keep these doses in perspective, the average UK background radiation is 2.2 mSv per year (varying from 1.5 to 7.5 mSv across the country). If we consider radiation doses from radiological procedures in these terms, a CT of the chest is approximately equivalent to 3.6 years of natural background radiation, a CT of the abdomen or pelvis 4.5 years.

The current risk estimate published by the International Commission on Radiological Protection (ICRP) suggests a total cancer risk of 3 – 4 in 100,000 per mSv. The risk of a serious genetic defect is estimated to be about 1 in 100,000 per mSv when considering the next two generations.

What are the implications of knowing the radiation dose and hence risks involved in such diagnostic radiological examinations and what are the implications for our clinical practice?

Germ cell tumours (GCTs) are primarily a disease of young men. They are highly chemo- and radio-sensitive and with current advances in therapy have an excellent prognosis particularly for early stage disease. These men are likely to survive the 12 to 25 years it takes for a secondary solid tumour such as a sarcoma or breast cancer, or a leukaemia or lymphoma to occur as a consequence of radiation exposure. We do not want to cure them of one malignancy only to put them at risk of developing another.

Once a histological diagnosis of a GCT has been made, formal radiological staging is required. The Royal Marsden Hospital staging system, which takes into account both tumour site and bulk, is used in the UK and Europe, and has been adopted by the EORTC [Table 60.1]. CT has been the workhorse of oncological imaging and is the most widely used imaging modality for staging testicular tumours. Nodal enlargement is the main criterion for assessing metastatic disease and knowledge of patterns of disease spread helps interpretation of equivocal findings. Lymphatic drainage from right-sided GCTs is primarily to the inter-aorticocaval, pre- and para-caval nodes between L1 and L3, whereas left sided tumours drain to the pre- and para-aortic groups just below the left renal vascular pedicle [3]. Crossover does occur, particularly with right-sided tumours, but only subsequent to bulky ipsilateral disease [3]. Pelvic nodal disease is uncommon in the absence of identifiable risk factors. These include bulky retroperitoneal disease (over 5 cm) where there is consequent retrograde spread down lymphatic channels into the iliac chains, past history of maldescent, orchidopexy or other scrotal surgery, or invasion of tumour through the tunica vaginalis [4]. There are always exceptions to the rules and occasionally pelvic lymphadenopathy is found without such risk factors, hence the pelvis should be examined at initial staging.

Seminomas metastasise in a relatively predictable fashion via lymphatic channels to contiguous nodal groups. Non seminomatous germ cell tumours (NSGCTs) have a more variable, haematogenous route of spread. Supradiaphragmatic disease in seminomas tends to be near contiguous spread from the retroperitoneum through the retrocrural groups and into the posterior mediastinum where the perioesophageal and subcarinal nodes are most frequently involved. Pulmonary metastases without such adenopathy are rare [5]. NSGCTs have a more random pattern of nodal involvement in the thorax and pulmonary metastases in the absence of any lymphadenopathy in the retroperitoneum or mediastinum is well recognized [5].

Table 60.1: The Royal Marsden Hospital Staging Classification for Testicular Germ Cell Tumours.

Stage	Definition
I	No evidence of metastases
IM	Rising serum markers with no other evidence of metastases
II	Abdominal node metastases
A	< 2 cm in diameter
B	2–5 cm in diameter
C	> 5 cm in diameter
III	Supradiaphragmatic node metastases
M	Mediastinal
N	Supraclavicular cervical axillary
0	No abdominal node metastases
ABC	Node size defined as in Stage II
IV	Extralymphatic metastases
	Lung:
L1	< 3 metastases
L2	> 3 metastases all < 2 cm in diameter
L3	> 3 metastases, one or more > 2 cm in diameter
H+	Liver metastases
Br+	Brain metastases
Bo+	Bone metastases

How Can We Use This Knowledge of Likely Pattern of Disease?

The thorax, abdomen and pelvis need to be imaged at initial staging. Routine scanning of the pelvis at follow up, however, is contentious and there is evidence in the radiological literature to support pelvic surveillance only in those men with a known risk factor for pelvic disease [4,6]. In addition omission of the pelvic CT would significantly reduce the radiation dose to the patient. The potential cost of omitting pelvic surveillance in such men is the risk of delayed detection of pelvic relapse. This is particularly pertinent when there have been reports of increased incidence of pelvic relapse in men with seminoma since the introduction of para-aortic radiotherapy alone rather than the para-aortic and ipsilateral pelvic field [7]. It may be that we are going to have to accept this as a trade off. Whilst it is desirable to detect disease as early as possible when the bulk is small in order to allow more treatment options, the cumulative radiation risk from repeated CT surveillance must be taken into account.

The difference in behaviour between seminomas and NSGCTs above the diaphragm also has implications for thoracic imaging in surveillance. Studies suggest that the frequent, variable and unpredictable nature of supradiaphragmatic disease in NSGCTs warrants CT of the thorax both at staging and at follow-up. Interval CXRs, however, are unnecessary in patients undergoing regular CT assessment, as there is low additional information yield from these examinations and they have limited impact on patient management. Conversely CXR alone probably is sufficient for thoracic surveillance in men with pure seminoma where there is a low pre-test probability of intrathoracic metastases i.e. negative CT abdomen and negative serum tumour markers, and CT of the thorax can then be avoided [8].

Which Imaging Modality Should We Use?

CT is currently the most widely used imaging modality in oncological radiology for initial staging of cancer, monitoring response to therapy, assessing development of complications and suspected disease relapse. It is now a widely available tool, and the images produced in such studies are usually of high quality and reproducible. Its use is rising, and the radiation dose from CT now contributes approximately half the collective dose from all radiological examinations [2]. There have also been dramatic advances in CT technology in recent years with a resultant broadening of applications. The development of spiral and now multislice CT has allowed an increase in body coverage for markedly reduced time penalty, but these advances have also brought with them the potential for increased radiation dose to patients. This aspect of cumulative dose is particularly relevant to young patients with potentially curable tumours such as the GCTs and lymphomas [9].

What Are the Alternatives?

Ultrasound (US) involves no ionising radiation. It is widely available and relatively cheap. It is excellent for assessment of parenchymal solid organ disease and upper abdominal adenopathy. However it is an operator dependent modality, not all patient are optimal US candidates for reasons of body habitus and the retroperitoneum cannot be reliably fully assessed. This makes it an inadequate tool for formal staging patients with GCTs.

Magnetic Resonance Imaging (MRI) does not involve ionising radiation and is becoming increasingly available. It is now established as the imaging modality of choice for staging certain pelvic cancers such as carcinoma of the cervix and prostate where it is used for both local tumour staging but also for assessing the retroperitoneum for nodal metastases (Figs 60.1, 60.2). There is evidence in the radiological literature which indicates that MRI is as accurate as CT for detecting nodal disease and it has also been shown to have an appropriate and cost effective role in the management of pelvic malignancy [10,11]. Continual improvements in MRI technology have allowed much shortened acquisition times for most sequences, and the current development of ultrasmall super-paramagnetic iron oxide lymphangiographic contrast agents may give radiologists an alternative to size as the only criterion for nodal involvement. These agents may have the potential to allow us to detect disease in non-enlarged lymph nodes.

MRI is currently limited in its assessment of the pulmonary parenchyma. This is an important short coming in staging and follow-up of GCTs, however a spiral CT of the chest combined with MRI of the abdomen and pelvis would clearly be a huge step forward in reducing radiation dose in this patient group.

Positron Emission Tomography (PET) is a functional imaging technique utilising glucose metabolism by active tissue via the labelled glucose analogue 18-fluoro-2-deoxyglucose (FDG). There are reports, albeit some conflicting, suggesting FDG-PET has the potential to improve staging, detection of relapse and management of residual masses in GCTs. A continual challenge for imaging is to differentiate active from inactive disease in residual masses, but, as yet, no technique has proved entirely reliable in this regard. In practice a common approach is serial monitoring, and in the absence of clinical parameters suggestive of relapse, lesions remaining unchanged over a year are considered inactive. It was hoped that the signal characteristics from

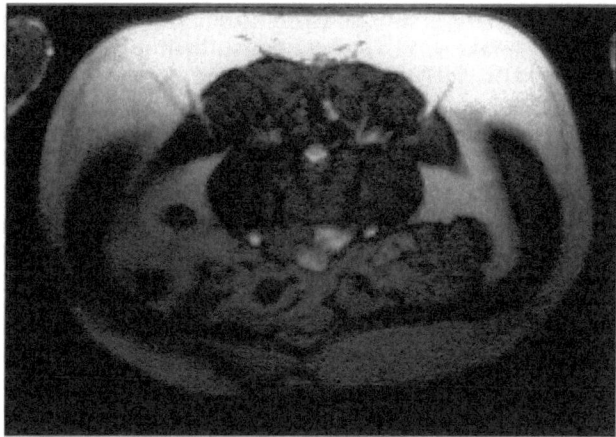

Figure 60.1: MRI of retropritoneal lymph nodes

Axial FISP sequence at the level of the bifurcation showing left sided intermediate signal intensity nodes. The aorta and IVC are high signal intensity on this sequence.

the differing MRI sequences would be able to give information regarding tumour activity, but there is much debate over this. There is some agreement from studies on residual masses in lymphoma that the demonstration of high signal intensity on T2

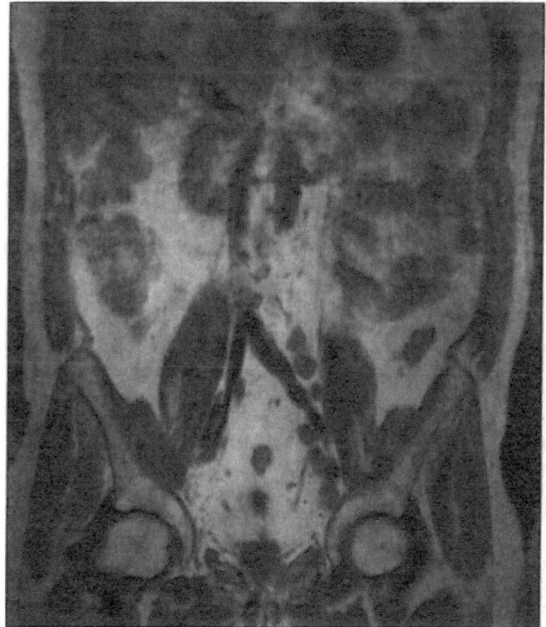

Figure 60.2: MRI of pelvic lymph nodes

Coronal TI weighted image demonstrsating a chain of abnormally enlarged nodes in the left common and external iliac chains.

weighted sequences correlates with poorer outcome [12]. A study from Europe found significantly higher uptake of FDG in seminoma than in NSGCTs. It also described excellent results for FDG-PET in the assessment of seminomatous residual masses, provided the study was performed at least two weeks after the completion of chemotherapy to avoid false positive uptake in inflammatory tissues. Their results showed a PET negative seminomatous residual mass had a 90 per cent probability of containing necrosis or fibrosis only, whereas the probability of residual tumour for a positive PET scan was approximately 80 per cent [13]. These are clearly exciting and promising results, particularly as the alternatives are monitoring with CT and its consequent radiation burden, or surgical excision. The main draw back to PET scanning is that it is an expensive and limited resource in the UK, as relatively few clinical PET scanners are available. PET scanning also is not without radiation dose, a PET scan of the head having an effective dose of 5 mSv.

What Next?

We need to tailor the imaging to the patient, the disease process and the information requirement. The wider use of MRI and FDG-PET in staging and follow-up in oncological radiology needs to be considered and more studies are required to look at their accuracy in a wider range of malignancies. These modalities however, will probably remain a relatively limited resource, and where there is no access to them, appropriate CT protocols should be applied. To do this, the responsibility will be placed on the referring clinician to supply the relevant and necessary clinical details to allow the radiologists to perform a more selective study where possible. This will enable us to avoid unnecessary radiation exposure and reduce cumulative radiation dose, which will ultimately benefit the patient.

References

1. http:www.legislation.hmso.gov.uk/si/si2000/20001059.htm
2. Royal College of Radiologists. *Making the best use of a Department of Clinical Radiology: Guidelines for Doctors.* 4th ed. London: Royal College of Radiologists, 1998
3. Dixon AK, Ellis M, Sikora K. Computed Tomography of Testicular Tumours: Distribution of Abdominal Lymphadenopathy. *Clin Radiol* 1986;37:519–523
4. White PM, Howard GCW, Best JJK, Wright AR. The Role of Computed Tomographic Examination of the Pelvis in the Management of Testicular Germ Cell Tumours. *Clin Radiol* 1997;52:124–129
5. Wood A, Robson N, Tung K, Mead G. Patterns of Supradiaphragmatic Metastases in Germ Cell Tumours. *Clin Radiol* 1996;51:273–276
6. Wright AR, White PM. Testicular Cancer – who needs surveillance pelvic CT? *Clin Radiol* 1999;54:78
7. Taylor MB, Carrington BM, Livsey JE, Logue JP. The Effect of Radiotherapy Treatment Changes on Sites of Relapse in Stage I Testicular Seminoma. *Clin Radiol* 2001;56:116–119
8. White PM, Adamson DJA, Howard GCW, Wright AR. Imaging of the thorax in the Management of Germ Cell Testicular Tumours. *Clin Radiol* 1999;54:207–211
9. Rehani MM, Berry M. Radiation doses in computed tomography. *Br Med J* 2000;342: 593–594
10. Subak LL, Hricak H, Powell CB, Azizi L, Stern JL. Cervical Carcinoma: Computed Tomography and Magnetic Resonance Imaging for Preoperative Staging. *Obstet Gynecol* 1995;86:43–50
11. Hricak H, Powell CB, Kyle KY et al: Invasive cervical carcinoma: role of MR imaging in pre-treatment work-up – cost minimisation and diagnostic efficacy analysis. *Radiology* 1996;198:403–409
12. Hill M, Cunningham D, MacVicar D. The Role of Magnetic Resonance Imaging in Predicting Relapse in Residual Masses after Treatment of lymphoma. *J Clin Oncol* 1993;11:2273–2278
13. Cremerius U, Effert PJ, Adam G et al. FDG PET for Detection and Therapy Control of Metastatic Germ Cell Tumor. *J Nucl Med* 1998;39:815–822

61. FDG PET Scanning in Germ Cell Tumours

R.A. Huddart, S.F. Hain

The Royal Marsden Hospital and. The Institute of Cancer Research, Sutton, Surrey, SM2 5PT, UK

Introduction

Cross sectional imaging plays a key role (in combination with tumour markers) in the management of men presenting with testicular germ cell tumours (TGCT). The most commonly used imaging modality is computerised tomography (CT) scanning. CT is routinely used in the initial staging of patients, in assessment of disease response and detection of relapse. CT, however, suffers from a number of limitations mainly due to its reliance on structural abnormalities to identify disease. This means CT cannot, for instance, detect disease in 'normal sized lymph nodes' or tell whether there is active tumour in residual masses after chemotherapy. These difficulties limit the accuracy of CT in assessing TGCT. A prime example of this is the knowledge that approximately 25 per cent of patients will have normal sized para-aortic nodes containing tumour and a proportion patients with enlarged nodes will not [1, 2].

In an effort to improve the sensitivity and specificity of disease detection, attention has turned to functional imaging modalities. Foremost amongst these has been the study of [18]Fluoro-deoxy glucose Positron Emission Tomography (FDG PET). Experience of this modality in TGCT has been limited. This review aims to provide an assessment of the current status of knowledge and highlight areas requiring further study.

PET Imaging with FDG

Proton rich isotopes undergo radioactive decay in which protons convert into neutrons with emission of positrons. Positrons are inherently unstable and rapidly undergo an annihilation reaction with electrons. The energy released from this reaction is emitted as two 511 KeV photons released at 180° relative to each other. This can be detected by a ring detector that can integrate the radiation emitted to produce an image of isotope distribution.

The most commonly used isotope is [18]Fluorine, substituted into deoxyglucose to make [18]FDG. FDG is taken into cells in a similar way to glucose, but because it is not metabolised, it accumulates in metabolically active tissues (Figure 61.1). FDG PET uses differences in glucose metabolism between tumour cells and normal tissues to identify tumour tissue independent of its size. These differences include increases in the uptake of glucose related to the increase of glucose transporters on the cell surface (GLUT 1–5; SGLT1), increased concentration and activity of hexokinases and the decreased production of the phosphorylase enzymes.

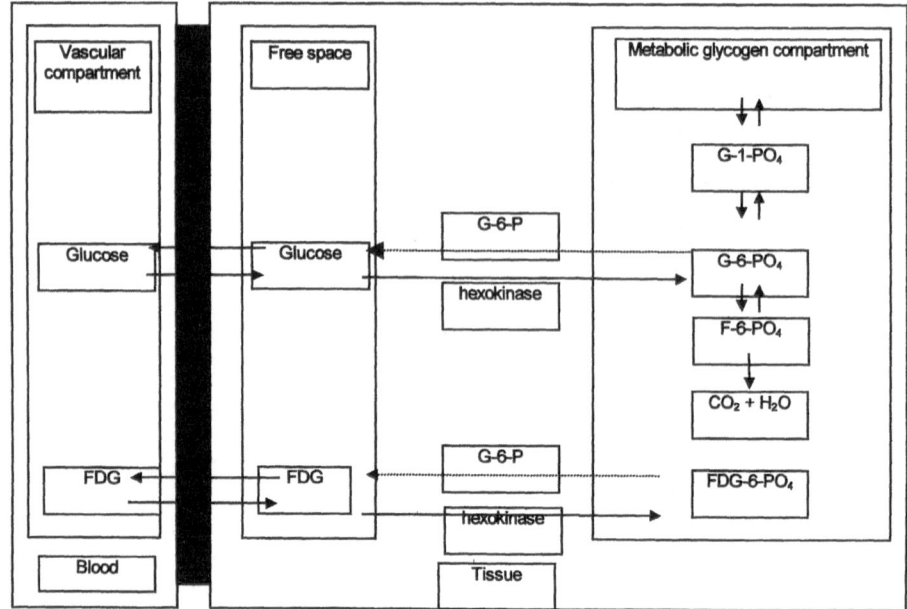

Figure 61.1: The metabolism of glucose and ^{18}Fluorodeoxyglucose (FDG).

The role of FDG PET is currently being evaluated for the localisation and staging of tumours, (e.g. in lung cancer [3–5]). For many tumours including breast cancer [6, 7], melanoma [8, 9], carcinoma of the large bowel [10, 11], carcinoma of the oesophagus [12] and soft tissue sarcomas [13–16], more disease is identified than at CT staging.

There is also the potential for the grading and monitoring of the treatment response [17] and the detection of viable tumour in areas of previously treated disease (e.g. in lymphoma and in rectal carcinoma), which may not be possible with conventional imaging techniques.

Uptake of FDG in GCT

Available data confirm that FDG is preferentially taken up into active GCT. A number of investigators have quantified this in terms of standard uptake values (SUV). SUVs quantify the amount of activity in a defined volume (pixel) and allow comparison of normal and pathological tissue. Results of some of these studies are summarised in Table 61.1. Both seminomas and non-seminomatous germ cell tumours (NSGCT) concentrate FDG with mean SUVs between 4.4–9.2 with, in one study, uptake being greater in seminoma than non-seminoma [18]. Stephens et al. [19] demonstrated that uptake in active tumour was significantly greater than in masses containing either necrotic tissue or differentiated teratoma (TD). The relative lack of uptake in residual masses containing TD has been noted in a number of series.

Table 61.1: Summary of studies investigating standard uptake values (SUV) in TGCT

Author	Mean Standard uptake value (range)			
	Seminoma	NSGCT	Teratoma differentiated	Necrosis/ fibrosis
Wilson et al 1995 [24]	7.3 (5.5–9.1)	6.0 (1.9–9.1)	–	–
Stephens et al 1996 [17]	–	8.82 (3.2–12.7)	3.07 (1.26–4.8)	2.86 (2.16–5.01)
Cremerius et al 1998 [16]	9.2 (7.l2–13.5)	4.4 (3.4–7)	–	–

NSGCT - Non seminomatous germ cell tumour
SUV = Tissue concentration (NBq/g) x Patient weight/injected dose (MBQ)

Application of PET to Clinical Practice

The increasing clinical availability of commercial PET scanning has led to increasing interest in the application of this technology to the management of patients with TGCT. A number of areas where PET may have an impact on management of patients can be envisaged. Possible roles are highlighted in Table 61.2.

Relapsed Disease

The outcome of patients with relapsed disease remains unsatisfactory. The management of such patients involves the use of intensive salvage chemotherapy and the ability to apply local treatment can be important part of this strategy. Our experience at the Royal Marsden has identified two clinical scenarios where information from PET scanning has been useful. The first is in the clinical situation where the tumour markers are rising and CT is either negative or shows stable disease. PET can often identify the site of disease and direct local treatment (Figure 61.2). The second scenario is where localised disease is identified on CT and surgery is being considered. PET can help to exclude the presence of active disease at other sites (Figure 61.3). We have performed a review of patients referred to St Thomas's Hospital for assessment of disease at time of relapse [20]. A total of 41 patients who had had PET scans were identified. Twenty-eight scans were positive including 12 with negative CT scans and 27 of these were proven to be true positives. The single false positive was an amoebic abscess. Thirteen patients had negative scans, seven of which proved to be correct. There were six false negatives. In two patients, PET missed a focus of active tumour in a large residual mass. Three patients had repeat PET scans and in all three, PET was the first modality to identify the site of disease. These results equate to a sensitivity of 71 per cent and specificity of 83 per cent. Analysis of the results

Table 61.2: Possible roles for FDG PET in TGCT

- Detection of subclinical disease in CS Stage I disease
- Confirmation of disease in patients with equivocal nodes
- Staging disease extent at presentation
- Response to treatment
- Staging disease extent at relapse
- Identification of disease site in patients with rising markers and negative CT
- Determination of patients with active disease/TD in residual masses

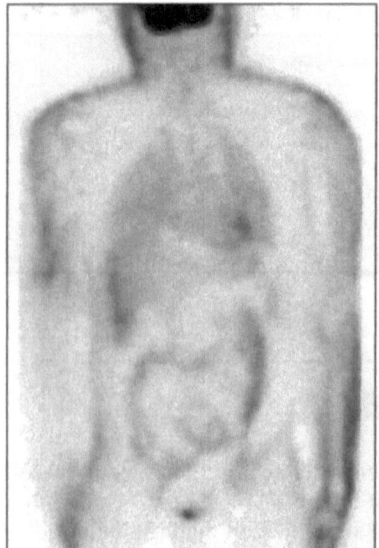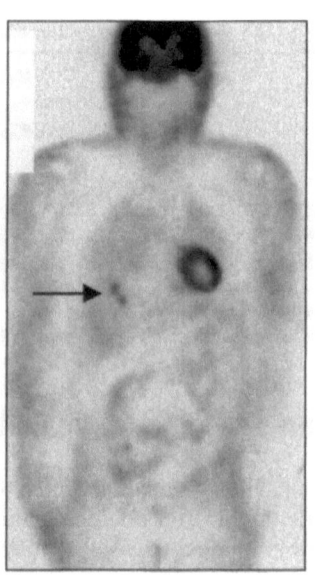

a   b

Figure 61.2: A patient with raised markers and normal CT had a normal PET scan (**a**). The markers continued to rise, the CT remained normal and the follow-up PET scan was the first imaging technology to identify the site of the disease (**b**, arrow). (Hain et al *BJC* 2000 ;83:863–869 with permission).

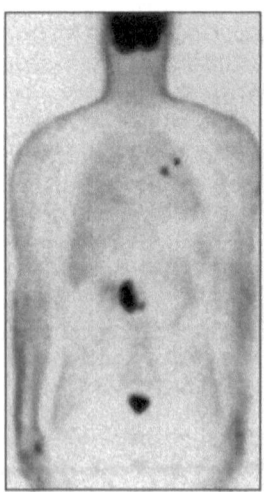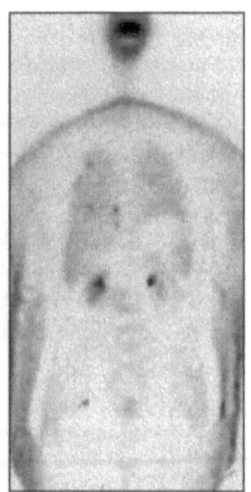

Figure 61.3: FDG-PET scan in a patient with a right para-aortic residual mass on CT and raised markers. He was being considered for laparotomy as definitive treatment if this was the only site of disease. CT of the abdomen and chest was otherwise normal although he previously had lung metastases. He was referred for a PET scan to exclude other sites of disease and thereby enable surgery. The images show increased uptake in the known mass as well as disease in the lungs and mediastinum. All sites were malignant. This directly altered the patient's management.

indicated that PET influenced patient management in 57 per cent of cases. This suggests that PET has promise in this area, although these results need confirmation by other groups. Further data on the benefits of PET, particularly with respect to long-term outcome, should be collected, ideally in a prospective manner or in the context of well designed clinical studies.

Assessment of Residual Masses

Following chemotherapy, residual masses frequently remain. Often (especially in seminoma), these masses consist of necrotic and/or fibrotic material only, but they may harbour active TGCT and, in NSGCTs, differentiated teratoma. Standard management in non-seminoma patients is to undertake surgical resection. Several groups have investigated whether PET can help differentiate between active TGCT, TD and necrosis. The experience of most workers is that TD TGCT (usually) does not take up FDG and thus FDG PET cannot distinguish reliably between TD and fibrotic masses. Its role in deciding who should undergo post chemotherapy resection is therefore likely to be limited. It has been suggested in one study that differentiated TGCT has beencan be successfully distinguished from fibrosis and necrosis in PET scans using kinetic rate constants, an interesting and important observation that needs further evaluation. [21].

The experience of St Thomas's PET centre suggests that PET can identify residual active NSGCT with a higher sensitivity and specificity than CT (Figure 61.4), although small foci of disease can be missed. Overall the positive predictive value for PET was 96 per cent compared to 56 per cent for CT scanning [20].

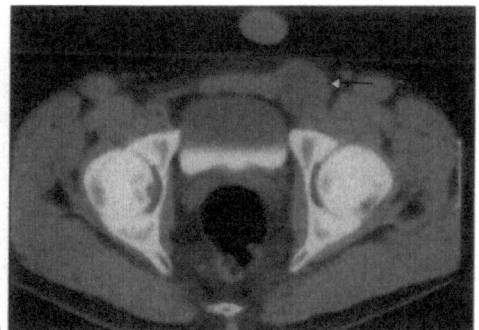
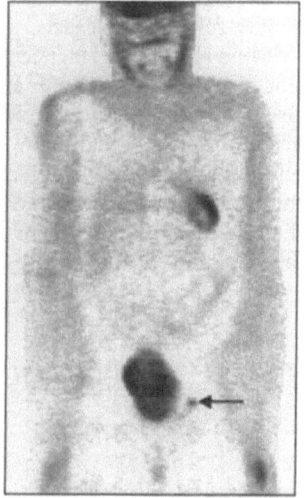
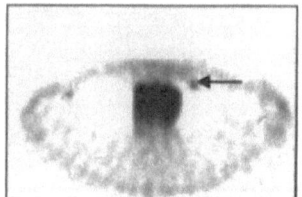

Figure 61.4: (a) A CT scan of the groin in a patient following chemotherapy and retroperitoneal radiotherapy for seminoma. The CT shows a node in the left groin (arrow) but is unable to distinguish viable tumour from fibrosis. (b) TheFDG-PET scan in the same patient clearly showing 18FDG accumulation in the left groin node (arrow). Biopsy showed this mass to contain seminoma. (Hain et al *BJC* 2000;83:863–869 with permission).

Other groups have reproduced this experience, showing that PET was more accurate than CT (86 per cent v 59 per cent) [22]. Results of available studies are summarised in Table 61.3. The value of this observation is likely to be limited in routine practice if surgical excision is planned to remove possible TD. However, PET could play a role in patients with widespread residual abnormalities where complete excision is not feasible, or if for other reasons, routine surgery is not planned. In such circumstances, PET may add security to an observation policy or direct surgical intervention to areas most likely to contain disease.

The potential for PET to play a role in the assessment of post chemotherapy residual masses in seminoma may be greater. These are common and there has been debate as to the optimum management. Most such masses consist of fibrotic/necrotic tissue but some can harbour active tumour, which can lead to disease relapse. Surgery in these circumstances is hazardous and is not advised. Some groups have practised routine postoperative radiotherapy but a review of MRC experience suggested this produced little benefit [23]. Identification of active disease sites and more targeted radiotherapy may be a better approach. The success of PET in this area has been mixed. Ganjoo et al. [24] scanned 29 patients with seminoma after chemotherapy. PET missed the only patient with active disease and produced one false positive result. However, in the study of Cremerius et al. [18], PET successfully identified all five patients with active disease. De Santis et al. reported at the Germ Cell Tumour Conference the results of a large well conducted Austrian study ("SEMPET"), in which PET successfully identified eight of nine patients with active residual disease. A small volume of disease, in a lymph node less that 2 cm in size, was missed in one patient. The authors have concluded that PET is a helpful tool to investigate residual masses in seminoma especially when they are over 3 cm in diameter. The one criticism of this study is the high level of positive residual masses probably due to the inclusion of patients with relapsed disease.

Two lessons have been learned from these studies. Firstly, false-positive results can occur. For instance, Nuutinen et al. [25] found that three of their positive scan results were false positives due to inflammatory processes either in the residual a masses or in adjacent tissues (e.g. due to pneumonitis). Other investigators report similar experiences, although this problem may be reduced if if sufficient interval from is left between the end of treatment and undertaking the scan. Thus false positives were not a major problem in the Austrian study when there was a minimum 4 week interval from the end of treatment. The second major lesson learnt is the importance of

Table 61.3: Summary of results of studies investigating PET following chemotherpy for residual masses or relapse disease

Author	Group	n	Sensitivity	Specificity	Accuracy of PET	Accuracy of CT
Nuutinen	Post chemotherapy	15	86%	77%	80%	
De Santis	Seminoma post chemotherapy	37	89%	100%		
Gunjoo	Post chemotherapy seminoma	29	0/1	96%		
Harns	Post chemotherapy	18	71%	90%		
Cremerius	Post chemotherapy					
	Seminoma	19	100	86%	90%	79%
	Non Seminoma	21	67%	92%	81%	52%
Hain	Residual masses	47	88%	95%	91%	
Hain	Raised markers	23	71%	83%	74%	

leaving such an interval. Undertaking a PET scan too soon after chemotherapy can also increase the risk of obtaining a false negative results. This was best documented by Cremerius et al. [18], who showed that the sensitivity of PET for residual disease fell from 78 per cent to 44 per cent if the scan was performed within 2 weeks of chemotherapy.

Further investigations into the details of scanning protocols may improve sensitivity. Different tumour types are known to have varying uptakes depending on the grade of malignancy and possibly the timing of the scan after injection of FDG. Patients are currently scanned at 60 minutes post injection and SUV measured at 90 minutes. In soft tissue tumours, FDG uptake reaches a peak at about 1 hour in benign tumours and then rapidly decreases, whereas a plateau of FDG uptake is not seen until 4–6 hours post injection for malignant tumours [16]. This indicates that a later scanning time provides better differentiation between benign and malignant soft tissue lesions. This has also been seen in breast cancer at 3 hours [26]. Further study of time to peak of FDG uptake in testicular cancer may lead to even better differentiation between benign and malignant disease. Recently, scanning times of 2 hours for half body FDG scans have been proposed to demonstrate metastases [27].

Staging of Disease

Sensitivity and specificity data of PET in the staging of disease are summarised in Table 61.4. In patients with established metastatic disease, it is unlikely that PET will have a routine role, although it may aid clinicians in difficult cases. Experience at the St Thomas's PET centre [28] has shown that PET will show that disease is more extensive than visualised on CT in a proportion of patients (4 out of 10 with positive scans). However, most patients with metastatic TGCT are treated with chemotherapy, the selection of which is based more on prognostic factors than on anatomical site [29]. Thus PET is only likely to affect treatment if unsuspected visceral metastases are detected, which occurred in one patient in the study of Hain et al [28]. An exception to this may be patients with seminoma and enlarged retroperitoneal nodes. For patients with smaller volume disease radiotherapy is usually advocated. Approximately 10–20 per cent will experience an out of field relapse and it is possible that PET could add additional security in the decision to use radiotherapy rather than chemotherapy. There are currently no data on this issue to guide practice.

PET may be useful in determining the nature of equivocal retroperitoneal lymph nodes. Series of patients undergoing retroperitoneal lymph node dissection have shown that a proportion of lymph nodes (25 per cent or more) considered pathological by CT criteria may be benign [1, 2]. Few data pertain to this area but in the series of Hain et al [20], 12 patients with suspicious CT scans had negative PET

Table 61.4: Summary of studies investigating the diagnostic accuracy of PET scanning

Author	Diagnostic group	n	Sensitivity	Specificity
Albers	Stage I/II	37	70%	100%
Hain	Metastatic disease at diagnosis	31	67–83%	100%
LOassen	Stage I	40	70%	100%
Cremerius	Any at diagnosis	50	87%	94%

scans. Seven patients received treatment so are difficult to evaluate, but there was no change on treatment. In two cases, biopsy demonstrated disease, proving the PET to be a false negative, but the three remaining patients had no disease progression on observation. Albers et al. [30] studied 12 patients with stage II seminoma (n = 3) and NSGCT (n = 9). Pathological examination of the nodes showed that in six of these patients (50 per cent), no disease was present. All these nodes were negative on PET supporting a role for PET in this area. However one of the limitations of PET was illustrated in that a large (4.8cm) lymph node containing TD did not take up FDG. Further work is required in this area but PET could have a role in preventing inappropriate treatment.

Approximately 30 per cent of clinical stage I patients (CSI) NSGCT patients and 20 per cent of CSI seminoma patients will relapse on surveillance. Although salvage treatment is very successful, the process of surveillance is associated with considerable organisational and financial implications for the treating centre and psychological morbidity for patients. For these reasons, surgical staging or adjuvant treatment have been advocated to either improve diagnostic accuracy or prevent relapse. Both approaches lead to significant over treatment of patients, which is especially important as appreciation is growing of the long-term risks, particularly of chemotherapy and radiotherapy.

The issue as to whether PET can detect subclinical disease in this situation and improve diagnostic accuracy has been tested in two studies to date. Lassen et al [31] undertook PET scans in 40 patients with CSI NSGCTs. Patients then underwent surveillance and 10 (25 per cent) relapsed, seven of which had had positive PET scans, suggesting that PET has a sensitivity of 70 per cent for occult disease in this setting. No false positive scans where found. Similar findings were observed in the study of Albers et al described above. In this study, 15 patients with CSI NSGCT and 10 patients with CSI seminoma underwent PET scanning. Six NSGCT patients with negative CT scans had pathologically involved lymph nodes. PET scan identified four of these patients. The two false negatives were in patients with involved nodes measuring less than 0.5cm. The sensitivity of PET in this study was thus 66 per cent. The inability of PET to detect very small lymph nodes involved with TGCT led to the authors to question the value of PET in this scenario. Nevertheless, even with a sensitivity at this level, the effect on clinical management of stage I disease may be considerable. As illustrated in Table 61.5, PET with a sensitivity as low as 50 per cent both reduces the amount of chemotherapy administered and ensures that it is targeted at patients who definitely require it. However, both studies were relatively small and the confidence intervals of the derived sensitivity are wide. To address these issues, a multi-centre study to investigate PET in high risk stage I NSGCT will be launched in the UK in 2001. This study (TE22), which will be the largest study to investigate PET in TGCT. It is organised by the MRC clinical trials office and supported by the Cancer Research Campaign and aims to recruit 135 patients and investigate the negative predictive value of PET scanning with a high degree of precision. Following a PET scan, patients with evidence of disease will undergo chemotherapy (or other treatment as defined by their clinician) whilst patients with a negative scan will undergo surveillance. This study should, if successful, answer clearly whether PET has a role in this setting. Any interested clinicians can obtain more details from MRC clinical trials website (www.mrc.ctu.ac.uk) or the MRC clinical trials unit (sharon.naylor@ctu.mrc.ac.uk).

Surprisingly, given the equivalent or high SUV's of seminoma, the question of a role in clinical stage I seminoma has been addressed in only one study, in which 21 patients had PET scans but no additional disease was revealed [32]. However, it is

Table 61.5: Theoretical effect of PET scanning relapses and chemotherapy in stage I NSGCT

Group	No. in group	No. of relapses	Courses of BEP/group	Total chemotherapy
Adjuvent BEP high risk	100	0	100	75
Surveillance low risk	50	7.5	22.5	122.5
PET 70% sensitivity:				57
Scan + ve	18	0	36	
Scan – ve	82	7	21	
PET 50% sensitivity:				62
Scan + ve	13	0	26	
Scan – ve	87	12	36	
High risk patients scanned (PET 70% sensitivity):				39*
Scan + ve	12	0	24	
Scan – ve	38	5	15	
(+ surveilance for low risk)	(50)	(7.5)	(22.5)	(Total for group 61.5)

* for 50 patients

The outcome of treating 100 patients in terms of chemotherapy used and relapse associated with different current treatment policies is shown if PET scanning was to be used in different sensitivities. A 25% overall risk of relapse in the surveillance group with 15% for low risk patients and 35% for high risk is assumed. It is also assumed patients with occult disease are to be treated with 2 cycles of BEP as per current high risk management and patients relapsing from surveillance will receive 3 cycles of BEP. Treatment of post chemotherapy relapses is not included (assumed same in all groups), (specificity is assumed close to 100%).

unclear whether this was due to lack of sensitivity or lack of disease. The slower and less defined relapse pattern may put into question the value of PET in this setting. Also, with a lower relapse rate, the diagnostic rate is likely to be lower. However given the excellent prognosis, the difficulties of surveillance and concerns over long term toxicity of adjuvant treatment, we believe this area deserves exploration.

Overview and Future Prospects

The current data on PET in TGCT are promising and suggest that FDG is taken up avidly into active TGCT and this uptake can be used to distinguish active tumour from normal tissues or fibrosis. In most studies, PET has a higher sensitivity and specificity than CT. A number of studies have suggested that PET may have a role in the management of TGCT in number of different settings. It should be noted that most of these studies have been small and often retrospective. The conclusions reached in these circumstances should be regarded as provisional and need to be confirmed by larger, well-designed prospective studies, in which the confidence limits of the parameters studied can be clearly defined. The recently reported Austrian study of post chemotherapy seminoma masses and the planned CRC/MRC study in stage I NSGCT should be seen as steps to obtain these data. Until such studies are completed, caution should be used before advocating wide spread adoption of this technology.

When using PET in TGCT, it is wise to consider the limitations of the technology. Assessment by PET of TD is especially difficult. Low grade uptake can occur risking the confusion between TD and active tumour but most often PET is negative so TD cannot be reliably distinguished from necrosis and fibrosis. PET has limited sensitivity and can miss small volume active tumour especially if within a large residual mass. PET is also unreliable within the first few weeks following chemotherapy and a gap of at least four weeks from the end of treatment should be left before undertaking evaluations.

In conclusion, FDG PET is a promising new tool in TGCT, particularly in the assessment of patients with negative CT staging, residual post chemotherapy masses and in relapsed disease. Further prospective studies are required to assess its value in patient management in these areas and to evaluate new applications such as assessing disease response.

References

1. Nichols C. Testicular cancer. *Curr Probl Cancer* 1998;22:187–274
2. Aass N, Fossa S, Ous S et al. Is routine primary retroperitoneal lymph node dissection still justified in patients with low stage non-seminomatous testicular cancer? *Br J Urol* 1990;65:385–90
3. Lewis P, Griffin S, Marsden P et al. Whole-body 18F-fluorodeoxyglucose positron emission tomography in preoperative evaluation of lung cancer. *Lancet* 1994;344:1265–6
4. Sazon DA, Santiago SM, Soo Hoo GW et al. Fluorodeoxyglucose-positron emission tomography in the detection and staging of lung cancer. *Am J Respir Crit Care Med* 1996;153:417–21
5. White P, Adams H, Crane M, Butchart E. Preoperative staging of carcinoma of the bronchus: Can computed tomographic scanning reliably identify stage III tumors? *Thorax* 1994;49:951–7
6. Avril N, Dose J, Janicke F et al. Assessment of axillary lymph node involvement in breast cancer patients with positron emission tomography using radiolabeled 2-(fluorine-18)- fluoro-2-deoxy-D-glucose. *J Natl Cancer Inst* 1996;88:1204–9
7. Utech CI, Young CS, Winter PF. Prospective evaluation of fluorine-18 fluorodeoxyclucose positron emission tomography in breast cancer for staging of the axilla related to surgery and immunocytochemistry. *Eur J Nucl Med* 1996;23:1588–93

8. Steinert HC, Huch Boni RA, Buck A et al. Malignant melanoma: staging with whole-body positron emission tomography and 2-[F-18]-fluoro-2-deoxy-D-glucose. *Radiology* 1995;195:705–9

9. Boni R, Boni RA, Steinert H et al. Staging of metastatic melanoma by whole-body positron emission tomography using 2-fluorine-18-fluoro-2-deoxy-D-glucose. *Br J Dermatol* 1995;132:556–62

10. Schiepers C, Penninckx F, De Vadder N et al. Contribution of PET in the diagnosis of recurrent colorectal cancer: comparison with conventional imaging. *Eur J Surg Oncol* 1995;21:517–22

11. Delbeke D, Vitola JV, Sandler MP et al. Staging recurrent metastatic colorectal carcinoma with PET. *J Nucl Med* 1997;38:1196–201

12. Flanagan FL, Dehdashti F, Siegel BA et al. Staging of esophageal cancer with 18F-fluorodeoxyglucose positron emission tomography. *Am J Roentgenol* 1997;168:417–24

13. Lucas JD, O'Doherty MJ, Wong JC et al. Evaluation of fluorodeoxyglucose positron emission tomography in the management of soft-tissue sarcomas. *J Bone Joint Surg Br* 1998;80:441–7

14. Eary JF, Conrad EU, Bruckner JD et al. Quantitative [F-18]fluorodeoxyglucose positron emission tomography in pretreatment and grading of sarcoma. *Clin Cancer Res* 1998;4:1215–20

15. Adler LP, Blair HF, Williams RP et al. Grading liposarcomas with PET using [18F]FDG. *J Comput Assist Tomogr* 1990;14:960–2

16. Lodge MA, Lucas JD, Marsden PK, Cronin BF, O'Doherty MJ, Smith MA. A PET study of 18FDG uptake in soft tissue masses. *Eur J Nucl Med* 1999;26:22–30

17. Romer W, Hanauske AR, Ziegler S et al. Positron emission tomography in non-Hodgkin's lymphoma: assessment of chemotherapy with fluorodeoxyglucose. *Blood* 1998;91:4464–71

18. Cremerius U, Effert PJ, Adam G et al. FDG PET for detection and therapy control of metastatic germ cell tumor. *J Nucl Med* 1998;39:815–22

19. Stephens A, Gonin R, Hutchins G, Einhorn L. Positron Emission Tomography Evaluation of Residual Radiographic Abnormalities in Postchemotherapy Germ Cell Tumor Patients. *J Clin Oncol* 1996;14:1637–41

20. Hain S, O'Doherty M, Timothy A, Leslie M, Harper P, Huddart R. Fluorodeoxyglucose positron emission tomography in the evaluation of germ cell tumours at relapse. *Brit J Cancer* 2000;83:863–9

21. Sugawara Y, Zasadny K, Grossman H, Francis I, Clarke M, Wahl R. Germ cell tumor: differentiation of viable tumor, mature teratoma, and necrotic tissue with FDG PET and kinetic modeling. *Radiology* 1999;211:249–56

22. Cremerius U, Bares R, Weis J et al. Fasting improves discrimination of grade 1 and atypical or malignant meningioma in FDG-PET. *J Nucl Med* 1997;38:26–30

23. Duchesne GM, Stenning SP, Aass N et al. Radiotherapy after chemotherapy for metastatic seminoma – a diminishing role. MRC Testicular Tumour Working Party. *Eur J Cancer* 1997;33:829–35

24. Ganjoo KN, Chan RJ, Sharma M, Einhorn LH. Positron emission tomography scans in the evaluation of postchemotherapy residual masses in patients with seminoma. *J Clin Oncol* 1999;17:3457–60

25. Nuutinen JM, Leskinen S, Elomaa I et al. Detection of residual tumours in postchemotherapy testicular cancer by FDG-PET. *Eur J Cancer* 1997;33:1234–41

26. Boerner AR, Weckesser M, Herzog H et al. Optimal scan time for fluorine-18 fluorodeoxyglucose positron emission tomography in breast cancer. *Eur J Nucl Med* 1999;26:226–30

27. Kubota K, Itoh M, Ozaki K et al. Advantage of delayed whole-body FDG-PET imaging for tumour detection. *Eur J Nucl Med* 2001;28:696–703

28. Hain S, O'Doherty M, Timothy A, Leslie M, Partridge S, Huddart R. Fluorodeoxyglucose (PET) in the initial staging of germ cell tumours. *Eur J Nucl Med* 2000;27:590–4

29. International Germ Cell Consensus Classification. International Germ Cell Consensus Classification: A prognostic factor-based staging system for metastatic germ cell cancers. *J Clin Oncol* 1997;15:594–603

30. Albers P, Bender H, Yilmaz H, Schoeneich G, Biersack H-J, Mueller S. Positron emission tomography in the clinical staging of patients with stage I and II testicular germ cell tumors. *Urology* 1998;53:808–11

31. Lassen U, Daugaard G, Rorth M, Eigtved A, Friberg L. Detection of metastatic disease with postron emission tomography negative non-seminomatous ger cell tumors (Abstract No. 1142). *Proc Am Soc Clin Oncol* 1997;16:321a

32. Muller-Mattheis V, Reinhardt M, Gerharz C et al. Positron emission tomography with (18 F)-2-fluoro-2-deoxy-D-glucose (18FDG-PET) in diagnosis of retroperitoneal lymph node metastases of testicular tumors. *Urology* 1998;37:609–20

33. Wilson CB, Young HE, Ott RJ et al. Imaging metastatic testicular germ cell tumours with 18FDG positron emission tomography: prospects for detection and management. *Eur J Nucl Med* 1995;22:508–13

34. Harns W, Bares R, Kamps H et al. Therapy control of metastatic testicular carcinoma with F18-DOG PET. *J Nucl Med* 1995;Suppl. 36:198P

62. Vascular Anomalies in Patients Undergoing Retroperitoneal Lymph Node Dissection (RPLND) for Testicular Germ Cell Tumours (TGCT)

A. Heidenreich, A. Elert

Department of Urology, Philipps-Universität, Baldingerstrasse, 35043 Marburg, Germany

Introduction and Objectives

Primary and secondary RPLND is an established staging and therapeutic procedure for the management of clinical stage I – IIB TGCT and for the resection of residual retroperitoneal masses post chemotherapy. However, RPLND might be complicated by vascular anomalies in the retroperitoneum. Anomalies of the renal vessels usually are clinically silent and might be demonstrated during CT scanning of the abdomen for staging of urological malignancies. Awareness of these rare anomalies is crucial especially in patients undergoing staging for TGCT in order to avoid over-staging and unnecessary therapy. In patients with advanced TGCT, the inferior vena cava (IVC) may be partially or completely occluded by extrinsic compression by lymph nodes or by direct invasion by metastases. Knowledge of the presence and extent of IVC thrombosis is essential to plan the surgical approach. We therefore report on the incidence of renal vessel anomalies and IVC changes in an unselected group of patients undergoing RPLND for testis cancer.

Patients and Methods

245 patients with TGCTs underwent primary or secondary RPLND following inductive chemotherapy. Prior to RPLND, all patients underwent abdominal staging by CT scans or by MRI. CT scans were reviewed with regard to the detection of vascular anomalies of the IVC, renal veins, renal arteries and iliac vessels. CT findings were correlated with intra-operative findings.

Results

Overall, vascular anomalies were encountered in 39 patients (15.9 per cent): a retro-aortic left renal vein in 10 (4.1 per cent), circumaortic left renal vein in 2 (0.8 per cent), reduplication of the common iliac vein in 1 (0.4 per cent), accessory renal arteries in 14 (5.7 per cent), thrombosis of the IVC in 12 (4.9 per cent) patients with IIC disease. Anomalies of the renal vein were detected in 10/12 (83 per cent). In two cases venous anomalies were falsely diagnosed as lymph node disease in stage I TGCT. All arterial anomalies were identified preoperatively. CT scan identified caval thrombosis in only 8 cases (68 per cent); four cases were identified by an additional MRI of the abdomen.

Conclusions

Vascular anomalies are frequently encountered in patients requiring RPLND for testis cancer and have to be recognised during surgery even with negative imaging studies. Retro-aortic renal vein is a common anomaly, detected in about 3 per cent of all autopsies and in approximately 3.7 per cent of retroperitoneal surgeries [1]. This anomaly may be misinterpreted by CT imaging as lymph nodes, resulting in unnecessary therapy [2]. It should be suspected when the suspicious lymph nodes are caudal to the renal hilum; in those cases a MRI seems to be appropriate. IVC thrombosis is encountered in 4 per cent to 11 per cent of advanced testis cancer patients and is best diagnosed by MRI of the abdomen, to assess the presence and cranial extension of the thrombus [3, 4]. The surgical approach involves cavotomy, caval resection and/or replacement.

References

1. Höltl W, Hruby W, Aharinejad S. Renal vein anatomy and its implications for retroperitoneal surgery. *J Urol* 1990;143:1108.
2. Moul JW, Maggio MI, Hardy MR, Hartman DS. Retroaortic left renal vein in testicular cancer patient: potential staging and treatment pitfall. *J Urol* 1992;147: 454.
3. Husband JES, Padhani AR, Long MA, Horwich A, Hendry WF, Dearnaley DP. Evaluation by magnetic resonance imaging of the inferior vena cava in patients with non-seminomatous germ cell tumors of the testis metastatic to the retroperitoneum. *Brit J Urol* 1997;79: 942.
4. Heidenreich A, Derakshani P, Neubauer S, Krug B, Engelmann UH. Evaluation of the inferior vena cava by magnetic resonance imaging in advanced testicular germ cell tumors. *Eur Urol* 1998;33 (Suppl 1): S49, #196.

63. The 5 Year Experience of a Rapid Access Diagnostic Testicular Swelling Clinic

C.J. Luscombe, A.P. Doherty, A. Elves, D.M.A. Wallace

Queen Elizabeth Hospital, Birmingham, UK

Introduction and Methods

Rapid access diagnostic clinics are widely used by many medical specialities to ensure early diagnosis of serious pathology. Urologists are familiar with haematuria and prostate assessment clinics, but diagnostic testicular swelling clinics are unusual. We report the 5 year experience of such a clinic. Patients were referred to the clinic as either urgent or routine. From December 1, 2000, in line with UK government guidelines, attempts were made to see urgent cases within 14 days. All patients had a clinical examination and scrotal ultrasound.

Results

A total of 1,928 patients attended clinic between August 1995 and May 2001. There were 472 diagnoses of epididymal cysts (24.5 per cent), 321 epididymal swellings (16.6 per cent), 148 hydroceles (7.7 per cent), 167 with post-vasectomy pain (8.7 per cent), 73 testicular tumours (3.8 per cent), 139 varicoceles (1.0 per cent) and 742 with normal scrotal contents or other diagnoses (38.5 per cent). For all patients, the median time from referral to appointment was 15 days (interquartile range in days (IQR) = 8–36). However, the median time for confirmed testicular tumour cases was only 11 days (IQR = 6–17). All but two of the 56 patients urgently referred to the clinic since December 1, were seen within 14 days (median 8, IQR = 8–14), and one had a testicular tumour (waiting time 13 days). During this period, four further tumours were diagnosed in the 168 patients referred routinely.

Discussion

The proportion of patients referred to a scrotal swelling clinic with a testicular tumour is small (3.8 per cent). Prioritisation into urgent or routine was not accurate (only one of the five testicular tumours detected was in a patient classified as urgent). Despite this, the rapid access diagnostic clinic provides early diagnosis in all cases.

64. Negative Predictive Value of "Clean Retroperitoneum" by Ultrasound in Patients with Testicular Cancer

Z. Mezvrishvili, T. Toidze, N. Turmanidze, A. Dzneladze,
M. Managadze, Z. Chanturaia, L. Managadze

National Center of Urology, Tbilisi, Georgia

Introduction

The assessment of retroperitoneum is of utmost importance in the management of patients with testicular germ cell tumours (TGCTs). Surgery is often the preferred option for patients with nonseminoma, normal serum markers, no distant metastasis, and low volume retroperitoneal disease. We analyzed the results of retroperitoneal ultrasound for its ability to exclude bulky disease.

Patients and Methods

We compared the retroperitoneal ultrasound and CT-scans (the "gold standard") of 86 men with TGCT. We assessed the effectiveness of ultrasound in detecting retroperitoneal bulky disease using three cut-offs: 5cm (conventional staging), 3cm (based on the minimal sonographical dimension of actual bulky disease) and nil ("clean retroperitoneum").

Results

The CT-scan classified 64 patients as non-bulky and 22 as bulky. The sensitivity of ultrasound for the 5cm, 3cm and nil cut-off points was 82, 100 and 100 per cent respectively, specificity was 95, 91 and 66 per cent, positive predictive value (PPV) 86, 79 and 50 per cent, negative predictive value (NPV) 94, 100 and 100 per cent, and accuracy 92, 93 and 74 per cent.

Discussion

The sensitivity and specificity of ultrasound with the 5cm cut-off were good, though bulky disease was underestimated in four of 22 patients. The minimal sonographical dimension in these patients was 3.4 cm, so by reducing the cut-off to the 3cm, the sensitivity and NPV became 100 per cent. Using the cut-off of 3cm therefore, ultrasound should be sufficient to exclude the presence of bulky disease and lymph node surgery could be performed without CT-scan evaluation. By decreasing the cut-off to zero, we retained a 100 per cent sensitivity and NPV. The specificity, PPV and accuracy were altered, but this may be outweighed by the ability to exclude bulky disease much more safely on ultrasound result of the "clean retroperitoneum", though in case of positive findings, it should be checked by CT-scan before choosing any treatment modality.

Conclusion

In low stage nonseminomas treatment decision depends on physician's experience and preference. If the treatment strategy is surgery, and our results are confirmed in a larger series of patients, ultrasound may facilitate the selection process for retroperitoneal lymphadenectomy, although a CT-scan should be performed in case of positive findings.

65. Multivariate Analysis of Predictive Factors of Late Relapse in 1264 Patients with Testicular Germ Cell Tumours

M. Shahidi, A.R. Norman, J. Nicholls, D.P. Dearnaley, A. Horwich, R.A. Huddart

1. The Royal Marsden Hospital and 2. The Institute of Cancer Research, Sutton, Surrey, SM2 5PT, UK

Background

10–30 per cent of patients with testicular germ cell tumours (GCTs) relapse after initial treatment. Most of these relapses happen in the first two years after treatment.

Table 65.1

	Patients	Relapses	Months to relapse	RFS % 95% CI (number at risk)			Relapse after	
				2 years	5 years	10 years	2 years	5 years
Seminoma								
Stage I	393	32	4–56	93.7 90.7–95.7 (344)	91.4 88.1–93.9 (314)	91.4 88.1–93.9 (158)	8	0
Stage II	135	28	4–72	84.1 76.6–89.3 (107)	79.2 71.2–85.3 (93)	78.4 70.2–84.5 (60)	7	1
Stage III, IV	60	13	3–20	76.8 63.4–85.8 (41)	76.8 63.4–85.8 (38)	76.8 63.4–85.8 (23)	0	0
Non-seminoma								
Stage I	373	84	1–82	80.5 76.1–84.2 (287)	77.3 72.6–81.3 (245)	76.9 72.2–80.9 (141)	12	1
Stage II	222	25	1–166	91.7 87.2–94.7 (189)	89.7 84.8–93.1 (165)	88.0 82.7–91.7 (95)	7	3
Stage III, IV	293	73	2–169	79.4 73.9–83.8 (198)	79.4 73.9–83.8 (198)	72.6 66.5–77.7 (109)	19	9

The time course and pattern of relapse after 2 years have implications for long-term follow up. This study was undertaken to identify patients at higher risk of late relapse.

Materials and Methods

A review was performed of 1264 patients with primary testicular GCTs presenting to the Royal Marsden Hospital between December 1979 and December 1993. In all, 255 episodes of relapse were documented (including 44 patients with multiple relapses). Relapse-free survivals were calculated (Table 65.1).

Results

Fifty-three patients (15 seminoma; 38 non-seminomatous GCT) relapsed more than 2 years after initial presentation. Significant predictors of risk of relapse after 2 years on multivariate analysis were positive tumour markers at presentation ($p = 0.035$; hazard ratio = 1.97) and the presence of differentiated teratoma in post-chemotherapy surgical specimen ($p < 0.001$; hazard ratio = 3.42). Stage at presentation was a significant factor on univariate analysis ($p = 0.037$; hazard ratio = 1.82). In the 14 patients (1 seminoma; 13 non-seminomatous GCT) relapsing after 5 years, 13 had metastatic disease at presentation; 9 were detected at routine follow up visits while 5 relapsed with symptoms leading to an unscheduled clinic visit.

Conclusion

Late relapses are rare in testicular GCTs and follow up to detect recurrence may not be needed beyond 5 years except in those presenting with metastatic non-seminomatous GCTs.

66. Risks and Benefits of Follow-up of Early Germ Cell Tumours – a Survey of Current Practice

J.K. Joffe

Cookridge Hospital, Leeds and Huddersfield Royal Infirmary, Huddersfield, UK

The vast majority of patients with early stage and good-prognosis advanced stage testicular germ cell tumours (GCTs) are cured of their disease by surgery with or without the application of non-surgical treatments. There is increasing concern about the amount of potentially harmful diagnostic irradiation that is used during follow-up and there is also recognition of the potential psychological harm that some patients may experience from prolonged follow-up. The COIN and SIGN guidance documents within the UK do not recommend follow-up beyond 5 years for uncomplicated good prognosis early stage tumours [1].

Within the Leeds Cancer Centre, the radiological follow-up protocols differ from most departments, in that plain chest radiographs (CXR) are not used routinely, but thoracic Computed Tomography (CT) is included. This policy resulted from an audit of the detection of relapse during follow-up of advanced testicular GCTs [2]. There is little evidence in the literature that pelvic CT adds to the detection of relapse in patients with normal anatomy and without evidence of pelvic disease at diagnosis.

A survey of practising oncologists was undertaken to identify common patterns of practice and evaluate the local follow-up policy. Respondents were asked to complete tables of their follow-up policies (clinical, biochemical and radiological activities) for stage I seminoma and non-seminoma with or without adjuvant therapies, and advanced patients with low risk (good prognosis disease) [3] following chemotherapy and surgery for residual disease.

Out of twenty enquiries only six respondents replied, one from North America, one from Eastern Europe, three from Western Europe and two from the UK. However, the differences in practice were sufficiently varied to warrant discussion.

It was not possible to identify any standard or "best" practice, although patterns of clinical follow-up were similar in the first five years. The duration of routine follow-up in all clinical circumstances varied between 5–15 years or longer. CT was not available for routine follow-up in Eastern Europe. CXR was employed routinely in each unit except Leeds. Pelvic CT was employed universally where CT was undertaken. There was a huge variation in the numbers of CT scans performed in each clinical situation. In stage I seminoma undergoing surveillance, between five and 23; following adjuvant therapy for stage I seminoma, from one to 10; in surveillance of Stage I non-seminoma between four and 14 over 5 years; in follow-up of good prognosis advanced disease with no evidence of disease after therapy from one to 14 CTs were performed. Radiological exposure varied between four and five times the lowest intensity.

It is not possible to conclude from these data any best practice for follow-up. However, there must be concern that some patients will suffer from excessive exposure to diagnostic irradiation, which may increase their chances of increased long-term morbidity. There is a need to evaluate less toxic modalities of imaging in these clinical situations and a need to develop a consensus of what constitutes "normal" or best practice. Furthermore, the role of imaging techniques in follow-up should be further evaluated in prospective clinical trials, as is being undertaken by the Medical Research Council in the TE08 Trial, which assesses CT follow-up in stage I non-seminoma.

Within Leeds, the omission of pelvic CT and a change to CXR from CT thorax, could reduce exposure in surveillance of stage I non-seminoma by 66 per cent. TE08 will inform our local decision making process in this indication only.

References

1. Guidelines on the management of adult testicular germ cell tumours. Clinical Oncology Information Network in partnership with Scottish Intercollegiate Guidelines Network. *Clin. Oncol.* 2000;12: S172–S210
2. Rathmell AJ, Brand IR, Carey BM, Jones WG. Early Detection of relapse after treatment for metastatic germ cell tumour of the testis: An exercise in medical audit. *Clin Oncol* 1993;5:34–38
3. International Germ Cell Consensus Classification: A prognostic factor-based staging system for metastatic germ cell cancers. The International Germ Cell Cancer Collaborative Group. *J. Clin. Oncol.* 1997;15:594–603

67. Survey of the Management of Brain Metastases from Malignant Germ Cell Tumours on Clinical Presentation

H. Charalambous, I.D. Pedley, J.T. Roberts

Northern Centre for Cancer Treatment, Newcastle General Hospital, Westgate Road, Newcastle upon Tyne, NE4 6BE

Aims

The management of patients with brain metastases from malignant germ cell tumours (MGCT) is controversial, due to the lack of randomised controlled trials in this setting. A national survey of all UK Cancer centres, as well as all previous collaborators to MRC Testicular Trials, was undertaken to establish patterns of treatment of brain metastases on presentation.

Results

Forty of 57 (70 per cent) of UK Cancer centres responded, 32 of which treated poor prognosis MGCT. Additionally, 69 MRC collaborators replied. Thirty seven percent of respondents screen routinely for brain metastases patients with poor prognosis disease, whilst 43 per cent screen only in the presence of other risk factors.

Twelve different main chemotherapy regimes are being used, with further variations regarding duration, dose intensity and numbers of cycles administered for each regimen. The most common regimen is BEP (36 per cent), followed by POMB ACE (16 per cent), EP OMB (11 per cent), C BOP BEP (7 per cent) and GAMEC (4 per cent). A further 4 per cent would use intrathecal or high dose methotrexate. Nine percent would consider entry into the EORTC trial. Seven percent would use high dose chemotherapy.

Forty-five percent of respondents always use radiotherapy for brain metastases and 31 per cent use radiotherapy only under specific conditions, e.g. when surgery is not feasible or for residual disease after chemotherapy. Eighty two percent use radiotherapy after chemotherapy and 15 different fractionation regimes are in use. The most popular fractionation regime was 40 Gy in 20 fractions (35 per cent). Eighty-four percent use whole brain fields, with 28 per cent treating in 2 phases. Twelve percent use a field including the lesion with a margin and 30 per cent would use a boost.

Thirty-nine percent always refer for surgery, whilst 47 per cent refer under certain circumstances only, e.g. single metastasis. Sixty-three refer after chemotherapy. Only 42 per cent would manage single and multiple lesions the same way regarding referral for surgical excision, whilst 89 per cent would not refer for tumour bed excision, if there has been a complete remission achieved on radiological grounds.

Only 49 per cent of centres have a standardised policy for treating MGCT with brain metastases on presentation.

Conclusion

These results highlight the variation in all aspects of treatment of these patients.

Suggestions

(a) Patients with brain metastases on presentation are treated in a few selected centres only or to consensus guidelines. (b) A workshop is organised to discuss the variation in clinical practice and to set up a prospective study protocol/consensus guidelines. (c) There is agreement at a national level to screen all patients with poor prognosis disease, to allow identification of patients with brain metastases at presentation and facilitate entry into a national register. This register would allow us to look prospectively at outcomes of these patients, especially the pattern of relapse (whether systemic or isolated CNS relapse) and accordingly modify our local or systemic treatment.

Index